Arthritis Sourcebook

Basic Information about Specific Forms of Arthritis and Related Rheumatic Disorders, Including Rheumatoid Arthritis, Osteoarthritis, Gout, Polymyalgia Rheumatica, Psoriatic Arthritis, Spondyloarthropathies, Juvenile Rheumatoid Arthritis, and Juvenile Ankylosing Spondylitis; Along with Information about Medical, Surgical, and Alternative Treatment Options and Including Strategies for Coping with Pain, Fatigue, and Stress

Edited by Allan R. Cook. 600 pages. 1998. 0-7808-0201-2. $78.

Back & Neck Disorders Sourcebook

Basic Information about Disorders and Injuries of the Spinal Cord and Vertebrae, Including Facts on Chiropractic Treatment, Surgical Interventions, Paralysis, and Rehabilitation, Along with Advice for Preventing Back Trouble

Edited by Karen Bellenir. 548 pages. 1997. 0-7808-0202-0. $78.

"The strength of this work is its basic, easy-to-read format. Recommended."
— *Reference and User Services Quarterly, Winter '97*

Blood & Circulatory Disorders Sourcebook

Basic Information about Blood and Its Components, Anemias, Leukemias, Bleeding Disorders, and Circulatory Disorders, Including Aplastic Anemia, Thalassemia, Sickle-Cell Disease, Hemochromatosis, Hemophilia, Von Willebrand Disease, and Vascular Diseases; Along with a Special Section on Blood Transfusions and Blood Supply Safety, a Glossary, and Source Listings for Further Help and Information

Edited by Karen Bellenir and Linda M. Shin. 575 pages. 1998. 0-7808-0203-9. $78.

Burns Sourcebook

Basic Information about Various Types of Burns and Scalds, Including Flame, Heat, Electrical, Chemical, and Sun; Along with Short- and Long-Term Treatments, Tissue Reconstruction, Plastic Surgery, Prevention Suggestions, and First Aid

Edited by Allan R. Cook. 600 pages. 1998. 0-7808-0204-7. $78.

Cancer Sourcebook, 1st Edition

Basic Information on Cancer Types, Symptoms, Diagnostic Methods, and Treatments, Including Statistics on Cancer Occurrences Worldwide and the Risks Associated with Known Carcinogens and Activities

Edited by Frank E. Bair. 932 pages. 1990. 1-55888-888-8.

Useful for patients

of reliable information for helping patients and the first steps in cancer."
— *Medical Reference Services Quarterly, Winter '91*

"Specifically created for the nontechnical reader . . . an important resource for the general reader trying to understand the complexities of cancer."
— *American Reference Books Annual, '91*

"This publication's nontechnical nature and very comprehensive format make it useful for both the general public and undergraduate students." — *Choice, Oct '90*

New Cancer Sourcebook, 2nd Edition

Basic Information about Major Forms and Stages of Cancer, Featuring Facts about Primary and Secondary Tumors of the Respiratory, Nervous, Lymphatic, Circulatory, Skeletal, and Gastrointestinal Systems, and Specific Organs; Statistical and Demographic Data; Treatment Options; and Strategies for Coping

Edited by Allan R. Cook. 1,313 pages. 1996. 0-7808-0041-9. $78.

"This book is an excellent resource for patients with newly diagnosed cancer and their families. The dialogue is simple, direct, and comprehensive. Highly recommended for patients and families to aid in their understanding of cancer and its treatment"
— *Booklist Health Sciences Supplement, Oct '97*

"The amount of factual and useful information is extensive. The writing is very clear, geared to general readers. Recommended for all levels." — *Choice, Jan '97*

Cancer Sourcebook for Women

Basic Information about Specific Forms of Cancer That Affect Women, Featuring Facts about Breast Cancer, Cervical Cancer, Ovarian Cancer, Cancer of the Uterus and Uterine Sarcoma, Cancer of the Vagina, and Cancer of the Vulva; Statistical and Demographic Data; Treatments, Self-Help Management Suggestions, and Current Research Initiatives

Edited by Allan R. Cook and Peter D. Dresser. 524 pages. 1996. 0-7808-0076-1. $78.

". . . written in easily understandable, non-technical language. Recommended for public libraries or hospital and academic libraries that collect patient education or consumer health materials."
— *Medical Reference Services Quarterly, Spring '97*

Cancer Sourcebook for Women *(Continued)*

"Would be of value in a consumer health library. . . . written with the health care consumer in mind. Medical jargon is at a minimum, and medical terms are explained in clear, understandable sentences."
— *Bulletin of the MLA, Oct '96*

"The availability under one cover of all these pertinent publications, grouped under cohesive headings, makes this certainly a most useful sourcebook."
— *Choice, Jun '96*

"Presents a comprehensive knowledge base for general readers. Men and women both benefit from the gold mine of information nestled between the two covers of this book. Recommended."
— *Academic Library Book Review, Summer '96*

"This timely book is highly recommended for consumer health and patient education collections in all libraries."
— *Library Journal, Apr '96*

Cardiovascular Diseases & Disorders Sourcebook

Basic Information about Cardiovascular Diseases and Disorders, Featuring Facts about the Cardiovascular System, Demographic and Statistical Data, Descriptions of Pharmacological and Surgical Interventions, Lifestyle Modifications, and a Special Section Focusing on Heart Disorders in Children

Edited by Karen Bellenir and Peter D. Dresser. 683 pages. 1995. 0-7808-0032-X. $78.

". . . comprehensive format provides an extensive overview on this subject."
— *Choice, Jun '96*

". . . an easily understood, complete, up-to-date resource. This well executed public health tool will make valuable information available to those that need it most, patients and their families. The typeface, sturdy non-reflective paper, and library binding add a feel of quality found wanting in other publications. Highly recommended for academic and general libraries. "
— *Academic Library Book Review, Summer '96*

Communication Disorders Sourcebook

Basic Information about Deafness and Hearing Loss, Speech and Language Disorders, Voice Disorders, Balance and Vestibular Disorders, and Disorders of Smell, Taste, and Touch

Edited by Linda M. Ross. 533 pages. 1996. 0-7808-0077-X. $78.

"This is skillfully edited and is a welcome resource for the layperson. It should be found in every public and medical library."
— *Booklist Health Sciences Supplement, Oct '97*

Congenital Disorders Sourcebook

Basic Information about Disorders Acquired during Gestation, Including Spina Bifida, Hydrocephalus, Cerebral Palsy, Heart Defects, Craniofacial Abnormalities, Fetal Alcohol Syndrome, and More, Along with Current Treatment Options and Statistical Data

Edited by Karen Bellenir. 607 pages. 1997. 0-7808-0205-5. $78.

"Recommended reference source." — *Booklist, Oct '97*

Consumer Issues in Health Care Sourcebook

Basic Information about Health Care Fundamentals and Related Consumer Issues, Including Exams and Screening Tests, Physician Specialties, Choosing a Doctor, Using Prescription and Over-the-Counter Medications Safely, Avoiding Health Scams, Managing Common Health Risks in the Home, Care Options for Chronically or Terminally Ill Patients, and a List of Resources for Obtaining Help and Further Information

Edited by Karen Bellenir. 592 pages. 1998. 0-7808-0221-7. $78.

Contagious & Non-Contagious Infectious Diseases Sourcebook

Basic Information about Contagious Diseases like Measles, Polio, Hepatitis B, and Infectious Mononucleosis, and Non-Contagious Infectious Diseases like Tetanus and Toxic Shock Syndrome, and Diseases Occurring as Secondary Infections Such as Shingles and Reye Syndrome, Along with Vaccination, Prevention, and Treatment Information, and a Section Describing Emerging Infectious Disease Threats

Edited by Karen Bellenir and Peter D. Dresser. 566 pages. 1996. 0-7808-0075-3. $78.

Diabetes Sourcebook, 1st Edition

Basic Information about Insulin-Dependent and Noninsulin-Dependent Diabetes Mellitus, Gestational Diabetes, and Diabetic Complications, Symptoms, Treatment, and Research Results, Including Statistics on Prevalence, Morbidity, and Mortality, Along with Source Listings for Further Help and Information

Edited by Karen Bellenir and Peter D. Dresser. 827 pages. 1994. 1-55888-751-2. $78.

. . . very informative and understandable for the layperson without being simplistic. It provides a comprehensive overview for laypersons who want a general understanding of the disease or who want to focus on various aspects of the disease." — *Bulletin of the MLA, Jan '96*

Arthritis
SOURCEBOOK

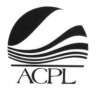

Health Reference Series

AIDS Sourcebook, 1st Edition
AIDS Sourcebook, 2nd Edition
Allergies Sourcebook
Alternative Medicine Sourcebook
Alzheimer's, Stroke & 29 Other Neurological Disorders Sourcebook
Alzheimer's Disease Sourcebook, 2nd Edition
Arthritis Sourcebook
Back & Neck Disorders Sourcebook
Blood & Circulatory Disorders Sourcebook
Burns Sourcebook
Cancer Sourcebook, 1st Edition
New Cancer Sourcebook, 2nd Edition
Cancer Sourcebook for Women
Cardiovascular Diseases & Disorders Sourcebook
Communication Disorders Sourcebook
Congenital Disorders Sourcebook
Consumer Issues in Health Care Sourcebook
Contagious & Non-Contagious Infectious Diseases Sourcebook
Diabetes Sourcebook, 1st Edition
Diabetes Sourcebook, 2nd Edition
Diet & Nutrition Sourcebook, 1st Edition
Diet & Nutrition Sourcebook, 2nd Edition
Ear, Nose & Throat Disorders Sourcebook
Endocrine & Metabolic Disorders Sourcebook
Environmentally Induced Disorders Sourcebook
Fitness & Exercise Sourcebook
Food & Animal Borne Diseases Sourcebook
Gastrointestinal Diseases & Disorders Sourcebook
Genetic Disorders Sourcebook
Head Trauma Sourcebook
Health Insurance Sourcebook
Immune System Disorders Sourcebook
Kidney & Urinary Tract Diseases & Disorders Sourcebook
Learning Disabilities Sourcebook
Men's Health Concerns Sourcebook
Mental Health Disorders Sourcebook
Ophthalmic Disorders Sourcebook
Oral Health Sourcebook
Pain Sourcebook
Pregnancy & Birth Sourcebook
Public Health Sourcebook
Rehabilitation Sourcebook
Respiratory Diseases & Disorders Sourcebook
Sexually Transmitted Diseases Sourcebook
Skin Disorders Sourcebook
Sleep Disorders Sourcebook
Sports Injuries Sourcebook
Substance Abuse Sourcebook
Women's Health Concerns Sourcebook

Health Reference Series

First Edition

Arthritis
SOURCEBOOK

*Basic Consumer Health Information
about Specific Forms of Arthritis and
Related Disorders, Including Rheumatoid
Arthritis, Osteoarthritis, Gout, Polymyalgia
Rheumatica, Psoriatic Arthritis,
Spondyloarthropathies, Juvenile Rheumatoid
Arthritis, and Juvenile Ankylosing
Spondylitis; Along with Information
about Medical, Surgical, and Alternative
Treatment Options, and Including Strategies
for Coping with Pain, Fatigue, and Stress*

Edited by
Allan R. Cook

Omnigraphics, Inc.

Penobscot Building / Detroit, MI 48226

BIBLIOGRAPHIC NOTE

Beginning with books published in 1999, each new volume of the *Health Reference Series* will be individually titled and called a "First Edition." Subsequent updates will carry sequential edition numbers. To help avoid confusion and to provide maximum flexibility in our ability to respond to informational needs, the practice of consecutively numbering each volume will be discontinued.

Edited by Allan R. Cook

Peter D. Dresser, Managing Editor, *Health Reference Series*
Karen Bellenir, Series Editor, *Health Reference Series*

Omnigraphics, Inc.

Tamekia N. Ashford, *Production Associate*
Matthew P. Barbour, *Manager, Production and Fulfillment*
Laurie Lanzen Harris, *Vice President, Editorial Director*
Peter E. Ruffner, *Vice President, Administration*
James A. Sellgren, *Vice President, Operations and Finance*
Jane J. Steele, *Marketing Consultant*

Robert R. Tyler, Executive Vice President and Associate Publisher
Frederick G. Ruffner, Jr., Publisher

© Copyright 1999, Omnigraphics, Inc.

Library of Congress Cataloging-in-Publication Data

Arthritis sourcebook : basic information about specific forms of arthritis and related disorders including rheumatoid arthritis, osteoarthritis, gout, polymyalgia rheumatica, psoriatic arthritis, spondyloarthropathies, juvenile rheumatoid arthritis, and juvenile ankylosing spondylitis along with treatment options from over-the-counter and prescription drugs to surgery and alternative measures and coping strategies to ease pain, fatigue, and stress / edited by Allan R. Cook.— 1st ed.
    p. cm. — (Health reference series ; v. 46)
    Includes bibliographical references and index.
    ISBN 0-7808-0201-2 (lib. bdg. : alk. paper)
    1. Arthritis. I. Cook, Allan R. II. Series.
RC933.A66526   1998   98-42073
616.7'22—dc21   CIP

∞

This book is printed on acid-free paper meeting the ANSI Z39.48 Standard. The infinity symbol that appears above indicates that the paper in this book meets that standard.

Printed in the United States of America

Table of Contents

Part IV: Arthritis-like Pains in Specific Joints

Part V: Osteoporosis: Not Another Form of Arthritis

Part VI: Arthritis Treatments

Part VII: Living with Arthritis

Part VIII: Additional Help and Information

Preface

About this Book

Arthritis and other rheumatic disorders are the most common self-reported, chronic conditions in the United States, affecting some 50 million persons and projected to affect more than 60 million by 2020. While the three main types—osteoarthritis, rheumatoid arthritis, and gout—account for the majority of cases, the affliction can take any of over 100 different forms. Pain, swelling, and stiffness most commonly affect wrists, hands, and feet but any synovial joint, the liquid-filled capsule of fibrous connective tissue attaching adjoining moveable bones, can be susceptible to arthritic deterioration. The effects can range from mildly irritating to debilitating and deforming. Most arthritis cannot be prevented or cured, so treatment seeks to relieve pain and either maintain or restore the function of the arthritic joint.

The articles in this volume offer introductory and basic information on the most common forms of arthritis along with prevention, treatment, and coping strategies.

How to Use this Book

This book is divided into parts and chapters. Parts focus on broad areas of interest and chapters on specific topics within those areas.

Part I: Understanding Arthritis offers statistics and important facts about arthritis and some advances in current research.

Part II: Major Forms of Arthritis identifies the three main forms of arthritis.

Part III: Other Forms of Arthritis and Related Disorders introduces some of the more than 100 different types of arthritis as well as disorders that are often associated with arthritis or other rheumatic disorders.

Part IV: Arthritis-like Pains in Specific Joints considers specific areas of complaint that are often associated with arthritis.

Part V: Osteoporosis: Not Another Form of Arthritis draws an important distinction between arthritis and osteoporosis and presents some basic facts about osteoporosis as it relates to arthritis. More complete information about osteoporosis can be found in the upcoming volume of the Health Reference Series, *Osteoporosis Sourcebook*.

Part VI: Arthritis Treatments focuses on the many different treatments that can be applied to alleviate the effects of arthritis.

Part VII: Living with Arthritis offers some strategies and advice on how to cope with chronic arthritis.

Part VIII: Additional Help and Information collects useful contact information and lists sources of additional help.

Bibliographic Note

This volume contains individual documents and excerpts from periodic publications issued by the National Institutes of Health (NIH), its sister agencies and subagencies, and the Centers for Disease Control and Prevention.

It also includes copyrighted articles, reprinted with permission, from the American College of Rheumatology, the Arthritis Foundation, the Mayo Foundation for Medical Education and Research, the National Osteoporosis Foundation, *Scientific American*, and the Spondylitis Association of America.

All copyrighted material is reprinted with permission. Document numbers where applicable and specific source citations are provided on the appropriate page of each chapter. Every effort has been made to secure all necessary rights to reprint the copyrighted material. If any omissions have been made, please contact Omnigraphics to make corrections for future editions.

Acknowledgements

Many people and organizations have contributed the material in this volume. The editor gratefully acknowledges the assistance and cooperation of the American College of Rheumatology, the Arthritis Foundation, the Mayo Foundation for Medical Education and Research, the National Osteoporosis Foundation, *Scientific American*, and the Spondylitis Association of America.

Special thanks to Margaret Mary Missar for her patient search for the documents that make up this volume, Karen Bellenir for her technical assistance and advice, Bruce the Scanman for his discriminating digital displacements, and David Cook for helping putting it all in place.

Note from the Editor

This book is part of Omnigraphics' Health Reference Series. The series provides basic information about a broad range of medical concerns. It is not intended to serve as a tool for diagnosing illness, in prescribing treatments, or as a substitute for the physician/patient relationship. All persons concerned about medical symptoms or the possibility of disease are encouraged to seek professional care from an appropriate health care provider.

Health Reference Series *Update Policy*

The inaugural book in the *Health Reference Series* was the first edition of *Cancer Sourcebook* published in 1992. Since then, the *Series* has been enthusiastically received by libraries and in the medical community. In order to maintain the standard of providing high-quality health information for the lay person, the editorial staff at Omnigraphics felt it was necessary to implement a policy of updating volumes when warranted.

Medical researchers have been making tremendous strides, and the challenge to stay current with the most recent advances is one our editors take seriously. Each decision to update a volume will be made on an individual basis. Some of the considerations will include how much new information is available and the feedback we receive from people who use the books. If there's a topic you would like to see added to the update list, or an area of medical concern you feel has not been adequately addressed, please write to:

Editor
Health Reference Series
Omnigraphics, Inc.
2500 Penobscot Bldg.
Detroit, MI 48226

The commitment to providing on-going coverage of important medical developments has also led to some technical changes in the *Health Reference Series*. Beginning with books published in 1999, each new volume will be individually titled and called a "First Edition." Subsequent updates will carry sequential edition numbers. To help avoid confusion and to provide maximum flexibility in our ability to respond to informational needs, the practice of consecutively numbering each volume will be discontinued.

Part One

Understanding Arthritis

Chapter 1

Arthritis:
The Cumulative Impact of a
Common Chronic Condition

Objective. To document the extent of disability related to arthritis among working-age (18-64-year-old) and elderly (≥ 70-year-old) individuals.

Methods. Data from the 1970-1987 National Health Interview Surveys were used to determine the prevalence of arthritis-related disability among working-age adults. The Longitudinal Study on Aging was used to determine the prevalence of arthritis-related disability among the elderly.

Results. Among working-age persons, 3.734 million men and 5.649 million women reported having arthritis, of whom in excess of two million and three million, respectively, reported activity limitation (the definition of disability in the National Health Interview Survey). Labor force participation among men with arthritis was ~20 percent lower than among those without arthritis and ~25 percent lower among women with arthritis than among those without. Among elderly individuals, 55 percent reported having arthritis and, of these, more than three-quarters were limited in a physical activity and more than one-third were limited in an activity of daily living. Moreover, disability rates for persons with arthritis were found to be increasing, even on an age-adjusted basis.

Conclusion. The impact of arthritis in terms of disability was shown to be high and was probably underestimated, given the high prevalence of the disease among women and elderly persons, and the limitations in the methods used in contemporary social surveys to establish the extent of disability, in these two population groups in particular.

Arthritis: The Cumulative Impact of a Common Problem

In 1990 Congress passed, and President Bush signed into law, the Americans with Disabilities Act, or ADA (1), the culmination of a 2-decade-long effort to extend the application of Civil Rights legislation to persons denied access to employment, housing, education, transportation, or leisure pursuits because of a limitation in activities due to chronic disease. As part of the effort to pass the ADA and as part of the subsequent effort to write and then enforce its regulations, Congress, the Executive branch, and private foundations have commissioned several studies to enumerate the population covered by the law and the number of such persons experiencing discrimination.

The current report has two purposes:

1. to contribute to this enumeration effort by estimating the number of persons with arthritis who meet the ADA's criteria for disability (defined as a limitation in one's ability to carry out major activities of daily life); and

2. to set forth the argument that these enumeration efforts are insufficient because the methods currently available to enumerate the population of persons with arthritis and disability have inherent shortcomings which discriminate against these persons.

The first part of the article describes the extent of arthritis-related disability, using data from national community-based studies to estimate the prevalence cross-sectionally and longitudinally (*see note below). These data show that persons with arthritis experience a disproportionate amount of disability even relative to those with other chronic conditions and that by most definitions, the prevalence of arthritis-related disability is rising. The second part of the article presents information supporting the contention that the prevalence of arthritis among older persons and women results in a severe underestimation of its impacts, primarily because its impacts, particularly in these two population groups, are not easily counted and when counted are not easily priced in economic terms.

4

Note: *Studies of the impact of arthritis can be divided into two general categories: those relying on clinical samples of persons with discrete conditions generally living in a defined small area (2-13) and those relying on community-based studies of persons with a broad range of arthritides living in the nation as a whole (14-30). I will cite both kinds of studies, but the data presented in the tables derive only from the latter, specifically, from the author's analysis of the 1970-1987 National Health Interview Surveys (NHIS) (31) and the Longitudinal Study on Aging (LSOA) (32). The results are presented separately for persons under age 65 and those 70 and over, since persons in these two age groups would be expected to perform different activities, with the measures of disability in the NHIS more reflective of the activities of working-age persons and those in the LSOA more reflective of the activities of elderly persons.

The National Health Interview Survey is an annual survey of the non-institutionalized population of the continental US. In the NHIS, arthritis is defined by self-report of symptoms and diagnoses (respondents are asked if a physician told them the specific names of their medical conditions). Studies comparing prevalence estimates from self-reports and examinations indicate that the former yields a more accurate estimate of those with symptoms and the latter, of disease in the absence of symptoms (22,31). Both contribute to an understanding of the population impact of the arthritides. The Longitudinal Study on Aging, begun in 1984, used the National Health Interview Survey sampling frame to select individuals over age 55. Individuals age 70 or over in the 1984 LSOA survey were reinterviewed in 1986.

In the National Health Interview Survey and the Longitudinal Study on Aging, the definition of disability, an inability to carry out major activities of daily living, is consistent with the definition of disability in the ADA. The data in Table 1.1 have not been presented elsewhere. The data in Tables 1.2-1.5 summarize information presented in references 33 and 34.

The Role of Arthritis in the Health of the Population

Slightly more than a decade ago, a debate began about the implications of declining mortality rates, in terms of the overall health of the population. One school of thought was that there would be a pandemic of chronic disease and disability, as frail individuals were kept alive longer (35); another was that the period of morbidity would be compressed as the age at onset of chronic disease rose, pushing against the natural limits of the human life span (36). There is now wide agree-

Table 1.1. Number (in millions) of working-age persons (age 18-64) and rate of activity limitation among such persons, by arthritis status and sex, United States, 1987*

	Men					Women				
	All		With limitation			All		With limitation		
Arthritis status group	No.	Column %	No.	Row %	Column %	No.	Column %	No.	Row %	Column %
Arthritis only	1.430	2	0.641	45	7	1.896	3	0.769	41	8
Arthritis and comorbidities	2.304	3	1.567	68	18	3.753	5	2.621	70	27
Both of above	3.734	5	2.208	55	25	5.649	8	3.390	60	35
Other conditions	22.417	31	6.555	29	75	26.850	36	6.332	24	65
No conditions	45.278	63				43.190	57			
All persons	71.429	100	8.763	12	100	75.689	100	9.722	13	100

* Row % is the percent with limitation in relation to all persons in the given arthritis status group, i.e., for men with arthritis only, 0.641 million (those with limitation) is 45% of the total 1.430 million with arthritis only. Column % is the percent in the given arthritis status group in relation to the total for all arthritis status groups, i.e., for men with limitation, 0.641 million (those with arthritis only) is 7% of the total 8.763 million with limitation. Source: author's analysis of data from the 1987 National Health Interview Survey.

ment that the data are more consistent with the former theory, with disability rates having risen even on an age-adjusted basis during the 1970s and early 1980s (29-37), although there is reason to believe that compression could occur in the future as we learn to prevent or more effectively treat various illnesses (38,39). Because arthritis is the most prevalent condition among the elderly, it is central to this debate.

However, arthritis is an important public health problem among adults of working ages (18-64 years), as well. Approximately one-fifth of men ages 45-64 report having arthritis, and ~3 percent of them experience activity limitation. Arthritis is the second most common disease and cause of activity limitation among men in this age range. Among women ages 45-64, approximately one-third have arthritis and 5 percent experience some form of limitation as a result; arthritis is the most common disease and cause of activity limitation among women in this age group (29).

The public health importance of arthritis will grow even if these prevalence rates stagnate in the years to come, because the US population is aging to the point at which the median age is getting closer to the usual age range for onset of arthritis. Between 1960 and 1990, for example, the proportion of the population over age 55 increased by about 12 percent, the proportion over 65 by 35 percent, and the proportion over 75 by 65 percent (40). However, the prevalence of arthritis has not stagnated. Published series covering the period until the mid-1980s show age-adjusted rates of arthritis rising (22-29), suggesting that the extent of arthritis and arthritis-related disability will grow faster than the growth in the population.*

Note: *Author's analysis of the National Health Interview Survey data shows a moderation in the rate of increase in the period 1982 through 1987.

Arthritis and the Working-age Population

Table 1.1 presents data on the prevalence of self-reported arthritis, stratified by co-morbidity status, as well as data on the extent of arthritis-related activity limitation, among working-age adults for 1987. Also shown is the number of persons with other chronic conditions. Several points are noteworthy. First, even among working-age adults, more individuals experience arthritis in conjunction with other conditions than arthritis alone. Fifty percent more men have arthritis and other conditions, than have arthritis alone (3 percent versus 2 percent), as do two-thirds more women (5 percent versus 3 percent).

Second, the prevalence rate of arthritis is higher among women than among men, and the difference is greater for the prevalence of arthritis with other conditions than for arthritis alone. Thus, the prevalence of arthritis alone among women (3 percent) exceeds that among men (2 percent) by half. The prevalence of arthritis with co-morbidities among women (5 percent) exceeds that among men (3 percent) by two-thirds. The overall prevalence of arthritis among women (8 percent) is 60 percent higher than the rate among men (5 percent).

Third, in the setting of arthritis, the probability of activity limitation is similar for men and women (55 percent of men and 60 percent of women report such limitation).

Fourth, the probability of activity limitation in persons with arthritis is much higher than the probability in those with other chronic conditions. Activity limitation rates among persons with other chronic conditions are approximately 40 percent lower than those among persons with arthritis alone (29 percent versus 45 percent among men, 24 percent versus 41 percent among women), and approximately 60 percent lower than those among persons with arthritis along with other conditions (29 percent versus 68 percent among men, 24 percent versus 70 percent among women). Thus, persons with arthritis are disproportionately represented among the ranks of those reporting limitation in their activities. Men with arthritis alone are only 2 percent of all working-age men, but are 7 percent of all men with activity limitation. Men with arthritis and co-morbidities represent only

Table 1.2. Labor force participation rates (percent), by arthritis status and sex, United States, 1987*

	Men		Women	
Arthritis status group	All	With limitations	All	With limitations
Arthritis only	83	74	58	48
Arthritis and comorbidities	62	50	44	32
Both of above	70	57	49	36
Other conditions	82	59	64	44
No conditions	90	–	70	–
All persons	86	59	66	41

* Values are the percent participating in the labor force. Source: author's analysis of data from the 1987 National Health Interview Survey.

3 percent of all working-age men, but constitute almost one-fifth of those with limitation. Women with arthritis alone are 3 percent of working-age women, but 8 percent of those with limitation, and women with arthritis and co-morbidities represent 27 percent of those reporting limitation in activities.

Fifth, the absolute number of working-age persons with arthritis and arthritis-related disability belies the notion that these are conditions of the elderly population. In 1987, over 9 million working-age adults (3.734 million men and 5.649 million women) reported having arthritis, of whom more than 5 1/2 million experienced activity limitation.

Persons with arthritis appear to have relatively low labor force participation rates, especially when there are co-morbidities and when there is activity limitation (Table 1.2). In 1987, 86 percent of all working-age men and 66 percent of all working-age women reported being in the labor force. In the absence of co-morbidity and activity limitation, labor force participation rates among persons with arthritis approached these levels: 83 percent of men and 58 percent of women with arthritis alone but without activity limitation reported being in the labor force.

However, in the presence of either co-morbidity or limitation, the labor force participation rate among persons with arthritis drops sharply, and the combination of co-morbidity and activity limitation can be devastating. Thus, men with arthritis only and activity limitation had a labor force participation rate of 74 percent, 11 percent lower than the rate among such men without limitation. The rate among men with arthritis and co-morbidities, but without limitation, was 16 percent lower than that among men with arthritis alone and limitation, and 25 percent lower than that among men with arthritis alone who reported no limitation. Finally, men with arthritis, co-morbidity, and limitation had 40 percent lower labor force participation rates than men with arthritis alone and no limitation, 42 percent lower rates than all working-age men, and 45 percent lower rates than men with no chronic conditions.

The relative impact of arthritis on labor force participation may be even greater for women. Women with arthritis, co-morbidity, and limitation experienced 45 percent lower labor force participation rates than women with arthritis alone but no limitation, 52 percent lower rates than all women, and 54 percent lower rates than women without chronic conditions. Women with arthritis, co-morbidity, and limitation also have much lower labor force participation rates than women limited by other chronic conditions, an effect not replicated

9

among men, suggesting again that arthritis has a more severe effect on the employment of women.

The combination of high rates of activity limitation and low rates of labor force participation when activity limitation is present makes arthritis the first-ranked cause of work loss in the working-age population (41,42). Men with arthritis represent 5 percent of working-age men overall, but 11 percent of all such men not in the labor force and 26 percent of all such men not in the labor force due to activity limitation. Likewise, women with arthritis represent 8 percent of all working-age women overall, but 11 percent of all such women not in the labor force and 38 percent of all such women not in the labor force due to activity limitation (not shown in tables).

Unfortunately, rates of labor force participation among persons with arthritis seem to be declining. Table 1.3 shows the labor force participation rates among persons with arthritis for three 6-year intervals, 1970-1975, 1976-1981, and 1982-1987. There were two major trends in labor force participation during this period: the exit of older male workers and the entrance of female workers (43). Accordingly, the table highlights the change in labor force participation for these older men and younger women, as well as the change in the overall labor force participation rate among all working-age men and women with arthritis.*

Table 1.3. Labor force participation rates (percent) among all persons and among those with arthritis and limitations in activity, by age and sex, United States, 1970-1975, 1976-1981, and 1982-1987*

	Men				Women			
	All		With arthritis and limitations		All		With arthritis and limitations	
Years	Ages 55–64	All working ages	Ages 55–64	All working ages	Ages 18–44	All working ages	Ages 18–44	All working ages
1970–1975	79	88	54	69	54	51	41	33
1976–1981	72	86	46	67	63	58	53	41
1982–1987	68	86	38	57	69	63	55	35

* Values are the percent participating in the labor force. Source: author's analysis of data from the National Health Interview Survey, 1970–1987.

10

Note: *Even with more than 100,000 observations per year, the National Health Interview Survey is not large enough to yield statistically reliable estimates of labor force participation for persons with discrete conditions. To obtain such estimates, it is necessary to merge data from several years and use broad disease classifications, in this instance by merging data from six years and combining persons with arthritis with and without co-morbidity into one group.

The labor force participation of men with arthritis follows the general trend experienced by all men, albeit in a more exaggerated form. That is, labor force participation rates among all working-age men with arthritis have declined over time and the rate of decline is accelerating, with a 3 percent change between the first and second 6-year periods and a 15 percent change in the last interval. The decline in the labor force participation of men ages 55-64 with arthritis was more severe: 15 percent between the first and second 6-year intervals, and 17 percent between the second and third.

Labor force participation of women with arthritis deviates from the pattern seen with the total group of working-age women. Whereas the labor force participation rate among all working-age women continued to increase throughout the 18 years studied, the rate among all working-age women with arthritis surged 24 percent between the first

Table 1.4. Number (in millions) and percent of community-dwelling elderly persons (age 70) with limitations in physical activities of daily living (ADL), by arthritis status, United States, 1984*

Arthritis status group	Total no. in group	% of all respondents	Limitations in physical activities (%)		Limitations in ADL (%)	
			Any	5 or more	Any	5 or more
Arthritis only	2.209	14	65	21	22	3
Arthritis and comorbidities	6.340	41	82	39	41	7
Both of above	8.549	55	78	34	36	6
Other conditions	4.259	27	55	18	20	5
No conditions	2.805	18				
All persons	15.613	100	63	25	26	5

* Source: author's analysis of data from the Longitudinal Study on Aging.

and second 6-year intervals, only to decline by 15 percent subsequently, almost reverting to the earlier levels. Moreover, whereas the group of all 18-44-year-old women continued to experience a dramatic increase in labor force participation, the increase slackened among such women with arthritis, from a 29 percent increase between the first and second 6-year intervals to a 4 percent increase between the second and third.

Thus, older male workers with arthritis experienced a disproportionate decline in labor force participation rates relative to all older male workers, and younger female workers with arthritis did not experience the same rate of increase in labor force participation as did all such younger female workers.

Arthritis and the Elderly Population

Most working-age adults have no chronic conditions, and only 5 percent report having arthritis (Table 1.1). Most community-dwelling persons age 70 and over (referred to hereinafter as community-dwelling elderly persons) report having arthritis, and three-quarters of those who do also have other chronic conditions (Table 1.4), placing arthritis at the center of the health issues facing the elderly. All told, 8.549 million of the 15.613 million community-dwelling elderly persons in the nation in 1984 experienced arthritis, of whom 6.340 million also had other conditions. The number with arthritis alone, though small relative to those with arthritis and other conditions, was still almost as large as the number with all other conditions combined. Most of those with arthritis reported being limited in one or more physical activities; significant proportions were limited in five or more.* Among persons with arthritis, regardless of co-morbidity status, 78 percent reported a limitation in a physical activity, and 34 percent reported limitation in five or more.

Note: *Physical limitations include walking 10 steps, walking a quarter of a mile, standing for two hours, sitting for two hours, stooping, reaching over head, reaching to shake hands, using fingers to grasp, lifting 25 pounds, and lifting 10 pounds.

Limitation in activities of daily living (ADL),† though common, occurred less frequently among persons with arthritis than did limitation in physical activities, suggesting that individuals with arthritis learn to function despite impairment. Nevertheless, more than one-third of community-dwelling elderly persons with arthritis reported being limited in an ADL, and 6 percent reported being limited in five or more.

Note: †Activities of daily living (ADL) include bathing, dressing, eating, rising from a chair, walking, getting out of the house, and toileting. One can pair individual physical activities with the individual ADLs (for example, using fingers to grasp with dressing), to note that limitations in physical activities are more common than limitations in ADL, suggesting that individuals learn to cope with their limitations. The Longitudinal Study on Aging also asked respondents to report limitations in instrumental activities of daily living (IADL), including preparing meals, shopping, managing money, using the phone, and completing heavy and light housework. Rates of limitation in IADL were similar to rates of limitation of ADL and, for the sake of brevity, are not reported here.

Persons with arthritis, representing 55 percent of all community-dwelling elderly persons, constitute just under 70 percent of those with one or more limitations in physical activities and three-quarters of those with five or more such limitations; they also constitute about two-thirds of those with five or more ADL limitations (not shown in tables).

Table 1.5. Status, in 1986, of elderly persons with arthritis who were first interviewed in 1984 (when all were living in the community)*

	1984 status		1986 status†				
Measure	No.	% of all respondents	No limitation	Some limitation	Nursing home	Deceased	Total
Limitation in physical activities							
None	1.791	21	39	53	1	8	100
Some	6.758	79	8	77	4	12	100
Total	8.549	100	14	72	3	11	100
Limitation in ADL							
None	5.454	64	61	31	1	7	100
Some	3.007	36	18	60	5	17	100
Total	8.461	100	46	42	2	11	100

* Source: author's analysis of data from the Longitudinal Survey on Aging. ADL = activities of daily living.
† Values are the percent in the given status group in relation to the total in the 1984 status group, i.e., 53% of the 1.791 million respondents who in 1984 had no limitation in physical activities, had some limitation in physical activities in 1986.

The Longitudinal Study on Aging allows us to evaluate how the health status of community-dwelling elderly persons changes over time as they age: Respondents were first interviewed in 1984, and in 1986, they or their proxies were contacted again. An analysis of the LSOA data indicates that the extent of arthritis-related disability increases with the passage of time, although significant numbers of elderly persons with arthritis reported an improvement in functional status (Table 1.5). In 1984, 21 percent of community-dwelling elderly persons with arthritis reported no limitation in any physical activities and 64 percent reported no ADL limitations. By 1986, only 14 percent of these persons were free of a limitation in a physical activity, and fewer than half (46 percent) reported no ADL limitations.

These overall figures, however, mask a very dynamic situation. Of those who had no limitation in physical activities in 1984, only 39 percent were free of such limitation in 1986, over half were limited in one or more physical activities, 8 percent had died, and 1 percent had moved to a nursing home. On the other hand, 8 percent of those who did have a physical limitation in 1984 no longer reported having one in 1986. Still, 4 percent and 12 percent, respectively, of those with physical limitations in 1984, were in a nursing home or had died by 1986, and both of these percentages exceeded those among persons who were without physical limitations in 1984.

The proportion of community-dwelling elderly persons with arthritis who had no limitation in an ADL decreased substantially between 1984 and 1986, from 64 percent to 46 percent. Almost one-third of such persons without an ADL limitation in 1984 reported limitation in one or more ADL in 1986, and another 1 percent and 7 percent, respectively were in a nursing home or had died. About one-fifth of those with an ADL limitation in 1984 reported that they were free of such limitation in 1986. However, almost as many (17 percent) had died, and another 5 percent were in a nursing home.

Baseline disability among persons with arthritis is a strong risk factor for adverse outcomes two years down the road. Community-dwelling elderly persons with arthritis and with one or more physical limitations in 1984 were 50 percent more likely to have died by 1986, and four times as likely to be in a nursing home, as those without such limitation. ADL limitation appears to be a stronger risk factor for adverse outcomes than does physical limitation: Community-dwelling elderly persons with one or more ADL limitation were about 2 1/2 times more likely to have died and five times as likely to end up in a nursing home, compared with those without such limitation.

14

Summary

This report documents:

1. that persons with arthritis experience a disproportionate amount of disability relative to persons with other chronic conditions,

2. that for reasons that by and large remain unknown, disability rates (including work disability rates) among such persons seem to be on the rise, and

3. that high proportions of community-dwelling elderly persons with arthritis experience worsening health status, which is manifested in as little as two years of follow up.

These findings derive from a series of cross-sectional surveys of the working-age population and a longitudinal study of one cohort of elderly persons.

As of yet, however, there are no national, community-based longitudinal studies of working-age adults with sufficient sample sizes to estimate the prognosis for persons with arthritis, in terms of broad-based measures of function and in terms of work.

Additionally, the one study of functional decline among the elderly needs to be replicated, to determine if the experience of the current cohort of elderly persons will apply to the baby-boom generation soon to approach the ages of high prevalence for arthritis. The literature is rife with claims about the future health status of this group; the experience of those who reached old age more than a decade ago provides no clear implication for this next generation of elderly persons.

Methods Matter

Creation of a longitudinal version of the National Health Interview Survey would help us to understand how persons with arthritis who are of working ages withdraw from work; replication of the Longitudinal Study on Aging with a more contemporary cohort of elderly persons would go a long way toward addressing the issue of whether successive cohorts of elderly persons with arthritis will experience longer or shorter periods of disability. However, collection of these additional survey data will not solve a more fundamental set of problems which lead, I believe, to a serious underestimation of the impacts of arthritis.

Arthritis disproportionately affects women and the elderly. Current methods of counting the impacts of illness have a strong bias toward male subjects. Methods to translate counts of impacts into economic measures of cost are prone to an additional set of distortions, which are described in greater detail below.

Reisine and colleagues have written extensively on the sex bias in studies of arthritis-related disability (11,13). The usual, but incomplete, explanation for the bias is that women are less likely to work outside the home and, therefore, less likely to report being limited in their usual activity, even though they are unable to perform the myriad parts of their usual care-giving roles. Their under-reporting reflects their internalizing of the low value society places on unremunerated work. However, were they to venture into the labor market, they would suffer discrimination in the kinds of jobs for which they might be hired, and they are penalized by salary systems that are based on seniority. In the labor market, the nurturant, teaching, and, of course, housekeeping functions of the homemaker are poorly remunerated (44). Thus, even though methods have been established to set a value for homemakers' activities (4), these methods still place a relatively low value on the activities. Women who perform these activities for pay are poorly remunerated relative to women who perform other paid work requiring similar levels of skill; women who do them at home without pay are doubly discriminated against because they do not receive the seniority bonus they deserve.

Methods to count the impacts of arthritis among the elderly have a different set of biases. Population surveys ask the elderly whether they can dress themselves, manage money, etc. The work of the older woman extends far beyond taking care of herself, however. Usually she performs many of the activities of daily living, and instrumental activities of daily living (see footnote above) for her husband; frequently she performs them for her children, grandchildren, friends, and neighbors, as well (45). In fact, working-age adults often rely on their elderly mothers because more members of the younger generation are in 2-career couples and do not have the time to take care of the family and the home, let alone assure adequate child care. "Normal activities" for elderly women include these roles, but survey instruments have not quite caught up with this set of expectations. The elderly woman with arthritis feels disabled if her husband needs her to help him with his activities of daily living or if her children rely on her for shopping or child care. However, survey questions elicit the impact of arthritis on only her personal activities.

Methods devised to translate counts of impacts into measures of cost also discriminate against persons with arthritis (2). The most frequently used method of estimating the cost of illness, the human capital approach, sums expenditures for medical services and wages lost due to morbidity or mortality. The cost of medical care has been rising faster than the Consumer Price Index for more than two decades, due in part to open-ended reimbursement for medical bills. On the other hand, real wages have stagnated since 1973 (46).

Because of the decline in real wages, use of the human capital approach would show the economic cost of illnesses with high work disability rates to be declining even if the work disability rate were stagnant. In contrast, it would show the economic cost of illnesses with high medical care costs to be rising even if the mix of services used did not change. Both dynamics adversely affect arthritis, resulting in an underestimation of its impacts: Persons with arthritis have low medical care costs relative to those with most other chronic conditions because there are few expensive procedures for this set of conditions and arthritis is usually managed on an outpatient basis; moreover, as shown above, persons with arthritis have high rates of work disability.

The second common method of estimating the cost of illness is called the willingness-to-pay approach. This method sets the cost of illness as the amount individuals would be willing to pay to forego disability in all its dimensions, including disability in all parts of women's lives, not just those remunerated in the labor market. In practice, however, people have had a difficult time placing values on their activities, often refusing to answer interviewers' attempts to elicit such values and at other times providing unreliable and logically inconsistent responses. However, even if they could and would estimate the benefit of preserving good functionality, they would be forced to rely on the marketplace rather than their own values to make such estimates. We live in a market society, and most of us know no other way to estimate value than by market pricing. As discussed above, persons with arthritis do a disproportionate share of work that is not remunerated at all or, if remunerated, poorly so.

Thus, the impact of arthritis will be underestimated as long as working for pay is valued more than taking care of one's family without remuneration, as long as producing goods and trading in securities is valued more in the labor market than providing direct services to people, and as long as using expensive, invasive medical procedures is valued more than restoring function. The flaws in our methods of

17

estimating the costs of illness may very well reflect the values of our society, and these may result in less money being directed toward arthritis care.

— by Edward Yelin

References

1. The Americans with Disabilities Act of 1990, PL101-336

2. Lubeck D, Yelin E: A question of value: measuring the impact of chronic disease. Milbank Q 66:444-464, 1988

3. Thompson M, Read J, Liang M: Feasibility of willingness-to-pay measurements in chronic arthritis. Med Decis Making 4:195-215, 1984

4. Meenan RF, Yelin EH, Henke CJ, Curtis DL, Epstein WV: The costs of rheumatoid arthritis: a patient-oriented study of chronic disease costs. Arthritis Rheum 21:827-833, 1978

5. Lubeck DP, Spitz PW, Fries JF, Wolfe F, Mitchell DM, Roth SH: A multi-center study of annual health service utilization and costs in rheumatoid arthritis. Arthritis Rheum 29:488-493, 1986

6. Liang MH, Larson M, Thompson M, Eaton H, McNamara E, Katz R, Taylor J: Cost and outcomes in rheumatoid arthritis and osteoarthritis. Arthritis Rheum 27:522-529, 1984

7. Stone C: The lifetime costs of rheumatoid arthritis. J Rheumatol 11:819-827, 1984

8. Yelin E, Shearn M, Epstein W: Health outcomes for a chronic disease in prepaid group practice and fee for service settings: the case of rheumatoid arthritis. Med Care 24:236-247, 1986

9. Lubeck D, Brown B, Holman H: Chronic disease and health system performance: care of osteoarthritis across three health services. Med Care 23:266-277, 1985

10. Yelin E, Meenan R, Nevitt M, Epstein W: Work disability in rheumatoid arthritis: effects of disease, social, and work factors. Ann Intern Med 93:551-556, 1980

11. Reisine ST, Grady KE, Goodenow C, Fifield J: Work disability among women with rheumatoid arthritis: the relative

importance of disease, social, work, and family factors. Arthritis Rheum 32:538-543, 1989

12. Yelin E, Henke C, Epstein W: The work dynamics of the person with rheumatoid arthritis. Arthritis Rheum 30:507-512, 1987

13. Reisine S, Goodenow C, Grady K: The impact of rheumatoid arthritis on the homemaker. Soc Sci Med 25:89-95, 1987

14. Basic Data from the National Health and Nutrition Examination Survey on Arthritis: Knee, Hip, and Sacroiliac Joints in Adults Ages 25-74 Years, U.S., 19711975. DHEW publication no. 79-1661 (Vital and Health Statistics; series 11, no. 213). Rockville, MD, National Center for Health Statistics, 1979

15. The National Ambulatory Care Survey, U.S., 1975-1981 and 1985 Trends. DHHS publication no. 88-1754 (Vital and Health Statistics; series 13, no. 93). Rockville, MD, National Center for Health Statistics, 1988

16. Detailed Diagnoses and Procedures for Patients Discharged from Short-Stay Hospitals, U.S., 1985: From the National Hospital Discharge Survey. DHHS publication no. 87-1751 (Vital and Health Statistics; series 13, no. 90). Rockville, MD, National Center for Health Statistics, 1987

17. Hing E: Use of Nursing Homes by the Elderly. Advance Data from Vital and Health Statistics, no. 135, 1987

18. Parsons P, Lichtenstein R, Berki S, Murt H, Lepkowski J, Stehouwer S, Landis J: Costs of illness, U.S., 1980, National Medical Care Utilization and Expenditures Survey. Series C, analytical report no. 3. DHHS publication no. 86-0403. US Dept. Health and Human Services, 1986

19. Kasper J, Rossiter L, Wilson R: A Summary of Expenditures and Sources of Payment for Personal Health Services from the National Medical Care Utilization and Expenditures Survey. DHHS publication no. 87-3411. US Dept. of Health and Human Services, 1987

20. Yelin E, Kramer J, Epstein W: Arthritis Policy and the Elderly: Report to the Administration on Aging through the Aging Health Policy Center, University of California, San Francisco. Policy paper no. 5, 1983

21. Prevalence of Osteoarthritis in Adults, U.S., 1960-1962. DHEW publication no. 1000 (Vital and Health Statistics; series 11, no. 15). Rockville, MD, National Center for Health Statistics, 1966

22. La Plante M: Data on Disability from the National Health Interview Survey, 1983-1985: Report to the National Institute on Disability and Rehabilitation Research. Washington, D.C., 1988

23. Rice D: Estimating the Cost of Illness. Health Economics Series, no. 6. Rockville, MD, National Center for Health Statistics, 1966

24. Cooper B, Rice D: The economic cost of illness revisited. Soc Secur Bull 39:21-35, 1976

25. Rice D, Hodgson T, Kopstein A: The economic costs of illness: a replication and update. Health Care Financing Rev 7:61-80, 1985

26. Rice D: Scope and Impact of Chronic Disease in the United States. NIH publication no. 79-1896, 1979

27. Murt H, Parsons P, Harlan W, Thomas J, Lepkowski J, Guire K, Berki S, Landis J: Disability, utilization, and costs associated with musculoskeletal conditions, U.S., 1980, National Medical Care Utilization and Expenditures Survey. Series C, analytical report no. 5. DHHS publication no. 86-20405, US Dept. of Health and Human Services, 1986

28. Pincus T, Mitchell J, Burkhauser R: Substantial work disability and earnings losses in individuals less than 65 with osteoarthritis: comparisons with rheumatoid arthritis. J Clin Epidemiol 42:449-457, 1989

29. Verbrugge L: Longer life but worsening health? Trends in health and mortality of middle-aged and older persons. Milbank Q 62:291-322, 1984

30. Burkhauser R, Butler J, Mitchell J, Pincus T: Effects of arthritis on wage earnings. J Gerontol 41:277-281, 1986

31. Kovar M, Poe G: The National Health Interview Survey Design 1973-1984 and Procedures 1975-1983 (Vital and Health Statistics; series I, no. 18). Rockville, MD, National Center for Health Statistics, 1985

32. Fitti J, Kovar M: A multi-mode longitudinal study: the longitudinal study of aging, Annual Meeting of the American Statistical Association, Survey Research Section. San Francisco, CA, August 1987

33. Yelin EH, Katz PP: Transitions in health status among community-dwelling elderly people with arthritis: a national, longitudinal study. Arthritis Rheum 33: 12051215, 1990

34. Yelin EH, Katz PP: Labor force participation among persons with musculoskeletal conditions, 1970-1987: national estimates derived from a series of cross-sections. Arthritis Rheum 34:1361-1370, 1991

35. Gruenberg E: The failures of success. Milbank Q 55:324, 1977

36. Fries J: Aging, natural death, and the compression of morbidity. N Engl J Med 303:130-135, 1980

37. Colvez A, Blanchet M: Disability trends in the United States population, 1966-1976. Am J Public Health 71: 464-471, 1981

38. Manton K: Changing concepts of morbidity and mortality in the elderly population. Milbank Q 60: 183-244, 1984

39. Olshansky S, Carnes B, Cassel C: In search of Methuselah: estimating the upper limits to human longevity. Science 250:634-640, 1990

40. Statistical Abstract of the U.S., 1990. US Bureau of the Census

41. Yelin EH, Henke CJ, Epstein WV: Work disability among persons with musculoskeletal conditions. Arthritis Rheum 29:1322-1333, 1986

42. Lando M, Cutler R, Gamber E: 1978 Survey of Disability and Work: Data Book Preliminary. Social Security Administration publication no. 13-11745, 1982

43. Osterman P: Employment Futures: Reorganization, Dislocation, and Public Policy. New York, Oxford University Press, 1988

44. Evans S, Nelson B: Wage Justice: Comparable Worth and the Paradox of Technocratic Reform. Chicago, University of Chicago Press, 1989

45. Kramer J: Who cares for the elderly: the relationship between formal and informal support (dissertation). University of California, Berkeley, 1988

46. Yelin E: Displaced concern: the social context of the work disability problem. Milbank Q 67(suppl 2): 114-165, 1989

Chapter 2

Prevalence and Impact of Arthritis among Women

Arthritis and other rheumatic conditions are among the most prevalent chronic conditions in the United States, affecting approximately 38 million persons (1). The self-reported prevalence of arthritis is greater among women than among men, and for women aged 45 years and older, arthritis is the leading cause of activity limitation (1,2). This report uses data from the National Health Interview Survey (NHIS) to provide estimates of the prevalence and impact of arthritis among women aged 15 years and older during 1989-1991, compares the prevalence estimates of arthritis to other chronic conditions affecting women during 1989-1991, and projects the prevalence of arthritis among women in 2020.

Prevalence and Impact Estimates

The NHIS is an annual national probability sample of the U.S. civilian, non-institutionalized population (3). Estimates of the prevalence of arthritis were based on a one-sixth random sample of women aged 15 years and older during 1989-1991 (n=24,201 of 145,832) who answered questions about the presence of any musculoskeletal condition during the preceding 12 months and details about these conditions. Each condition was assigned a code from the International Classification of Diseases, Ninth Revision, Clinical Modification (ICD-9-CM). This analysis used the definition of arthritis, which included

---

Morbidity and Mortality Weekly, May 1995.

Table 2.1. Estimated average annual prevalence of self-reported arthritis and activity limitation attributed to arthritis among women aged ≥15 years or more, by selected characteristics—National Health Inverview Survey (NHIS), United States, 1980-1991.

| | Self-reported arthritis | | | | | Self-reported activity limitation | | | | |
| | | Rate* | | | | | Rate* | | | |
Characteristic	No.†	Unadjusted	(95% CI§)	Age-adjusted	(95% CI)	No.†	Unadjusted	(95% CI)	Age-adjusted	(95% CI)
Age group (yrs)										
15-24	581	3.3	(±0.6)	—	—	62	0.4	(±0.1)	—	—
25-34	1,658	7.7	(±0.7)	—	—	163	0.8	(±0.3)	—	—
35-44	2,803	14.7	(±1.1)	—	—	342	1.8	(±0.4)	—	—
45-54	3,625	27.8	(±1.6)	—	—	572	4.4	(±0.8)	—	—
55-64	4,509	40.2	(±1.9)	—	—	989	8.8	(±1.4)	—	—
65-74	5,095	50.9	(±2.1)	—	—	1,238	12.4	(±1.4)	—	—
75-84	3,433	60.7	(±2.8)	—	—	893	15.5	(±2.1)	—	—
≥85	1,051	62.0	(±4.7)	—	—	339	21.3	(±4.5)	—	—
Race										
White	19,552	23.7	(±0.7)	22.1	(±0.5)	3,795	4.6	(±0.3)	4.2	(±0.1)
Black	2,459	20.6	(±1.4)	23.4	(±1.3)	659	5.5	(±0.9)	6.5	(±0.4)
American Indian/ Alaskan Native	180	22.7	(±6.6)	24.5	(±6.0)	45	5.7	(±2.8)	6.9	(±1.7)
Asian/ Pacific Islander	224	8.5	(±2.8)	10.8	(±2.9)	35	1.3	(±0.7)	2.0	(±0.5)
Other¶	339	14.6	(±3.5)	18.6	(±4.0)	63	3.0	(±2.4)	3.9	(±0.9)
Body mass index**										
≥27.3	11,379	32.7	(±1.0)	28.9	(±0.8)	2,718	7.8	(±0.3)	6.7	(±0.2)
<27.3	11,272	18.7	(±0.7)	20.5	(±0.6)	1,866	3.1	(±0.1)	3.4	(±0.1)
Education (yrs)										
≤8	3,965	41.3	(±2.3)	24.8	(±1.7)	1,216	12.7	(±1.6)	6.8	(±0.4)
9-11	3,474	23.0	(±1.5)	24.4	(±1.4)	866	5.6	(±0.8)	5.8	(±0.3)
12	8,406	21.7	(±1.1)	20.9	(±0.9)	1,489	3.9	(±0.5)	3.8	(±0.2)
13-15	3,781	19.3	(±1.2)	22.5	(±1.1)	595	3.0	(±0.5)	3.8	(±0.3)
16	1,635	16.9	(±1.5)	19.4	(±1.6)	238	2.4	(±0.7)	3.1	(±0.3)
≥17	1,276	20.6	(±2.1)	22.0	(±2.1)	152	2.4	(±0.8)	3.0	(±0.4)
Unknown	219	19.4	(±5.1)	15.7	(±4.8)	40	3.9	(±2.3)	2.6	(±0.8)
Annual household income										
<$10,000	3,866	32.8	(±2.1)	28.3	(±1.7)	1,221	10.3	(±1.2)	8.7	(±0.4)
$10,000-$19,999	4,730	27.9	(±1.6)	25.0	(±1.3)	1,064	6.4	(±0.9)	5.3	(±0.3)
$20,000-$34,999	4,224	19.9	(±1.1)	21.0	(±1.1)	697	3.3	(±0.5)	3.6	(±0.2)
$35,000-$49,999	2,445	16.7	(±1.4)	19.8	(±1.3)	321	2.2	(±0.5)	3.1	(±0.3)
≥$50,000	2,931	17.0	(±1.2)	20.2	(±1.4)	343	1.9	(±0.4)	2.7	(±0.3)
Unknown	4,559	25.1	(±1.4)	19.1	(±1.1)	952	5.3	(±0.8)	3.8	(±0.2)
Total	22,755	22.7	(±0.6)	21.9	(±0.5)	4,597	4.6	(±0.3)	4.4	(±0.1)

*Average annual rate in percentages in the 1989–1991 U.S. civilian, noninstitutionalized population. Age-adjusted rates use the eight listed age categories to adjust to the same population.
†In thousands. To generate national estimates, NHIS rates were applied to the U.S. civilian, noninstitutionalized population for age, race, education, and annual household income.
§Confidence interval.
¶Includes persons of unknown or multiple races.
**Calculated for women aged ≥18 years only.

arthritis and other rheumatic conditions, developed by the National Arthritis Data Workgroup (1). These data were weighted to provide average annual prevalence estimates.

Arthritis impact, defined as activity limitation caused by arthritis, was estimated using all women aged 15 years and older participating in NHIS. Respondents were asked whether they were limited in working, housekeeping, or performing other activities as a result of health condition(s) and the condition(s) they considered to be responsible for these activity limitations. Data from women who attributed their activity limitation to arthritis were weighted to provide average annual prevalence estimates of the impact of arthritis among women aged 15 years and older during 1989-1991.

An estimated 22.8 million (22.7 percent) women self-reported arthritis during 1989-1991 (Table 2.1). The prevalence of self-reported arthritis increased directly with age and was 8.6 percent for women aged 15-44 years, 33.5 percent for women aged 45-64 years, and 55.8 percent for women aged 65 years and older. Rates were higher for women who were overweight (body mass index BMI) equal to or greater than 27.3 (28.9 percent), had 11 or more years of education (30.0 percent), and resided in households with an annual income $20,000 or more (29.9 percent).

An estimated 4.6 million (4.6 percent) women reported arthritis as a major or contributing cause of activity limitation during 1989-1991 (Table 2.1). Activity limitation associated with arthritis increased directly with age and was 1.0 percent for women aged 15 to 44 years, 6.4 percent for women aged 45-64 years, and 14.2 percent for women aged 65 or older years. Age adjusted rates of activity limitation were higher for blacks (6.5 percent) and American Indians/Alaskan Natives (6.9 percent) than for whites (4.2 percent). Age-adjusted rates of activity limitation for women who were overweight were nearly twofold greater than for those who were not, and nearly threefold greater for women who resided in a household with an annual income equal to or greater than $10,000 per year than for those who resided in a household with an annual income equal to or greater than $35,000.

Comparison With Other Chronic Conditions Affecting Women

Average annual prevalence estimates of other chronic conditions affecting women were based on a one-sixth random sample of women who answered questions, on separate condition lists, regarding the presence of impairments; respiratory conditions; circulatory conditions; and selected conditions of the genitourinary, endocrine, and nervous systems. These data were weighted to provide average annual prevalence estimates of other chronic conditions among women aged 15 years or older during 1989-1991. Average annual prevalence estimates of activity limitation caused by these chronic conditions were determined as they were for arthritis.

Arthritis was the most common self-reported chronic condition affecting women (Table 2.2), ranking ahead of self-reported hypertension (15.7 million), ischemic heart disease (2.4 million), and other chronic conditions, including breast cancer and malignancy of the female reproductive tract (e.g., ovarian, endometrial, and cervical cancer). Among the conditions reported responsible for activity limitations, women most frequently mentioned arthritis (4.6 million), followed by orthopedic deformity (3.7 million) and ischemic heart disease (1.9 million).

Table 2.2. Estimated average annual prevalence of self-reported chronic conditions and activity limitations among women aged ≥15 years, by conditions—National Health Interview Survey (NHIS), United States, 1989-1991.

Condition	Overall No	No. with activity limitation*
Arthritis	22,755	4,597
Chronic Sinusitis	17,511	80
Hypertension	15,720	1.875
Orthopedic deformity	14,536	3,689
"Hay Fever," rhinitis	10,700	127
Hearing Impairment	9,199	479
Ischemic heart disease	2,421	874
Other selected conditions†	11,825	2,356

*In thousands. To generate national estimates, NIHS rates were applied to the U.S. civilian noninstutionalized population.

†Diabetes, thyroid disorder, bladder disorder, cerebrovascular disease, breast neoplasm, and female reproductive malignancy.

Projections for 2020

Arthritis among women aged 15 years or older was projected to 2020 by applying the average annual arthritis prevalence rate for 1989-1991, stratified by age and race to the relevant U.S. population projected by the Bureau of the Census (4). From 1989-1991 to 2020, the prevalence of self-reported arthritis among women aged 15 years or older is projected to increase from 22.8 million (22.7 percent) to 35.9 million (26.7 percent).

Reported by: Statistics Br, and Aging Studies Br, Div of Chronic Disease Control and Community Intervention, National Center for Chronic Disease Prevention and Health Promotion, CDC.

Editorial Note: The findings in this report indicate that during 1989-1991, arthritis was the most common self-reported chronic condition and cause of activity limitation among women aged 15 years and older. By 2020, an estimated 36 million women may be affected by arthritis—primarily reflecting the increasing average age of the population.

The analysis in this report also documents higher prevalences of self-reported arthritis and related activity limitation among older women, overweight women, and women with lower income and education levels. Older age and overweight are commonly recognized risk factors for arthritis. The cross-sectional analysis in this report precluded determination of whether overweight precedes or results from arthritis; however, overweight has been established as a risk factor for osteoarthritis of the knee (5). In addition, low socioeconomic status, for which income and education may be markers, has been associated with increased prevalence, mortality, and disability among persons with arthritis and other rheumatic conditions (6,7). Although prevalence rates for self-reported arthritis among blacks and American Indians/Alaskan Natives were similar to those among whites, activity limitation was more prevalent among both of these groups. Reasons for the increased activity limitation among blacks and American Indians/Alaskan Natives have not been determined but might reflect socio-cultural differences or access to health care.

Diseases considered to have particularly important public health ramifications for women include those that affect only women (e.g., endometrial, ovarian, and cervical cancers); are more prevalent among women (e.g., breast cancer and osteoporosis); are more prevalent overall (e.g., hypertension, diabetes, and cardiovascular disease); have different risk factors for women (e.g., menopause and cardiovascular disease or smoking and pregnancy); or require different interventions for women (e.g., infertility)(8). Although the prevalence of arthritis is approximately 60 percent greater among women than men (1), the public health importance of arthritis among women has not been emphasized previously.

The NHIS data enables a more accurate estimate of the prevalence and impact of arthritis than alternative data sources (e.g., Medicare, health maintenance organization databases, and hospital discharge data) because many persons with arthritis do not visit physicians for their condition. However, these self-reported conditions and the ICD-9-CM codes assigned to them have not been validated.

In addition to limitations in understanding the epidemiology of self-reported arthritis among women, the relation of arthritis to other chronic conditions among women has not been well characterized. To assist in reducing the public health impact of arthritis among women, priorities in the assessment of this problem include determining frequencies of the different types of arthritis and their natural histories among women, estimating more accurately the economic and societal burden of this condition in women, and evaluating the effectiveness of interventions, including supervised exercise programs, weight loss, and self-education courses (5,9,10). Additional strategies public health agencies and health-care providers can consider to reduce the impact of arthritis among women include 1) promoting primary prevention of arthritis through weight reduction and prevention of sports- or occupational-related joint injury and 2) encouraging early detection and appropriate management of women with arthritis through use of medical and physical therapy, exercise, and established educational programs such as the Arthritis Self-Management Course (9, 10).

References

1. CDC. Arthritis prevalence and activity limitations-United States, 1990. MMWR 1994;43:433-8.

2. Verbrugge LM, Patrick DL. Seven chronic conditions: their impact on U.S. adults' activity levels and use of medical services. Am J Public Health 1995,85-173-82

3. Massey JT, Moore TF, Parsons VL, Tadros W. Design and estimation for the National Health Interview Survey, 1985-1994. Vital Health Stat 1989;2:1-5.

4. Day JC. Population projections of the United States, by age, sex, race, and Hispanic origin: 1993 to 2050. Washington,

D.C.: US Department of Commerce, Bureau of the Census, 1993. (Current population reports; series P25, no. 1104).

5. Felson DT, Zhang Y, Anthony JM, Naimark A, Anderson JJ. Weight loss reduces the risk for symptomatic knee osteoarthritis in women: the Framingham Study. Ann Intern Med 1992, 116:536-9.

6. Leigh JP, Fries JF Occupation, income, and education, as independent covariates of arthritis in four national probability samples. Arthritis Rheum 1991;34:984-94.

7. Badley EM, Ibanez D. Socioeconomic risk factors and musculoskeletal disability. J Rheumatol 1994;21:515-22.

8. Merritt DH, Kirchstein RL. Women's health: report of the public health task force on women's health issues. Vol ll. Washington, D.C.: US Department of Health and Human Services, Public Health Service, 1987; DHHS publication no. (PHS)88-50506.

9. Kovar PA, Allegrante JP, MacKenzie CR, Peterson MGE, Gutin B, Charlson ME. Supervised fitness walking in patients with osteoarthritis of the knee: a randomized, controlled trial. Ann Intern Med 1992;116:529-34.

10. Lorig KR, Mazonson PD, Holman HR. Evidence suggesting that health education for self management in patients with chronic arthritis has sustained health benefits while reducing health care costs. Arthritis Rheum 1993;36:439-45.

Chapter 3

Prevalence and Impact of Arthritis by Race and Ethnicity

Arthritis and other rheumatic conditions are among the most prevalent chronic conditions in the United States, affecting an estimated 40 million persons in 1995 and a projected 60 million by 2020(1). Previous reports have documented marked differences in the prevalence rates of arthritis and related activity limitations by race and ethnicity(1,2), suggesting the relative importance of arthritis might vary among these groups. In addition, race and ethnicity are associated with important differences in health characteristics and must be addressed in efforts to reduce health disparities as specified by the national health objectives for the year 2000(3). To examine the relative importance of arthritis among these groups, data from the 1989-1991 National Health Interview Survey (NHIS) were used to estimate the prevalence of self-reported arthritis and related activity limitation by race and ethnicity, compare these estimates to those for other chronic conditions, and estimate these prevalences for 2020.

Prevalences of Arthritis and Activity Limitation

The NHIS is an annual national probability sample of the civilian, non-institutionalized population of the United States (4). Estimates of the prevalence of arthritis were based on a one-sixth random sample of 1989-1991 respondents (n=59,289) who answered questions about the presence of any musculoskeletal condition during the preceding 12

Morbidity and Mortality Weekly. May 1996.

months and provided details about these conditions. Each condition was assigned a code from the International Classification of Diseases, Ninth Revision (ICD-9). This analysis used the definition of arthritis, which included arthritis and other rheumatic conditions, developed by the National Arthritis Data Workgroup(1). Data were weighted to estimate the average annual number of cases and prevalence rates. Because age and sex are strongly associated with arthritis prevalence rates, adjusted rates were estimated using eight age categories (0-24, 25-34, 35-44, 45-54, 55-64, 65-74, 75-84, and 85 years and older) and by sex. Race (white, black, American Indian/Alaskan Native, and Asian/Pacific Islander) and ethnicity (Hispanic, non-Hispanic white, and non-Hispanic black) were determined by the respondent's description of his or her background.

Activity limitation caused by arthritis was estimated by using all respondents in the 1989-1991 NHIS (n=356,592). Respondents were asked if they were unable to perform, or were limited in, their major activity (play or school for children and adolescents; working or keeping house for persons aged 18-69 years; independent living for those aged 70 years and older) as a result of health condition(s), and if so, to specify the condition(s) they considered to be responsible for their limitations. Data from those attributing activity limitation to arthritis were weighted to estimate the average annual number of affected persons, prevalence rate, and age- and sex-adjusted rates.

Unadjusted race-specific prevalence rates for arthritis varied from 5.6 percent (Asians/ Pacific Islanders) to 16.0 percent (whites) (Table 3.1). Age- and sex-adjusted rates were significantly lower for Asians/ Pacific Islanders (7.2 percent [95 percent confidence interval (CI)=plus or minus 1.6 percent]) than for other races (15.2 percent [95 percent CI=plus or minus 0.3 percent] for whites, 15.3 percent [95 percent CI=plus or minus 0.8 percent] for blacks, and 16.5 percent [95 percent CI=plus or minus 3.3 percent] for American Indians/Alaskan Natives). The unadjusted population prevalence rates for activity limitation attributable to arthritis varied from 0.7 percent (Asians/ Pacific Islanders) to 3.0 percent (blacks and American Indians/Alaskan Natives). Age- and sex-adjusted rates were significantly higher for American Indians/ Alaskan Natives (4.2 percent [95 percent CI=plus or minus 1.0 percent]) and blacks (4.0 percent [95 percent CI=plus or minus 0.2 percent]) and significantly lower for Asians/ Pacific Islanders (1.1 percent [95 percent CI=plus or minus 0.3 percent]) than for whites (2.7 percent [95 percent CI=plus or minus 0.1 percent]). The proportion of persons with arthritis who had activity

32

Table 3.1. Estimated average annual numbers and prevalence rates* of persons with self-reported arthritis† and related activity limitation in the total population, by race and ethnicity§—National Health Interview Survey, United States, 1981-1991.

Characteristic	Race				Ethnicity		
	White	Black	American Indian/ Alaskan Native	Asian/ Pacific Islander	Hispanic	Non-Hispanic white	Non-Hispanic black
Self-reported arthritis							
No. (thousands)	31,864	3,672	270	401	1,412	30,662	3,533
Rate (95% CI)							
Unadjusted	16.0% (±0.5%)	12.3% (±0.7%)	13.4% (±3.5%)	5.6% (±1.4%)	6.5% (±0.8%)	16.9% (±0.4%)	12.4% (±0.7%)
Age- and sex-adjusted	15.2% (±0.3%)	15.3% (±0.8%)	16.5% (±3.3%)	7.2% (±1.6%)	11.2% (±1.0%)	15.5% (±0.3%)	15.4% (±0.8%)
Self-reported activity limitation attributable to arthritis							
No. (thousands)	5,620	899	61	52	314	5,364	858
Rate (95% CI)							
Unadjusted	2.8% (±0.1%)	3.0% (±0.2%)	3.0% (±0.8%)	0.7% (±0.2%)	1.4% (±0.2%)	3.0% (±0.1%)	3.0% (±0.2%)
Age- and sex-adjusted	2.7% (±0.1%)	4.0% (±0.2%)	4.2% (±1.0%)	1.1% (±0.3%)	2.7% (±0.3%)	2.7% (±0.1%)	3.9% (±0.2%)
Proportion of persons with arthritis who have activity limitation attributable to arthritis	17.6%	24.5%	22.6%	13.0%	22.2%	17.5%	24.3%

*Unadjusted rates are estimated for the 1989–1991 National Health Interview Survey (NHIS) civilian, noninstitutionalized population (CNI), using the appropriate weights. Age- and sex-adjusted rates use eight age categories (0–24, 25–34, 35–44, 45–54, 55–64, 65–74, 75–84, and ≥85 years) to adjust to the 1989–1991 CNI population. To generate national numbers, unadjusted NHIS rates were applied to the total population.

†Arthritis is defined by using the National Arthritis Data Workgroup's definition, which is based on the *International Classification of Diseases, Ninth Revision, Clinical Modification*, codes 95.6, 98.5, 99.3, 136.1, 274, 277.2, 287.0, 344.6, 353.0, 354.0, 355.5, 357.1, 390, 391, 437.4, 443.0, 446, 447.6, 696.0, 710–716, 719.0, 719.2–719.9, 720–721, 725–727, 728.0–728.3, 728.6–728.9, 729.0–729.1, and 729.4.

§Race and ethnicity are self-reported by the respondent.

¶Confidence interval. CIs were calculated using SUDAAN.

limitation attributable to arthritis was lower among whites (17.6 percent) and Asians/Pacific Islanders (13.0 percent) than among blacks (24.5 percent) and American Indians/Alaskan Natives (22.6 percent).

Unadjusted prevalence rates for arthritis by ethnicity were 6.5 percent for Hispanics, 12.4 percent for non-Hispanic blacks, and 16.9 percent for non-Hispanic whites (Table 3.1). Age- and sex-adjusted rates were significantly lower for Hispanics (11.2 percent [95 percent CI=plus or minus 1.0 percent]) than for non-Hispanic whites and non-Hispanic blacks (15.5 percent [95 percent CI=plus or minus 0.3 percent] and 15.4 percent [95 percent CI=plus or minus 0.8 percent], respectively). Unadjusted population prevalence rates for activity limitation were 1.4 percent for Hispanics and 3.0 percent for non-Hispanic whites and non-Hispanic blacks. Age- and sex-adjusted rates for activity limitation were similar for Hispanics and non-Hispanic whites (2.7 percent), and for both groups were significantly lower than for non-Hispanic blacks (3.9 percent [95 percent CI=plus or minus 0.2 percent]). The proportions of persons with arthritis who had activity limitation attributable to arthritis were similar for Hispanics (22.2 percent) and non-Hispanic blacks (24.3 percent) and were higher than that for non-Hispanic whites (17.5 percent).

Comparison with Other Chronic Conditions

Average Annual Prevalence Estimates of chronic conditions other than arthritis were based on a one-sixth random sample of NHIS respondents in 1989-1991 who answered questions (on six separate condition lists) regarding the presence of these conditions. Analyses included the 21 most common conditions in the NHIS that were defined as chronic (i.e., a condition lasting more then 3 months or assumed to be chronic [e.g., diabetes]). These data were weighted to estimate average annual numbers of persons affected. Average annual numbers of persons with activity limitation caused by these chronic conditions were estimated as they were for arthritis.

Arthritis was the most common self-reported chronic condition among whites, the second most common among American Indians/ Alaskan Natives and Hispanics, the third most common condition among blacks, and the fourth most common condition among Asian/ Pacific Islanders (Table 3.2). For all groups, arthritis prevalence was higher than self-reported hearing impairment, heart disease, chronic bronchitis, asthma, and diabetes. Among the conditions reported to account for activity limitations, arthritis ranked first among blacks and second among the other groups.

34

Table 3.2. Estimated average annual numbers* of persons with self-reported chronic conditions† and related activity limitations in the civilian, noninstutionalized population, by race, ethnicity§, and condition—National Health Interview Survey, United States—1989-1991.

	No. (thousands), by race/ethnicity				
Condition	White	Black	American Indian/ Alaskan Native	Asian/ Pacific Islander	Hispanic
Top five and selected self-reported conditions					
Arthritis¶	31,612	3,678	275	335	1,492
Chronic sinusitis	28,089	3,745	212	260	1,439
Deformity or orthopedic impairment	24,786	2,556	279	429	1,857
High blood pressure (hypertension)	22,516	4,185	188	338	1,315
Hearing impairment	19,780	1,486	156	329	979
Hay fever or allergic rhinitis without asthma	19,572	1,823	187	556	1,447
Heart disease	13,919	1,712	84	154	648
Chronic bronchitis	10,862	1,093	100	117	731
Asthma	9,064	1,578	140	205	926
Diabetes	5,163	1,082	91	109	491
Top five and selected self-reported conditions as a cause of activity limitation					
Deformity or orthopedic impairment	6,272	785	96	108	544
Arthritis	5,646	908	64	47	327
Heart disease	4,107	564	40	39	225
High blood pressure (hypertension)	1,972	797	32	36	205
Intervertebral disk disorders	1,831	170	20	14	115
Diabetes	1,733	497	31	26	216
Asthma	1,661	423	23	33	257
Visual impairment	1,027	151	21	18	87
Hearing impairment	954	79	11	14	66
Cerebrovascular disease	841	166	9	6	42

*The average annual number of persons affected in the civilian, noninstitutionalized population was estimated by using the appropriate weights in the 1989–1991 National Health Interview Survey (NHIS). Data in this table reflect the internal weights of the 1989–1991 NHIS, which are based on civilian, noninstitutionalized population estimates that differ slightly from those of the 1990 census total population estimates. Using the internal weights of the 1989–1991 NHIS allows easier comparison among the different chronic conditions.

†A condition lasting >3 months or that is assumed to be chronic (e.g., diabetes).

§Race and Hispanic ethnicity are self-reported by the respondent.

¶Arthritis is defined by using the National Arthritis Data Workgroup's definition, which is based on the *International Classification of Diseases, Ninth Revision, Clinical Modification*; other chronic conditions are defined by using NHIS chronic condition recode C. Impairments are coded according to a special classification system for the NHIS.

Projections for 2020

Arthritis prevalence was projected for 2020 by applying the average annual arthritis prevalence rate for 1989-1991, stratified by age and sex, to the relevant U.S. population projected by the Bureau of the Census(5). Based on these projections, in 2020, self-reported arthritis will affect an estimated 49.7 million whites, 7.0 million blacks, 442,000 American Indians/Alaskan Natives, 1.6 million Asian/Pacific Islanders, and 5.1 million Hispanics. In 2020, activity limitation attributable to arthritis will affect an estimated 9.3 million whites, 1.8 million blacks, 115,000 American Indians/Alaskan Natives, 264,000 Asians/Pacific Islanders, and 1.2 million Hispanics. Reported by: National Arthritis Data Workgroup. Div of Adult and Community Health, National Center for Chronic Disease Prevention and Health Promotion, CDC.

Editorial Note: The findings in this report indicate that during 1989-1991, arthritis was the first or among the top four self-reported chronic conditions among all racial/ethnic groups in the United States. As a cause of activity limitation, arthritis ranked either first or second within each group. For these racial groups and for Hispanics, both the large numbers and percentages of persons affected in 1989-1991 probably will increase markedly by 2020, reflecting projected increases in the average age of these populations. Potential explanations for group-specific differences may include variations in cultural thresholds for reporting arthritis(6) and group-specific differences in factors associated with the prevalence of arthritis (e.g., overweight, low socioeconomic status, and occupations involving knee-bending)(7,8). In addition, major histocompatibility genes—especially molecularly defined alleles—vary among ethnic groups and are associated with diseases such as rheumatoid arthritis(9).

Although NHIS self-reported data enable more accurate estimates of activity limitation attributable to arthritis than do other sources (e.g., physician-based data)(10), neither the self-reported data nor the assigned ICD-9 codes were validated by a healthcare provider. To improve understanding of arthritis and reduce its occurrence and activity limitation attributable to it, public health research and intervention efforts must focus on groups at greatest risk, better define the reasons for these differences among groups, better characterize the epidemiology and natural history of the different types of arthritis, more accurately estimate their economic and societal burden, and evaluate the effectiveness of interventions among these groups. In

1996, six state health departments have initiated use of an optional Behavioral Risk Factor Surveillance System arthritis module to obtain state-level information about arthritis, including data by race and ethnicity. Primary-care providers and state programs can decrease the impact of arthritis among affected groups by 1) promoting primary prevention of arthritis through weight reduction and prevention of sports- or occupational-associated joint injury and 2) encouraging early detection and appropriate education and exercise interventions.

References

1. CDC. Arthritis prevalence and activity limitations-United States, 1990. MMWR 1994;43:433-8.

2. CDC. Prevalence and impact of arthritis among women-United States, 1989-1991. MMWR 1995;44:329-34.

3. CDC. Chronic disease in minority populations. Atlanta, Georgia: US Department of Health and Human Services Public Health Service, CDC, National Center for Chronic Disease Prevention and Health Promotion, 1994:1-1.

4. Massey JT, Moore TF, Parsons VL, Tadros W. Design and estimation for the National Health Interview Survey, 1985-1994. Vital Health Stat [2] 1989;1-5.

5. Day JC. Population projections of the United States, by age, sex, race, and Hispanic origin: 1993-2050. Washington, D.C.: U.S. Department of Commerce, Bureau of the Census, 1993. (Current population reports; series P25, no. 1104).

6. Berkanovic E, Telesky C. Mexican-American, Black-American, and White-American differences in reporting illnesses, disability, and physician visits for illnesses. Soc Sci Med 1985;20:567-77.

7. Felson DT. Weight and osteoarthritis. J Rheumatol 1995;22(suppl 43):7-9.

8. Leigh JP, Fries JF Occupation, income, and education as independent covariates of arthritis in four national probability samples. Arthritis Rheum 1991;34:984-95.

9. Schumacher HR Jr, Klippel JG, Koopman WJ. Primer of the rheumatic diseases. 10th ed. Atlanta, Georgia: Arthritis Foundation, 1993:39-40.

10. Edwards S. Evaluation of the National Health Survey diagnostic reporting. Rockville, Maryland: Westat, Inc., December 21, 1992. [Report to NCHS].

Chapter 4

Research on Arthritis, Rheumatic Diseases, and Related Disorders

Highlights in Arthritis Research

"An explosion of science is having an impact on arthritis research, and these new findings will ultimately benefit the patient," said Dr. Stephen I. Katz, Director of NIAMS, at the opening of a Science Writers Briefing on Arthritis that was held at the NIH on May 30, 1997. The briefing was part of the first biennial Arthritis Research Conference, co-sponsored by NIAMS, NIAID, the American College of Rheumatology, and the Arthritis Foundation, that brought together established researchers and young investigators to discuss their research findings.

Dr. John J. McGowan, Deputy Director of NIAID, noted that there are many institutes at the NIH interested in arthritis. He explained the role of NIAID in studying and understanding the basic immune response in arthritis. McGowan said that the objective of NIAID is to improve the understanding of the molecular and immunologic mechanisms of these diseases in order to better prevent, diagnose and treat them.

"New information from the research bench will ultimately be translated into better diagnosis and better treatment for patients with rheumatic disease," said Dr. William Koopman, Chairman of the Department

National Institute of Arthritis and Musculoskeletal and Skin Diseases.
From the Science Writers Briefing on Arthritis, May 30, 1997. [http://www.nih.gov/niams/news/scibrief.htm].

of Medicine at the University of Alabama at Birmingham, and President of the American College of Rheumatology. He said that this is important because rheumatic diseases affect over 40 million Americans, and by the year 2020 it is estimated that 60 million Americans will be affected by some form of arthritis.

A session on the impact of arthritis and what can be done to reduce it was introduced by Dr. Doyt Conn, Senior Vice President for Medical Affairs, the Arthritis Foundation, He said that in the past 50 years we have come a long way. "With early diagnosis, many types of arthritis, especially rheumatoid arthritis, can be managed very well. The next few years will result in dramatic changes and improvements in the management of all types of arthritis," he said.

Debra Lappin, Esquire, Chair of the Arthritis Foundation, said that arthritis is not just minor aches and pains, but is a major public health issue. "It affects people of all ages and is the leading cause of disability in the Nation today. The estimated cost of arthritis in medical costs and lost wages is about $64 billion dollars each year." She said that people with arthritis need early aggressive therapy, referral to a specialist, and accurate information about their disease. Lappin stressed the importance of patient self-management. She added that good treatment, self-help programs, and exercise may prevent disability and improve the quality of life for the arthritis patient. Lappin also emphasized research results that dispel the myth that people with arthritis shouldn't exercise.

A personal experience with rheumatoid arthritis-related employment difficulties was discussed by Dr. Saralynn Allaire, Assistant Professor of Medicine at Boston University in Massachusetts. She said that arthritis is the leading cause of work loss in working-aged people and the second leading cause of Social Security disability payment. As a former nurse, Allaire said that she had to change occupations in order to keep working. She said that disability is a common outcome of arthritis and because of the large number of people with the disease, it is a serious problem for society. Allaire added that research studies have identified many risk factors associated with arthritis-related work disability. These include physical demands of the job, ability of the worker to control pace of work, self confidence in work ability, degree of physical limitation, and age. She discussed possible ways of coping with these problems, such as the need to identify suitable work and needed training, and the option to work at home. "Early medical and vocational rehabilitation treatments may reduce work disability and enable the person to keep their job," she said, although this still needs to be tested.

"Most people are not aware that chronic conditions, such as arthritis and musculoskeletal disorders, account for three out of every four deaths in the United States," said Dr. Matthew Liang, Director of the Multipurpose Arthritis and Musculoskeletal Diseases Center at Brigham and Women's Hospital in Boston, Massachusetts. Liang discussed the importance of prevention programs for arthritis and other disabling musculoskeletal disorders. "Primary prevention is only possible if the causes of rheumatic diseases are identified, but it requires additional research and vigilance to translate these discoveries into practice." He added that studies have shown that patients with arthritis may have improved quality of life from exercise training and arthritis self-help courses. These methods have been shown to reduce health costs, which is becoming more important in planning health care for individuals with arthritis. "For people with chronic disease, psychological and social factors and health policy are powerful determinants of their ability to maintain independence and general health," Liang said.

Scientists at the briefing also discussed genetic aspects of rheumatic diseases. Dr. Edward Wakeland, Professor of Pathology, Immunology and Laboratory Medicine, and Director of the Center for Mammalian Genetics at the University of Florida College of Medicine in Gainsville, said that susceptibility to many rheumatic diseases may be influenced by several genes. He added that since not everyone with these genes gets the disease, environmental factors may act as a trigger in the susceptible individual. Wakeland then discussed animal models of research. He said that researchers have developed models in which mice have specific genes that predispose them to get lupus. Scientists have identified the sites of some of these genes and are working on identifying the genes and finding ways to suppress their actions. "If we can understand the process by which mice develop lupus then we are better positioned to understand the disease in humans," he said.

Dr. Peter Gregersen, Chief of the Division of Biology and Human Genetics at North Shore University Hospital in Manhasset, New York, said that many rheumatic diseases have a genetic basis and multiple genes may contribute to these disorders. "In identical twins, if one twin gets a rheumatic disease, the other twin has a 30 to 50 percent chance of getting the same disease. In addition, having a relative with the disease puts other family members at risk," he added. Gregersen said that studies of fundamental mouse genetics have contributed to studies of human genetics. He added that we are currently in an era of extremely rapid change in biomedical research, where genetic studies

41

are making a major contribution to the understanding of disease. "In the future, a physician may be able to genetically map a patient and develop customized treatments for their disease," he said.

In a talk of promising therapies, Dr. Peter Lipsky, Director of the Specialized Center of Research in Rheumatoid Arthritis at the University of Texas Southwestern Medical Center in Dallas, said that rapidly identifying genes involved in disease and studying their biology can generate new treatments for patients. Lipsky said when arthritis patients see a doctor their primary concern is pain. The doctor will usually prescribe a nonsteroidal anti-inflammatory drug (NSAID) such as ibuprofen to suppress the inflammation and pain of arthritis. "NSAIDs are probably the largest selling drugs in the world and are taken by 15 to 30 million Americans," he said. However, Lipsky added, "between 2 and 4 percent of all patients taking NSAIDs will have a major gastrointestinal problem that may put them in the hospital." He said that researchers have been searching for drugs without this toxic side effect.

Lipsky said that researchers have discovered an inhibitor of inflammation and pain that has very few side effects. This substance, called a COX-2 inhibitor, affects the COX-2 enzyme that is only expressed in the body when you have inflammation. NSAIDs block the action of COX-2, but also inhibit a related enzyme, COX-1, which helps protect the stomach lining from irritation and has other housekeeping functions. "If you treat an animal model of arthritis with a COX-2 inhibitor, the animal gets better. We found that patients given a COX-2 inhibitor got the same relief as with an NSAID but without the stomach problems." Lipsky said that the COX-2 inhibitor is being developed by drug companies and will be available in the future.

In summing up the main themes of the conference, Dr. Koopman said, "An investment in science is a clear example of where new information holds great promise for future therapeutic targets, better understanding, and ultimately better health for the patient."

—by Barbara Weldon
7/11/97

Chapter 5

The Arthritis Gene

Researchers Report Arthritis Gene

A team of researchers reports finding a gene that causes osteoarthritis, the most common form of arthritis.

The report in the Sept. 4 *Proceedings of the National Academy of Sciences* discusses results of a study of 19 members of a three-generation family, including nine family members affected with osteoarthritis, a condition that causes protective cartilage to fray, wear, and, in extreme cases, disappear entirely, leaving a bone-on-bone joint.

Using techniques of molecular biology, researchers at Thomas Jefferson University in Philadelphia isolated and characterized a faulty gene for collagen II, a protein that strengthens the cartilage that cushions joints. The faulty gene directed the production of the amino acid cysteine, instead of the amino acid arginine, found in normal collagen II. The single amino acid mutation (among more than 1,000 amino acids in the protein) was found in all members of the family who had osteoarthritis, but not in any of the unaffected members tested or in 57 unrelated individuals.

The family members were initially examined for osteoarthritis by University Hospitals at Case Western Reserve University. Clinicians there performed research to rule out potential causes of the disorder

This chapter contains one document from *FDA Consumer*, December 1990, "Researchers Report Arthritis Gene," and two press releases from NIAMS Research News: Release dates June 1997 and September 4, 1997.

and collaborated with Thomas Jefferson researchers in their search for a causative gene. Research at both facilities was funded by the National Institute of Arthritis and Musculoskeletal Diseases.

Although it is known that secondary osteoarthritis can be caused by joint injuries and congenital bone defects, the cause of primary generalized osteoarthritis remained unknown. The condition can affect many parts of the body, including hands, feet, hips, and knees. Osteoarthritis is a major reason for the more than 150,000 total joint replacement procedures performed in this country every year.

Nationwide Hunt for Rheumatoid Arthritis Genes Launched: National Institutes of Health and Arthritis Foundation Announce Research Partnership

The National Institute of Arthritis and Musculoskeletal and Skin Diseases (NIAMS), the National Institute of Allergy and Infectious Diseases (NIAID) and the Arthritis Foundation announced at a press briefing that they were joining forces to support a national consortium of 12 research centers in the search for genes that determine susceptibility to rheumatoid arthritis. Genetic factors are known to play a role in predisposing people to the disease, in part because rheumatoid arthritis tends to run in families. But scientists do not yet know much about the specific genes that are involved.

In what is the largest such effort in the world, researchers participating in the North American Rheumatoid Arthritis Consortium (NARAC) hope to learn more about genes that play a role in the disease. They plan to collect medical information and genetic material (DNA) from 1,000 families nationwide in which two or more siblings have rheumatoid arthritis that began when they were between 18 and 60 years old. The project will be headed by Peter Gregersen, M.D., of North Shore University Hospital in Manhasset, NY. North Shore will serve as a central registry of information on sibling pairs with rheumatoid arthritis (including clinical, x-ray and laboratory data) and as a repository of serum, blood cells and DNA from patients.

"Findings from this project should give us a window onto the causes of rheumatoid arthritis, which opens up the possibility of developing new ways to diagnose and treat the disease," says Stephen I. Katz, M.D., Ph.D., director of the NIAMS. "We're very pleased to be participating in a partnership with the NIAID and the Arthritis Foundation to reach these common goals." Adds Anthony S. Fauci, M.D., director of the NIAID, "This collaborative effort promises to provide important new insights into a disease that exacts an enormous toll, both in terms of human suffering and economic costs. We look forward to participating in this important initiative to better understand this debilitating autoimmune disease."

Doyt L. Conn, M.D., Senior Vice President for Medical Affairs of the Arthritis Foundation, says: "The state of knowledge and technology today make this type of study possible. The Arthritis Foundation will not only provide financial support for the study, but through its chapters and publications will help in recruiting siblings with the disease." "This collaboration is a synergistic way to reach the goal of identifying these genes," says Debra Lappin, Esq., Chair of the Arthritis Foundation. "This is the first time in the history of the Foundation that we have joined in a partnership to support a collaborative research endeavor."

Rheumatoid arthritis, which affects over two million people in the United States, or about 1 percent of the adult population, is a potentially disabling inflammatory form of arthritis that causes pain, swelling, stiffness and loss of function in the joints, and may also affect other body systems. As rheumatoid arthritis progresses, the inflammation process—whose hallmarks include redness, swelling, warmth and pain—can cause erosion, or destruction, of bone and cartilage in the joints. The disease has a major impact on both the individual and society, causing significant pain, impaired function and disability, as well as costing millions of dollars in health-care expenses and lost wages.

Rheumatoid arthritis is an autoimmune disease, so-called because a person's immune system attacks his or her own body tissues. Scientists don't know the cause, but they believe it results from a combination of genetic factors that make a person susceptible to the disease and some type of environmental trigger—possibly an infectious agent such as a virus or bacterium.

Treatment for rheumatoid arthritis includes a variety of medications as well as lifestyle strategies such as exercise and self-management programs. No treatment is ideal, however, and there is no cure. Development of new treatments and even ways to prevent the disease are active areas of research supported by both the NIH and the Arthritis Foundation.

The consortium's first goal in the next three to five years is to find and begin to study 1,000 families with two or more siblings who have rheumatoid arthritis and, if possible, at least one surviving parent. With help from the Arthritis Foundation, the researchers will be looking for pairs of siblings in which at least one sibling has relatively severe disease, as indicated by a hand X-ray that shows some erosion of bone. Studies show that if a person has rheumatoid arthritis, his or her siblings are somewhere between 2 to 10 times more likely to develop the disease than other people in the population.

Researchers at 10 of the centers (listed below), including the NIAMS intramural Arthritis and Rheumatism Branch, will collect medical information and blood samples from each patient. (Two additional centers are participating in the project but not recruiting patients.) Blood samples will be sent to North Shore University Hospital, where researchers will prepare DNA from white blood cells. The researchers will analyze DNA from affected siblings to look for genetic regions that they share more frequently than would be expected by chance—that is, more than 50 percent of the time. These shared regions are likely to contain genes that are involved in the disease.

The researchers expect to find a number of genes that are involved in causing rheumatoid arthritis. "I think it's unlikely that the same genes are going to be involved in every person," says Gregersen. "It will probably be fairly complicated, with different gene combinations involved in different people." Scientists hope that by identifying genes that play a role in the disease, they will gain a better understanding of the disease itself, which Gregersen notes is still poorly understood. Explaining the long-term goals of studies such as this, Gregersen says: "Specific treatments for rheumatoid arthritis are what we all hope will ultimately come out of this."

People with rheumatoid arthritis who have a brother or sister with the disease and are interested in participating in the study can call the coordinating center at North Shore University Hospital toll free at **800-382-4827** or send e-mail to **narac@nshs.edu**. The Web site for the consortium can be found at http://www.medicine.ucsf.edu/narac/narac.html

The principal investigators and participating centers in the consortium are:

Peter K. Gregersen, M.D.
North Shore University Hospital
Manhasset, N.Y. (coordinating center)

David S. Pisetsky, M.D., Ph.D.
Duke University Medical Center
Durham, N.C.

Richard M. Pope, M.D.
Northwestern University
Chicago, Ill.

Lindsey A. Criswell, M.D., MPH
University of California San Francisco
San Francisco, Calif.

Salvatore Albani, M.D.
University of California San Diego (UCSD)
La Jolla, Calif.

Daniel O. Clegg, M.D.
University of Utah Health Sciences Center
Salt Lake City, Utah

J. Lee Nelson, M.D.
Fred Hutchinson Cancer Research Center
Seattle, Wash.

Harry W. Schroeder, M.D., Ph.D.
The University of Alabama at Birmingham
Birmingham, Ala.
(co-principal investigator S. Louis Bridges, Jr., M.D., Ph.D.)

Michael F. Seldin, M.D., Ph.D.
University of California Davis
Davis, Calif.

Ronald Wilder, M.D., Ph.D. and Daniel Kastner, M.D., Ph.D.
NIAMS, NIH
Bethesda, Md.

Mark H. Wener, M.D.*
University of Washington
Seattle, Wash.

Christopher Amos, Ph.D.*
University of Texas
M.D. Anderson Cancer Center
Houston, Texas

* Participating but not recruiting patients.

National Institutes of Health. National Institute of Arthritis and Musculoskeletal and Skin Diseases. Released Thursday, September 4, Elia Ben-Ari/Barbara Weldon, NIAMS (301) 496-8190 Patricia Randall, NIAID (301) 402-1663. [http://www.nih.gov/niams/news/genetx.htm].

Niams Awards Contracts for Gene Therapy Research on Skin and Rheumatic Diseases

The National Institute of Arthritis and Musculoskeletal and Skin Diseases (NIAMS) recently awarded contracts to eight research institutions in an effort to develop gene therapy technology in the areas of skin and rheumatic diseases. "Current gene therapy techniques are not always readily applicable to skin and rheumatic diseases," says Dr. Alan Moshell, Chief of the Skin Diseases Branch at NIAMS. The NIAMS initiative was designed to tailor developments in gene therapy to the field of skin and rheumatic diseases. The outcome of the research proposed through these contracts will set the stage for pursuing further goals.

Gene therapy involves technology that introduces a new, functional gene into the patient's own cells to correct a disease-causing defect or augment disease-fighting processes. To achieve this, various technical approaches have been designed over the years through advances in the fields of molecular biology and genetics. Most commonly the functional gene, also known as the "DNA insert," is introduced into cells through the use of viruses. A virus is capable of entering a cell where it expresses its genome—its own genetic material or DNA—to produce new virus particles. Scientists can insert the new gene of interest into the virus genome in place of non-essential viral DNA regions, and use this "recombinant" virus to infect the cell, thus delivering the therapeutic gene. The virus thus serves as a vector—an agent that transmits genetic material to a cell or organism.

Rheumatic Diseases. Although gene therapy has tremendous potential, much research and testing are still needed before it becomes a safe, effective and available method of treatment for a wide range of diseases. Application of gene therapy to rheumatic diseases and rheumatoid arthritis in particular has been limited. "The pathogenesis of these diseases is likely due to the concerted action of numerous genes with effects on the immune system as well as on the target organs," explains Dr. Susana Serrate-Sztein, Chief of the Rheumatic Diseases Branch at NIAMS. Normal function of the immune system depends on a finely tuned balance resulting from the multiple interactions of many different molecules that are part of a complex system. Potential gene therapy approaches for rheumatoid arthritis may therefore aim at modifying the immune response or the inflammatory reaction, rather than at correcting a single defective gene.

48

Rheumatoid arthritis is an autoimmune disease affecting more than two million people in the United States, more than 60 percent of whom are women. This chronic inflammatory disease causes pain, stiffness, swelling, and eventually loss of function in the joints. An unknown factor in the body, possibly an infectious agent, triggers an immune response that takes place in the joints. The joint lining, or synovium, becomes the site of an inflammatory reaction, where white blood cells migrate, macrophages proliferate, and cytokines are produced. (Macrophages are cells of the immune system that swallow up and destroy bacteria and other foreign cells, and cytokines are molecules that function as chemical messengers that regulate the immune response and cell growth.)

Six of the gene therapy contracts awarded by NIAMS are related to rheumatoid arthritis. At the **University of Pittsburgh in Pennsylvania, Dr. Paul D. Robbins**' team will create an animal model of rheumatoid arthritis and develop new viral vectors to deliver genes to the affected joints for therapeutic purposes. The researchers will produce a rabbit model of the disease by transplanting into the rabbit knee synovial cells genetically engineered to produce (or "express") various molecules known to play a role in the disease. These molecules will include interleukin-1 (IL-1), tumor necrosis factor alpha (TNF-alpha), and interleukin-6 (IL-6)—cytokines that are involved in the inflammatory response. This approach will allow the researchers to "reproduce features of rheumatoid arthritis and to dissect the cascade of events in the pathogenesis of this disease," says Dr. Sztein. Dr. Robbins' group will then use virus-based vectors to deliver genes coding for proteins such as the IL-1 receptor and TNF-alpha receptor, which inhibit the action of the very cytokines used to produce the animal model, and will test the effectiveness of this gene therapy approach on the rabbit knee model.

Another contract that revolves around the intricate network of immune system interactions in rheumatoid arthritis is the one headed by **Dr. C. Garrison Fathman at Stanford University in Stanford, California**. The Stanford group aims to counteract the abnormal immune response that takes place in the disease. The investigators will inhibit the actions of one subset of the T-cell population (a T cell is a type of white blood cell) that plays a key role in this abnormal immune response. They will do this by using genes encoding disease-regulating cytokines such as interleukin-4, interleukin-10, or transforming growth factor beta (TGF-beta). This is expected to "change the balance between the two T-cell populations which are involved in the immune response in rheumatoid arthritis," explains Dr. Sztein, in an attempt to stop the inflammatory process and ameliorate disease.

A critical aspect of effective gene therapy is the use of appropriate promoters (that is, special DNA sequence elements that regulate gene expression) that ensure high expression of the therapeutic gene in the target cell. **Dr. Richard M. Pope** and colleagues at **Northwestern University in Chicago, Illinois,** will focus on identifying promoters that are effective in driving gene expression in macrophages. The ultimate goal is to use these promoters to express genes that block productions of TNF-alpha, an inflammatory cytokine, in synovial tissues.

The research group led by **Dr. John D. Mountz,** at the **University of Alabama at Birmingham,** will base its gene therapy approach on Fas, a protein found on the surface of cells. When Fas is activated by certain molecules such as the "Fas ligand," it sets off a program of events within the cell leading to that cell's death (apoptosis). The body uses apoptosis to eliminate unnecessary or potentially harmful cells. Mountz and coworkers will construct viral vectors expressing either the mouse Fas or Fas ligand gene and will develop a way to target them to cell populations that are known to play a key role in rheumatoid arthritis, with the aim of inducing apoptosis in those cells. To test the potential therapeutic effect of these genes, the researchers will introduce them in Fas-deficient and Fas ligand-deficient mice, which are known to develop spontaneous arthritis, and will determine whether the constructs can reverse development of disease.

Three of the contracts have been awarded to laboratories developing new technologies for gene delivery in rheumatic or skin diseases. **Dr. Raphael Hirsch**, of **Children's Hospital Medical Center in Cincinnati, Ohio,** has developed a novel method of gene delivery known as antifection, which is short for "antibody-mediated transfection." An antibody that is targeted to a receptor present on the surface of a specific cell type is linked to a piece of DNA (that is, the therapeutic gene). Because the antibody-DNA complex enters the cell after binding to the cell receptor, this method delivers the therapeutic gene into the cell without use of a viral vector. In addition, antibodies are available that target a variety of cell receptors and cell types. Hirsch and colleagues will study various parameters, including different antibody-DNA coupling methods and an array of possible therapeutic genes and cell receptors, to identify the best cellular target for rheumatoid arthritis gene therapy in the synovium.

Another innovative delivery approach for gene therapy of rheumatoid arthritis comes from scientists at the **Virginia Mason Research Center in Seattle, Washington**. Their idea is to introduce in the target cell a piece of DNA (an "anti-gene" oligonucleotide) that specifically inactivates the target gene. **Dr. Gerald T. Nepom** and colleagues will focus on major histocompatibility (MHC) genes, which code for proteins on the cell surface that recognize and bind foreign proteins. Certain MHC genes are believed to play an as yet unknown but key role in development of rheumatoid arthritis.

Skin diseases. The third project focusing on a new methodology for gene delivery is that directed by **Dr. Blake J. Roessler** of the **University of Michigan in Ann Arbor**. This project deals with optimizing the use of liposomes for delivery of cytokine genes to perifollicular cells (cells near the hair follicles in skin). Liposomes are bubble-like membrane structures that can fuse with the membrane that forms the outside of a cell. For that reason, liposomes have already been successfully used to deliver DNA to some cells. "The hair follicle is an anatomical break in the rather impermeable stratum corneum [the tough outer layer] of the skin," explains Dr. Moshell, and thus represents a good target region for getting genes into the skin. If successful, this technique could be applicable to gene therapy for a variety of skin and systemic diseases.

Epidermolysis bullosa simplex (EBS) is an ideal candidate for gene therapy treatment. Because of the wealth of information that scientists have recently accumulated about EBS, it is also one of the most ready for gene therapy experimentation. EB is a group of hereditary disorders that affect the skin and mucous membranes. These skin diseases are characterized by the formation of blisters that occur upon mild injury and, in some cases, even spontaneously. EB is a rare disease that can seriously alter a person's everyday life. About 50,000 people in the United States are thought to have some form of EB.

In the case of EBS, scientists have shown that people with the disease carry a defect in one of the genes encoding keratin. Keratins are the most abundant proteins in the cells of the epidermis—the outermost layer of skin—and form an internal web-like network that ensures the integrity and structure of the skin. Abnormal keratins form abnormal networks, leading to skin fragility.

The project being done by **Dr. Dennis R. Roop** and colleagues of the **Baylor College of Medicine in Houston, Texas**, is "not at all far from human application if the technology works out" at each step, says Dr. Moshell. Of course, there will be safety issues to consider for humans. The researchers will develop mice that are affected by blistering disease similar to human EBS. The gene therapy approach proposed by Dr. Roop will involve the use of epidermal stem cells (cells in the epidermis from which epidermal cells derive). Targeting gene therapy to epidermal stem cells provides the best chance for a long-lasting effect of the therapy, since other epidermal cells are shorter-lived.

The researchers will introduce a normal copy of the keratin gene into epidermal stem cells in order to replace the defective gene. Then they will graft the "corrected" cells onto the skin of affected mice to confirm that this leads to formation of a normal epidermis. In this gene therapy approach the assumption is that, provided that epidermal stem cells can be corrected and put back into the patients in the blistered areas, the corrected cells will have a growth advantage over the defective ones, and will eventually repopulate the affected skin regions.

Gene therapy for human diseases continues to offer exciting opportunities for scientists and clinicians, and to inspire hope for patients. Much work is still to be done to overcome the complexity and possible pitfalls of this approach. "We will gain a lot of basic knowledge," says Dr. Sztein, "and we hope to promote interaction among the investigators," who will meet annually over the 5-year period of the contracts to share information on their progress. Through this initiative, NIAMS is supporting a systematic evaluation of the available tools and reagents and encouraging the search for new technologies and avenues of treatment for rheumatic and skin diseases.

Institute of Arthritis and Musculoskeletal and Skin Diseases. *NIAMS Research News*. Released June 1997. Contact: Elia Ben-Ari. (301) 496-8190 (media). (301) 496-8188 (public). Elia_Ben--Ari@nih.gov. [http://www.nih.gov/news/pr/sept97/niams-04.htm].

Part Two

Major Forms of Arthritis

Chapter 6

Arthritis in Brief

Is it Arthritis?

Chances are you or someone you know has arthritis. It causes pain, stiffness and sometimes swelling in or around joints. This can make it hard to do the movements you rely on every day for work or taking care of your family. But you can take steps now to avoid arthritis or to reduce pain and keep moving.

Arthritis affects one in every seven Americans. It affects people of all ages, but it most often comes on as a person gets older. It usually lasts a long time; for many people, it may not go away.

Warning Signs of Arthritis

Pain * Stiffness * Swelling (sometimes)

If you have any of these signs in or around a joint for more than two weeks, it's time to see your doctor. These symptoms can develop suddenly or slowly. Only a doctor can tell if it's arthritis.

Warning Signs

Pain from arthritis can be ongoing or can come and go. It may occur when you're moving or after you have been still for some time. You may feel pain in one spot or in many parts of your body.

Your joints may feel stiff and be hard to move. You may find that it's hard to do daily tasks you used to do easily, such as climbing stairs or opening a jar. Pain and stiffness may be more severe during certain times of the day or after you've done certain tasks.

Some types of arthritis cause swelling, or inflammation. The skin over the joint may appear swollen and red, and feel hot to the touch. Some types of arthritis can also cause fatigue.

Causes

There are more than 100 different types of arthritis. What causes most types is unknown. Because there are so many different types, there are likely to be many different causes.

Scientists are currently studying what roles three major factors play in certain types of arthritis. These include the genetic factors you inherit from your parents, what happens to you during your life and how you live. The importance of these factors varies for every type of arthritis.

Can You Prevent it?

There are things you can do to reduce your risk for getting certain types of arthritis or to reduce disability if you already have arthritis.

If You Don't Have Arthritis

People who are overweight have a higher frequency of arthritis. Excess weight increases your risk for developing osteoarthritis in the knees, and possibly in the hips and hands. Women are at special risk for this. In men, excess weight increases your risk for developing gout. It's important to maintain your recommended weight, especially as you get older.

What if you're already overweight? Research shows that middle-age and order women of average height who lose 11 pounds or more over 10 years cut their risk for developing knee osteoarthritis in half. To lose weight, try exercising and eating fewer calories. If you're having trouble with weight control, ask your doctor or a registered dietitian for help.

Joint injuries caused by accidents or overuse increase your risk for some types of arthritis. You can also inherit certain genes that may increase your risk for some types of arthritis. More research is needed to find out how to reduce your risk from these factors.

If You Have Arthritis

What can you do to maintain your independence if you already have arthritis? Studies show that exercise helps reduce the pain and fatigue of many different kinds of arthritis. Exercise keeps you moving, working and doing daily activities that help you remain independent. Read the chapter on exercise in this sourcebook (Chapter 53, "Exercise and Your Arthritis") for tips to help you start or maintain an exercise program.

It's also important to control your weight if you have knee osteoarthritis. Being overweight puts you at risk for worse disease, and for getting osteoarthritis in your other knee if only one is affected now.

How Does Your Doctor Diagnose Arthritis?

It's important to find out if you have arthritis and what type it is because treatments vary for each type. Early diagnosis and treatment are important to help slow or prevent joint damage that can occur during the first few years for several types.

Only a doctor can tell if you have arthritis and what type it is. When you see your doctor for the first time about arthritis, expect at least three things to happen. Your doctor will ask questions about your symptoms, examine you and take some tests or X-rays.

You can help your doctor by writing down information about your symptoms before your appointment. Bring your answers when you see your doctor.

What to Tell Your Doctor

- Where it hurts
- When it hurts
- When it first began to hurt
- How long it has hurt
- If you have seen any swelling
- What daily tasks are hard to do now
- If you have ever hurt the joint in an accident or overused it on the job or in a hobby
- If anyone in your family has had similar problems

Arthritis may limit how far and how easily you can move a joint. Your doctor may move the joint or ask you to move it. Your doctor may also check for swelling, tender points, skin rashes or problems with other parts of your body.

Finally, your doctor may conduct some tests. These may include tests of your blood, muscles, urine, or joint fluid. They may also include X-rays or scans of your body. The tests will depend on what type of arthritis your doctor suspects. They help confirm what type of arthritis your doctor suspects based on your medical history and physical exam and help rule out other diseases that cause similar symptoms.

What Your Doctor Should Tell You

- If it's arthritis
- What type it is
- What to expect
- What you can do about it

The overall results from your medical history, physical exam and tests help your doctor match your symptoms to the pattern for a specific type of arthritis. It may take several visits before your doctor can tell what type of arthritis you have. Symptoms for some types of arthritis develop slowly and may appear similar to other types in early stages. Your doctor may suspect a certain type of arthritis, but may watch how your symptoms develop over time to confirm it.

What type of doctor should you see for arthritis?

Your family doctor can diagnose and treat common types of arthritis. However, your doctor may need to refer you to an arthritis specialist for a difficult diagnosis or special care. Arthritis specialists are called rheumatologists. Ask your local Arthritis Foundation for a list of arthritis specialists.

What's Your Type?

Arthritis most often affects areas in or around joints. Joints are parts of the body where bones meet, such as your knee. The ends of the bones are covered by cartilage, a spongy material that acts as a shock absorber to keep bones from rubbing together. The joint is enclosed in a capsule called the synovium. The synovium's lining releases a slippery fluid that helps the joint move smoothly and easily. Muscles and tendons support the joint and help you move. Different types of arthritis can affect one or more parts of a joint. This often results in a change of shape and alignment in the joints.

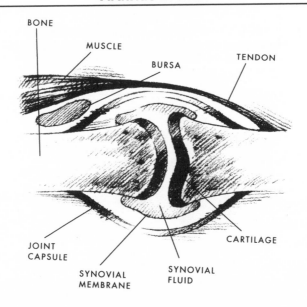

Figure 6.1. Arthritis can affect different parts of a joint.

Certain types of arthritis can also affect other parts of the body such as the skin and internal organs.

There are more than 100 different types of arthritis. It is important to know which type of arthritis you have so you can treat it properly. If you don't know which type you have, call your doctor or ask during your next visit.

Some common types of arthritis are described on the following pages.

Osteoarthritis

The most common type of arthritis is osteoarthritis. It affects many of us as we grow older. It is sometimes called degenerative arthritis because it involves the breakdown of cartilage and bones. This causes pain and stiffness. Osteoarthritis usually affects the fingers and weight-bearing joints, including the knees, feet, hips and back. It affects both men and women, and usually occurs after age 45. Treatments include pain relievers or anti-inflammatory drugs, exercise, heat or cold, joint protection, pacing your efforts, self-help skills and sometimes surgery.

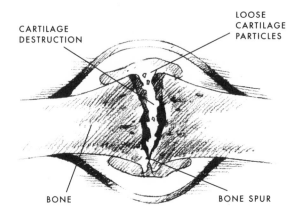

Figure 6.2. *Joint with osteoarthritis*

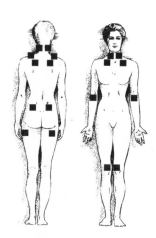

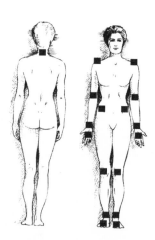

Figure 6.3. *"Tender points" that are common in fibromyalgia*

Figure 6.4. *Joints that may be affected by rheumatoid arthritis*

Fibromyalgia

Fibromyalgia affects muscles and their attachments to bone. It results in widespread pain and tender points, which are certain places on the body that are more sensitive to pain. It also may result in fatigue, disturbed sleep, stiffness and sometimes psychological distress. Fibromyalgia affects mostly women. It is common and often misdiagnosed. Treatments include exercise, relaxation techniques, pacing your activities and self-help skills.

Rheumatoid Arthritis

In rheumatoid arthritis, a fault in the body's defense or immune system causes inflammation or swelling. Inflammation begins in the joint lining and then damages both cartilage and bone. Rheumatoid arthritis often affects the same joints on both sides of the body. Hands, wrists, feet, knees, ankles, shoulders and elbows can be affected. Rheumatoid arthritis is more common in women than in men. Treatments include anti-inflammatory and disease-modifying drugs, exercise, heat or cold, saving energy, joint protection, self-help skills and sometimes surgery.

Gout

Gout results when the body is unable to get rid of a natural substance called uric acid. The uric acid forms needle-like crystals in the joint that cause severe pain and swelling. Gout usually affects the big toe, knees and wrists. More men than women have gout. Treatments include anti-inflammatory and special gout drugs, and sometimes a diet low in purines. Foods such as organ meats, beer, wine and certain types of fish contain high levels of purines.

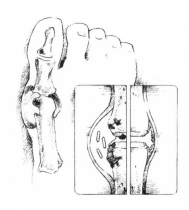

Figure 6.5. *Joint with gout*

Low Back Pain

Low back pain results from a back injury or certain types of arthritis. Back pain is one of the most common health problems in the United States. It can occur at any age in both men and women. Treatments include pain relievers or anti-inflammatory drugs, exercise, heat or cold, joint protection, pacing your activities and self-help skills.

Bursitis and Tendinitis

Bursitis and tendinitis result from irritation caused by injuring or overusing a joint. Bursitis affects a small sac that helps muscles move easily; tendinitis affects the tendons that attach muscle to bone. Refer to the illustration of a normal joint (Figure 6.1) to see where tendons and bursae are located. Treatments include anti-inflammatory drugs, heat or cold and exercise.

There are many more types of arthritis and related diseases, including ankylosing spondylitis, juvenile rheumatoid arthritis, polymyalgia rheumatica and systemic lupus erythematosus.

Chapter 7

Osteoarthritis

What Is Osteoarthritis?

Osteoarthritis (OS-tee-oh-ar-THRY-tis) is a disease that causes the breakdown of cartilage in joints, leading to joint pain and stiffness. Osteoarthritis (OA) is one of the oldest and most common diseases of man. It also is known by many other names, such as degenerative joint disease, arthrosis, osteoarthrosis or hypertrophic arthritis.

Osteoarthritis can affect any joint, but it commonly occurs in the hips, knees and spine. It also commonly affects finger joints, the joint at the base of the thumb and the joint at the base of the big toe (the "bunion joint"). It rarely affects the wrists, elbows, shoulders, ankles or jaw, except as a result of injury or unusual stress.

Almost 16 million people in the United States have osteoarthritis. The tendency to develop osteoarthritis increases with age, and it affects both men and women. Up to age 45, OA is more common in men; beyond age 55, it is more common in women.

What Happens in Osteoarthritis?

Osteoarthritis causes the breakdown of joint tissue. Cartilage becomes damaged in the process. As a result, bones rub together, causing pain. These joint changes can be seen by comparing the drawing of a normal joint with a drawing of a joint with osteoarthritis.

For a normal Joint, see Figure 6.1. in chapter 6.

In normal joints, a firm, rubbery material called cartilage (KAR-tih-lij) covers the end of each bone. Cartilage provides a smooth, gliding surface for joint motion and acts as a cushion, or shock absorber, between the bones.

See Figure 6.2. Joint with osteoarthritis

The breakdown of joint tissue caused by osteoarthritis occurs in several phases:

1. The smooth cartilage surface softens and becomes pitted and frayed. When this happens, the cartilage loses its elasticity and is more easily damaged by excess use or by injury.

2. With time, large sections of cartilage may wear away completely. As a result, the bones rub together, causing pain.

3. As the cartilage breaks down, the joint may lose its normal shape. The bone ends thicken and form bony growths, or spurs, where the ligaments and capsule attach to the bone. (Calcium intake has nothing to do with the formation of spurs.)

4. Fluid-filled cysts may form in the bone near the joint. Bits of bone or cartilage may float loosely in the joint space. All these changes can create pain when the joint is moved.

Symptoms

Osteoarthritis affects each joint somewhat differently. Osteoarthritis in the hands, for example, is different from osteoarthritis in the hips. No matter what joint it affects, the symptoms usually begin slowly and at first may not seem important. Most people feel mild aching and soreness, especially when they move. A few people develop constant nagging pain, even when they're resting.

General Symptoms. Usually the affected joint or joints hurt most after you've overused them or after long periods of inactivity. You probably will find it difficult to move the affected joint easily, but it usually will not become completely stiff. If you don't move and exercise the sore joint, the muscles surrounding the joint will become weaker and sometimes even smaller in size. Because the weak muscles won't be able to support the joint as well, you may have increased joint pain. You also may notice that your coordination and posture may not be as good as they were before.

In the Hips. You may feel pain around the groin or inner thigh. Some people feel referred pain in the buttocks, knee or along the side of the thigh. The pain may cause you to limp when you walk.

In the Knees. You may feel joint tenderness in the knee area and pain when you move your knee. You may feel a "grating" or "catching" sensation in your joint when you move. It may be painful to walk up or down stairs or to get up from a chair. If the pain prevents you

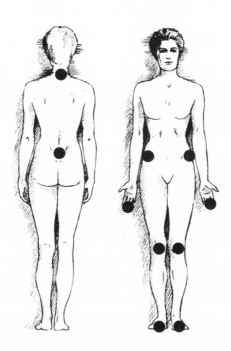

Figure 7.1. *Joints usually affected by osteoarthritis*

from moving or exercising your knee, the large muscles around the knee area will become weaker.

In the Fingers. The breakdown of joint tissue in the fingers causes bony growths (spurs) to form in these joints. If spurs occur in the end joints of the fingers, they are called Heberden's nodes. If they occur in the joints in the middle of the fingers, they are called Bouchard's nodes.

Heberden's nodes appear most often in women with OA and sometimes occur as early as age 40. They tend to run in families. Both Heberden's and Bouchard's nodes may appear first in one or a few fingers and then may develop in others. You may suddenly notice redness, swelling, tenderness and aching in the affected joints. Your fingertips may be numb and may tingle. Although these nodes may make your finger joints painful, you'll probably still have good use of your hands. Some people don't experience any pain, redness or tenderness and may never have serious problems in other joints.

In the Feet. You may feel pain and tenderness in the large joint at the base of the big toe. Wearing tight shoes and high heels can make this pain worse.

In the Spine. Breakdown of joint tissues in the spine may cause stiffness and pain in the neck and back and also may place extra pressure on the nerves in the spinal column. You may feel pain at the base of your head; in your neck, legs or lower back; or down your arms. You may feel stiffness in your neck or lower back. You also may feel weakness or numbness in your arms or legs and at times may have difficulty using your arms or walking.

Referred Pain. The pain of osteoarthritis usually occurs only in the joint or in the area around the joint. In rare cases, people feel pain far from the affected joint. This feeling is called referred pain. For example, it is possible to have osteoarthritis in your hip but feel referred pain in your thigh or near your knee.

Differences Between Osteoarthritis, Osteoporosis, and Rheumatoid Arthritis

Some people confuse osteoarthritis with osteoporosis. Although they sound similar, they are two distinctly different conditions. Osteoarthritis is a disease of joints, primarily affecting cartilage and resulting in joint pain and stiffness. Osteoporosis is a disease of bones, resulting from loss of bone mass. It causes broken bones in the wrist, spine and hip, primarily in older women.

Some people also confuse osteoarthritis with rheumatoid (ROO-mah-toyd) arthritis. As you'll see in the chart that follows, these diseases also are different. Some people can have both osteoarthritis and rheumatoid arthritis at the same time.

Table 7.1.

Osteoarthritis	Rheumatoid Arthritis
Usually begins after age 40	Usually begins between ages 25 and 50
Usually develops slowly, over many years	Often develops suddenly, within weeks or months
Often affects joints on only one side of the body at first	Usually affects same joint on both sides of the body (e.g., both knees)
Usually doesn't cause redness, warmth, swelling (inflammation) of joint	Causes redness, warmth and swelling of joints
Affects only certain joints; rarely affects elbows or shoulders	Affects many joints, including elbows and shoulders
Doesn't cause a general feeling of sickness	Often causes a general feeling of sickness, fatigue, weight loss and fever

What Causes Osteoarthritis?

Researchers now think there are several factors that increase your risk for developing osteoarthritis. These factors include heredity, obesity, injury and repeated overuse of certain joints.

Heredity

People born with slight defects that make their joints fit together incorrectly or move incorrectly, such as bow legs or a dislocated hip, may be more likely to develop osteoarthritis. Being born with laxity (double-jointedness) also increases the tendency to develop osteoarthritis.

In some families, Osteoarthritis may be the result of a hereditary defect in one of the genes responsible for a major protein component of cartilage called collagen. This leads to defective cartilage and more rapid deterioration. Such problems may not present any difficulty during youth, but may gradually wear down the joints over time. Women with a type of hereditary bony node usually present in the finger joints also maybe at increased risk for osteoarthritis.

Obesity

Studies indicate that obesity increases the risk for osteoarthritis of the knee. Researchers have found that body weight during mid or later years appears to have the greatest effect on a person's risk for developing knee osteoarthritis, particularly in the 8 to 12 years before symptoms appear.

Habitually overweight individuals can substantially lower their risk by losing weight. In one study, women who lost 11 pounds over a 10-year period reduced their risk for developing symptoms of knee OA by 50 percent.

Avoiding excess weight gain as you grow older or losing excess weight may help prevent osteoarthritis in the knee.

Injury or Overuse

Some people may develop osteoarthritis in certain joints due to an accidental injury or overuse. A history of an injury to the knee or hip increases your risk for developing osteoarthritis in these joints. For instance, football and soccer players who have knee-related injuries may be at higher risk. Avoiding trauma or accidental injury to a joint may help prevent the onset of osteoarthritis.

Joints that are used repeatedly in certain jobs may develop osteoarthritis because of an injury from overuse. Jobs that require repeated knee bending appear to increase the risk for osteoarthritis in the knees. For instance, some studies indicate that miners and shipyard or dock workers have higher rates of osteoarthritis in the knees. There are ways to modify jobs to prevent damage to joints from overuse. An occupational therapist can help you if osteoarthritis is affecting the way you perform your job.

How Is it Diagnosed?

Your doctor usually diagnoses osteoarthritis based upon your medical history and physical examination. However, your doctor also may require that some other procedures and/or tests, such as X-rays, be done to help confirm the diagnosis, determine how much joint damage has been done and help rule out other kinds of arthritis. Joint aspiration, a procedure in which fluid is drained from affected joints and examined, is routinely used, as are blood tests, to rule out other diseases. Your doctor can provide you with more information about these tests and procedures.

Chapter 8

Rheumatoid Arthritis

This chapter is for people who have rheumatoid arthritis, as well as for their family members, friends, and others who want to find out more about this disease. The chapter describes how rheumatoid arthritis develops, how it is diagnosed, and how it is treated, including what patients can do to help manage their disease. It also highlights current research efforts supported by the National Institute of Arthritis and Musculoskeletal and Skin Diseases (NIAMS) and other components of the National Institutes of Health (NIH). If you have further questions after reading this chapter, you may wish to discuss them with your doctor.

Features of Rheumatoid Arthritis

Rheumatoid arthritis is an inflammatory disease that causes pain, swelling, stiffness, and loss of function in the joints. It has several special features that make it different from other kinds of arthritis. For example, rheumatoid arthritis generally occurs in a symmetrical

NIH Publication. National Institutes of Health, National Institute of Arthritis and Musculoskeletal and Skin Diseases. Rheumatoid Arthritis. This chapter is not copyrighted. Readers are encouraged to duplicate and distribute as many copies as needed. Additional copies are available as a booklet from the National Arthritis and Musculoskeletal and Skin Diseases Information Clearinghouse, NIAMS, National Institutes of Health, 1 AMS Circle, Bethesda, Maryland 20892-3675, and on the NIAMS Web site at http://www.nih.gov/niams/healthinfo/.

pattern. This means that if one knee or hand is involved, the other one is also. The disease often affects the wrist joints and the finger joints closest to the hand. It can also affect other parts of the body besides the joints. In addition, people with the disease may have fatigue, occasional fever, and a general sense of not feeling well (malaise).

Another feature of rheumatoid arthritis is that it varies a lot from person to person. For some people, it lasts only a few months or a year or two and goes away without causing any noticeable damage. Other people have mild or moderate disease, with periods of worsening symptoms, called flares, and periods in which they feel better, called remissions. Still others have severe disease that is active most of the time, lasts for many years, and leads to serious joint damage and disability.

Although rheumatoid arthritis can have serious effects on a person's life and well-being, current treatment strategies—including pain relief and other medications, a balance between rest and exercise, and patient education and support programs—allow most people with the disease to lead active and productive lives. In recent years, research has led to a new understanding of rheumatoid arthritis and has increased the likelihood that, in time, researchers can find ways to greatly reduce the impact of this disease.

Common Features of Rheumatoid Arthritis

- Tender, warm, swollen joints.

- Symmetrical pattern. For example, of one knee is affected, the other is also.

- Joint inflammation often affecting the wrist and finger joints closest to the hand; other affected joints can include those of the neck, shoulders, elbows, hips, ankles, and feet.

- Fatigue, occasional fever, a general sense of not feeling well (malaise).

- Pain and stiffness lasting for more than 30 minutes in the morning or after a long rest.

- Symptoms that can last for many years.

- Symptoms in other parts of the body besides the joints.

- Variability of symptoms among people with the disease.

How Rheumatoid Arthritis Develops and Progresses

The Joints. A normal joint (the place where two bones meet) is surrounded by a joint capsule that protects and supports it (see Figure 8.1). Cartilage covers and cushions the ends of the two bones. The joint capsule is lined with a type of tissue called synovium, which produces synovial fluid. This clear fluid lubricates and nourishes the cartilage and bones inside the joint capsule.

In rheumatoid arthritis, the immune system, for unknown reasons, attacks a person's own cells inside the joint capsule. White blood cells that are part of the normal immune system travel to the synovium and cause a reaction. This reaction, or inflammation, is called synovitis, and it results in the warmth, redness, swelling, and pain that are typical symptoms of rheumatoid arthritis. During the inflammation process, the cells of the synovium grow and divide abnormally, making the normally thin synovium thick and resulting in a joint that is swollen and puffy to the touch (see Figure 8.2).

As rheumatoid arthritis progresses, these abnormal synovial cells begin to invade and destroy the cartilage and bone within the joint. The surrounding muscles, ligaments, and tendons that support and stabilize the joint become weak and unable to work normally. All of

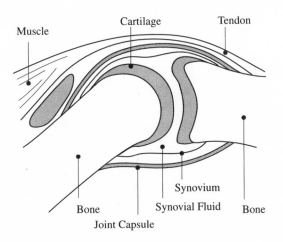

Figure 8.1. Normal Joint

73

these effects lead to the pain and deformities often seen in rheumatoid arthritis. Doctors studying rheumatoid arthritis now believe that damage to bones begins during the first year or two that a person has the disease. This is one reason early diagnosis and treatment are so important in the management of rheumatoid arthritis.

Other Parts of the Body. Some people also experience the effects of rheumatoid arthritis in places other than the joints. About one-quarter develop rheumatoid nodules. These are bumps under the skin that often form close to the joints. Many people with rheumatoid arthritis develop anemia, or a decrease in the normal number of red blood cells. Other effects, which occur less often, include neck pain and dry eyes and mouth. Very rarely, people may have inflammation of the blood vessels, the lining of the lungs, or the sac enclosing the heart.

Occurrence and Impact of Rheumatoid Arthritis. Scientists estimate that about 2.1 million people, or 1 percent of the U.S. adult population, have rheumatoid arthritis. Interestingly, some recent studies have suggested that the overall number of new cases of rheumatoid arthritis may actually be going down. Scientists are now investigating why this may be happening.

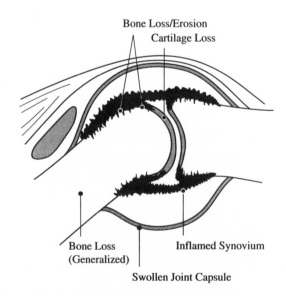

Figure 8.2. *Joint affected by Rheumatoid Arthritis*

Rheumatoid arthritis occurs in all races and ethnic groups. Although the disease often begins in middle age and occurs with increased frequency in older people, children and young adults also develop it. Like some other forms of arthritis, rheumatoid arthritis occurs much more frequently in women than in men. About two to three times as many women as men have the disease.

By all measures, the financial and social impact of all types of arthritis, including rheumatoid arthritis, is substantial, both for the Nation and for individuals. From an economic standpoint, the medical and surgical treatment for rheumatoid arthritis and the wages lost because of disability caused by the disease add up to millions of dollars. Daily joint pain is an inevitable consequence of the disease, and most patients also experience some degree of depression, anxiety, and feelings of helplessness. In some cases, rheumatoid arthritis can interfere with a person's ability to carry out normal daily activities, limit job opportunities, or disrupt the joys and responsibilities of family life. However, there are arthritis self-management programs that help people cope with the pain and other effects of the disease and help them lead independent and productive lives. These programs are described later in this chapter in the section Diagnosing and Treating Rheumatoid Arthritis.

Searching for the Cause of Rheumatoid Arthritis

Rheumatoid arthritis is one of several "autoimmune" diseases ("auto" means self), so-called because a person's immune system attacks his or her own body tissues. Scientists still do not know exactly what causes this to happen, but research over the last few years has begun to unravel the factors involved.

Genetic (Inherited) Factors

Scientists have found that certain genes that play a role in the immune system are associated with a tendency to develop rheumatoid arthritis. At the same time, some people with rheumatoid arthritis do not have these particular genes, and other people have these genes but never develop the disease. This suggests that a person's genetic makeup is an important part of the story but not the whole answer. It is clear, however, that more than one gene is involved in determining whether a person develops rheumatoid arthritis and, if so, how severe the disease will become.

Environmental Factors

Many scientists think that something must occur to trigger the disease process in people whose genetic makeup makes them susceptible to rheumatoid arthritis. An infectious agent such as a virus or bacterium appears likely, but the exact agent is not yet known. Note, however, that rheumatoid arthritis is not contagious: A person cannot "catch" it from someone else.

Other Factors

Some scientists also think that a variety of hormonal factors may be involved. These hormones, or possibly deficiencies or changes in certain hormones, may promote the development of rheumatoid arthritis in a genetically susceptible person who has been exposed to a triggering agent from the environment.

Even though all the answers aren't known, one thing is certain: Rheumatoid arthritis develops as a result of an interaction of many factors. Much research is going on now to understand these factors and how they work together (see the Current Research section of this chapter).

Diagnosing and Treating Rheumatoid Arthritis

Diagnosing and treating rheumatoid arthritis is a team effort between the patient and several types of health care professionals. A person can go to his or her family doctor or internist or to a rheumatologist. A rheumatologist is a doctor who specializes in arthritis and other diseases of the joints, bones, and muscles. As treatment progresses, other professionals often help. These may include nurses, physical or occupational therapists, orthopedic surgeons, psychologists, and social workers.

Studies have shown that people who are well informed and participate actively in their own care experience less pain and make fewer visits to the doctor than do other people with rheumatoid arthritis.

Patient education and arthritis self-management programs, as well as support groups, help people to become better informed and to participate in their own care. An example of a self-management program is the arthritis self-help course offered by the Arthritis Foundation and developed at one of the NIAMS-supported Multipurpose Arthritis and Musculoskeletal Diseases Centers. Self-management programs teach about rheumatoid arthritis and its treatments, exercise and relaxation approaches, patient/health care provider communication, and problem solving. Research on these programs has shown that they have the following clear and long-lasting benefits:

- They help people understand the disease.
- They help people reduce their pain while remaining active.
- They help people cope physically, emotionally, and mentally.
- They help people feel greater control over their disease and help build a sense of confidence in the ability to function and lead a full, active, and independent life.

Diagnosis

Rheumatoid arthritis can be difficult to diagnose in its early stages for several reasons. First, there is no single test for the disease. In addition, symptoms differ from person to person and can be more severe in some people than in others. Also, symptoms can be similar to those of other types of arthritis and joint conditions, and it may take some time for other conditions to be ruled out as possible diagnoses. Finally, the full range of symptoms develops over time, and only a few symptoms may be present in the early stages. As a result, doctors use a variety of tools to diagnose the disease and to rule out other conditions:

Medical history: This is the patient's description of symptoms and when and how they began. Good communication between patient and doctor is especially important here. For example, the patient's description of pain, stiffness, and joint function and how these change over time is critical to the doctor's initial assessment of the disease and his or her assessment of how the disease changes.

Physical examination: This includes the doctor's examination of the joints, skin, reflexes, and muscle strength.

Laboratory tests: One common test is for rheumatoid factor, an antibody that is eventually present in the blood of most rheumatoid arthritis patients. (An antibody is a special protein made by the immune system that normally helps fight foreign substances in the body.) Not all people with rheumatoid arthritis test positive for rheumatoid factor, however, especially early in the disease. And, some others who do test positive never develop the disease. Other common tests include one that indicates the presence of inflammation in the body (the erythrocyte sedimentation rate), a white blood cell count, and a blood test for anemia.

X-rays: X-rays are used to determine the degree of joint destruction. They are not useful in the early stages of rheumatoid arthritis before bone damage is evident, but they can be used later to monitor the progression of the disease.

Treatment

Doctors use a variety of approaches to treat rheumatoid arthritis. These are used in different combinations and at different times during the course of the disease and are chosen according to the patient's individual situation. No matter what treatment the doctor and patient choose, however, the goals are the same: relieve pain, reduce inflammation, slow down or stop joint damage, and improve the person's sense of well-being and ability to function.

Treatment is another key area for communication between patient and doctor. Talking to the doctor can help ensure that exercise and pain management programs are provided as needed and that drugs are prescribed appropriately. Talking can also help in making decisions about surgery.

Goals of Treatment

- Relieve pain
- Reduce inflammation
- Slow down or stop joint damage
- Improve a person's sense of well-being and ability to function

Current Treatment Approaches

- Lifestyle
- Medications
- Surgery
- Routine monitoring and ongoing care

Lifestyle

This approach includes several activities that help improve a person's ability to function independently and maintain a positive outlook.

Rest and exercise: Both rest and exercise help in important ways. People with rheumatoid arthritis need a good balance between the two, with more rest when the disease is active and more exercise when it is not. Rest helps to reduce active joint inflammation and pain and to fight fatigue. The length of time needed for rest will vary from person to person, but in general, shorter rest breaks every now and then are more helpful than long times spent in bed.

Exercise is important for maintaining healthy and strong muscles, preserving joint mobility, and maintaining flexibility. Exercise can also help people sleep well, reduce pain, maintain a positive attitude, and lose weight. Exercise programs should be planned and carried out to take into account the person's physical abilities, limitations, and changing needs.

Care of joints: Some people find that using a splint for a short time around a painful joint reduces pain and swelling by supporting the joint and letting it rest. Splints are used mostly on wrists and hands, but also on ankles and feet. A doctor or a physical or occupational therapist can help a patient get a splint and ensure that it fits properly. Other ways to reduce stress on joints include self-help devices (for example, zipper pullers, long-handled shoe horns); devices to help with getting on and off chairs, toilet seats, and beds; and changes in the ways that a person carries out daily activities.

Stress reduction: People with rheumatoid arthritis face emotional challenges as well as physical ones. The emotions they feel because of the disease—fear, anger, frustration—combined with any pain and physical limitations can increase their stress level. Although there is no evidence that stress plays a role in causing rheumatoid arthritis, it can make living with the disease difficult at times. Stress may also affect the amount of pain a person feels. There are a number of successful techniques for coping with stress. Regular rest periods can help, as can relaxation, distraction, or visualization exercises. Exercise programs, participation in support groups, and good communication with the health care team are other ways to reduce stress.

Healthful diet: With the exception of several specific types of oils (mentioned in the Current Research section), there is no scientific evidence that any specific food or nutrient helps or harms most people with rheumatoid arthritis. However, an overall nutritious diet with enough—but not an excess of—calories, protein, and calcium is important. Some people may need to be careful about drinking alcoholic beverages because of the medications they take for rheumatoid arthritis. Those taking methotrexate may need to avoid alcohol altogether. Patients should ask their doctors for guidance on this issue.

Climate: Some people notice that their arthritis gets worse when there is a sudden change in the weather. However, there is no evidence that a specific climate can prevent or reduce the effects of rheumatoid arthritis. Moving to a new place with a different climate usually does not make a long-term difference in a person's rheumatoid arthritis.

Medications

Most people who have rheumatoid arthritis take medications. Some medications are used only for pain relief; others are used to reduce inflammation. Still others—often called disease-modifying antirheumatic drugs, or DMARDs—are used to try to slow the course of the disease. The person's general condition, the current and predicted severity of the illness, the length of time he or she will take the drug, and the drug's effectiveness and potential side effects are important considerations in prescribing drugs for rheumatoid arthritis. The table below shows currently used rheumatoid arthritis medications, along with their effects, side effects, and monitoring requirements.

Traditionally, rheumatoid arthritis therapy has involved an approach in which doctors prescribed aspirin or similar drugs, rest, and physical therapy first, and prescribed more powerful drugs later only if the disease became much worse. Recently, many doctors have changed their approach, especially for patients with severe, rapidly progressing rheumatoid arthritis. This change is based on the belief that early treatment with more powerful drugs, and the use of drug combinations in place of single drugs, may be more effective ways to halt the progression of the disease and reduce or prevent joint damage.

Surgery

Several types of surgery are available to patients with severe joint damage. These procedures can help reduce pain, improve the affected joint's function and appearance, and improve the patient's ability to perform daily activities. Surgery is not for everyone, however, and the decision should be made only after careful consideration by patient and doctor. Together they should discuss the patient's overall health and the effects of a surgical procedure, the condition of the joint or tendon that will be operated on, and the reason for and cost of the surgery. Surgical procedures include joint replacement, tendon reconstruction, and synovectomy.

Joint replacement: This is the most frequently performed surgery for rheumatoid arthritis, and it is done to relieve pain, improve or preserve joint function, and improve appearance. In making a decision about replacing a joint, people with rheumatoid arthritis should consider that some artificial joints function more like normal human joints than do others. Also, artificial joints are not always permanent and may eventually have to be replaced. This may be an issue for younger people.

Tendon reconstruction: Rheumatoid arthritis can damage and even rupture tendons, the tissues that attach muscle to bone. This surgery, which is used most frequently on the hands, reconstructs the damaged tendon by attaching an intact tendon to it. This procedure can help to restore some hand function, particularly if it is done early, before the tendon is completely ruptured.

Synovectomy: In this surgery, the doctor actually removes the inflamed synovial tissue. Synovectomy by itself is seldom performed now because not all of the tissue can be removed, and it eventually grows back. Synovectomy is done as part of reconstructive surgery, especially tendon reconstruction.

Routine Monitoring and Ongoing Care

Regular medical care is important to monitor the course of the disease, determine the effectiveness and any negative effects of medications, and change therapies as needed. Monitoring typically includes regular visits to the doctor. It may also include blood, urine, and other laboratory tests and x-rays.

Osteoporosis prevention is one issue that patients may want to discuss with their doctors as part of their long-term, ongoing care. Osteoporosis is a condition in which bones lose calcium and become weakened and fragile. Many older women are at increased risk for osteoporosis, and their rheumatoid arthritis increases the risk further, particularly if they are taking corticosteroids such as prednisone. These patients may want to discuss with their doctors the potential benefits of calcium and vitamin D supplements, hormone replacement therapy, or other treatments for osteoporosis.

Alternative and Complementary Therapies

Special diets, vitamin supplements, and other alternative approaches have been suggested for the treatment of rheumatoid arthritis. Although many of these approaches may not be harmful in and of

81

Medications	Uses/Effects
Aspirin and other non-steroidal anti-inflammatory drugs (NSAIDs) Examples: • Plain aspirin • Buffered aspirin • Ibuprofen (Advil,* Motrin IB) • Ketoprofen (Orudis) • Naproxen (Naprosyn) • Diclofenac (Voltaren) • Diflunisal (Dolobid)	• Used to reduce pain, swelling, and inflammation, allowing patients to move more easily and carry out normal activities • Generally part of early and continuing therapy
Disease-modifying antirheumatic drugs (DMARDs) (also called slow-acting antirheumatic drugs [SAARDs] or second-line drugs) Examples: • Gold, injectable or oral (Myochrysine, Ridaura) • Antimalarials, such as hydroxychloroquine (Plaquenil) • Penicillamine (Cuprimine, Depen) • Sulfasalazine (Azulfidine)	• Used to alter the course of the disease and prevent joint and cartilage destruction • May produce significant improvement for many patients • Exactly how they work still unknown • Generally take a few weeks or months to have an effect • Patients may use several over the course of the disease

Table 8.1a. *Medications Commonly Used To Treat Rheumatoid Arthritis. Continued on following pages.*

Side Effects	Monitoring
<ul><li>Upset stomach</li><li>Tendency to bruise easily</li><li>Fluid retention (NSAIDs other than aspirin)</li><li>Ulcers</li><li>Possible kidney and liver damage (rare)</li></ul>	Patients should have periodic blood tests.
Toxicity is an issue– DMARDs can have serious side effects: <ul><li>Gold–skin rash, mouth sores, upset stomach, kidney problems, low blood count</li><li>Antimalarials–upset stomach, eye problems (rare)</li><li>Penicillamine–skin rashes, upset stomach, blood abnormalities, kidney problems</li><li>Sulfasalazine–upset stomach</li></ul>	Patients should be monitored carefully for continued effectiveness of medication and for side effects: <ul><li>Gold–blood and urine test monthly; more often in early use of drug</li><li>Antimalarials–eye exam every 6 months</li><li>Penicillamine–blood and urine test monthly; more often in early use of drug</li><li>Sulfasalazine–periodic blood and urine tests</li></ul>

Brand names included in this chapter are provided as examples only and their inclusion does not mean that these products are endorsed by the National Institutes of Health or any other Government agency or by Omnigraphics. Also, if a particular brand name is not mentioned, this does not mean or imply that the product is unsatisfactory.

Medications	Uses/Effects
Immunosuppressants (also considered DMARDs) Examples: ▪ Methotrexate (Rheumatrex) ▪ Azathioprine (Imuran) ▪ Cyclophosphamide (Cytoxan)	▪ Used to restrain the overly active immune system, which is key to the disease process ▪ Same concerns as with other DMARDs: potential toxicity and diminishing effectiveness over time ▪ Methotrexate can result in rapid improvement; appears to be very effective ▪ Azathioprine– first used in higher doses in cancer chemotherapy and organ transplantation; used in patients who have not responded to other drugs; used in combination therapy ▪ Cyclophosphamide– also used in higher doses in cancer chemotherapy; effective, but used only in very severe cases of rheumatoid arthritis because of potential toxicity

Table 8.1b. Medications Commonly Used To Treat Rheumatoid Arthritis. Continued from previous pages and continued on following pages.

Side Effects	Monitoring
Toxicity is an issue–immunosuppressants can have serious side effects:	Patients should be monitored carefully for continued effectiveness of medication and for side effects:
▪ Methotrexate–upset stomach, potential liver problems, low white blood cell count ▪ Azathioprine–potential blood abnormalities, low white blood cell count, possible increased cancer risk ▪ Cyclophosphamide–low white blood cell count, other blood abnormalities, increased cancer risk	▪ Methotrexate–regular blood tests, including liver function test; baseline chest x ray ▪ Azathioprine–regular blood and liver function tests ▪ Cyclophosphamide–regular blood, urine, and general medical tests

*Brand names included in this chapter are provided as examples only and their inclusion does not mean that these products are endorsed by the National Institutes of Health or any other Government agency or by Omnigraphics. Also, if a particular brand name is not mentioned, this does not mean or imply that the product is unsatisfactory.

Medications	Uses/Effects
Corticosteroids (also known as glucocorticoids) Examples: • Prednisone (Deltasone, Orasone) • Methylprednisolone (Medrol)	• Used for their anti-inflammatory and immunosuppressive effects • Given either in pill form or as an injection into a joint • Dramatic improvements in very short time • Potential for serious side effects, especially at high doses • Often used early while waiting for DMARDs to work • Also used for severe flares and when the disease does not respond to NSAIDs and DMARDs

Table 8.1c. Medications Commonly Used To Treat Rheumatoid Arthritis. Continued from previous pages.

Side Effects	Monitoring
• Osteoporosis • Mood changes • Fragile skin, easy bruising • Fluid retention • Weight gain • Muscle weakness • Onset or worsening of diabetes • Cataracts • Increased risk of infection • Hypertension (high blood pressure)	Patients should be monitored carefully for continued effectiveness of medication and for side effects.

*Brand names included in this chapter are provided as examples only and their inclusion does not mean that these products are endorsed by the National Institutes of Health or any other Government agency or by Omnigraphics. Also, if a particular brand name is not mentioned, this does not mean or imply that the product is unsatisfactory.

themselves, controlled scientific studies either have not been conducted or have found no definite benefit to these therapies. Some alternative or complementary approaches may help the patient cope or reduce some of the stress associated with living with a chronic illness. As with any therapy, patients should discuss the benefits and drawbacks with their doctors before beginning an alternative or new type of therapy. If the doctor feels the approach has value and will not be harmful, it can be incorporated into a patient's treatment plan. However, it is important not to neglect regular health care. The Arthritis Foundation publishes material on alternative therapies as well as established therapies, and patients may want to contact this organization for information. (See the For More Information section of this chapter and Part VIII of this sourcebook.)

Current Research

Over the last several decades, research has greatly increased our understanding of immunology, genetics, and cellular and molecular biology. This foundation in basic science is now showing results in several areas important to rheumatoid arthritis. Scientists are thinking about rheumatoid arthritis in exciting ways that were not possible even 10 years ago.

The National Institutes of Health funds a wide variety of medical research at its headquarters in Bethesda, Maryland, and at universities and medical centers across the United States. One of the NIH institutes, the National Institute of Arthritis and Musculoskeletal and Skin Diseases, is a major supporter of research and research training in rheumatoid arthritis through grants to individual scientists, Specialized Centers of Research, and Multipurpose Arthritis and Musculoskeletal Diseases Centers.

Following are examples of current research directions in rheumatoid arthritis supported by the Federal Government through the NIAMS and other parts of the NIH.

Scientists are looking at basic abnormalities in the immune systems of people with rheumatoid arthritis and in some animal models of the disease to understand why and how the disease develops. Findings from these studies may lead to precise, targeted therapies that could stop the inflammatory process in its earliest stages. They may even lead to a vaccine that could prevent rheumatoid arthritis.

Researchers are studying genetic factors that predispose some people to developing rheumatoid arthritis, as well as factors connected with disease severity. Findings from these studies should increase our understanding of the disease and will help develop new therapies as well as guide treatment decisions. In a major effort aimed at identifying genes involved in rheumatoid arthritis, the NIH and the Arthritis Foundation have joined together to support the North American Rheumatoid Arthritis Consortium. This group of 12 research centers around the United States is collecting medical information and genetic material from 1,000 families in which two or more siblings have rheumatoid arthritis. It will serve as a national resource for genetic studies of this disease.

Scientists are also gaining insights into the genetic basis of rheumatoid arthritis by studying rats with autoimmune inflammatory arthritis that resembles human disease. NIAMS researchers have identified several genetic regions that affect arthritis susceptibility and severity in these animal models of the disease, and found some striking similarities between rats and humans. Identifying disease genes in rats should provide important new information that may yield clues to the causes of rheumatoid arthritis in humans.

Scientists are studying the complex relationships among the hormonal, nervous, and immune systems in rheumatoid arthritis. For example, they are exploring whether and how the normal changes in the levels of steroid hormones (such as estrogen and testosterone) during a person's lifetime may be related to the development, improvement, or flares of the disease. Scientists are also looking at how these systems interact with environmental and genetic factors. Results from these studies may suggest new treatment strategies.

Researchers are exploring why so many more women than men develop rheumatoid arthritis. In hopes of finding clues, they are studying female and male hormones and other elements that differ between women and men, such as possible differences in their immune responses.

To find clues to new treatments, researchers are examining why rheumatoid arthritis often improves during pregnancy. Results of one study suggest that the explanation may be related to differences in certain special proteins between a mother and her unborn child. These proteins help the immune system distinguish between the body's own cells and foreign cells. Such differences, the scientists speculate, may change the activity of the mother's immune system during pregnancy.

A growing body of evidence indicates that infectious agents, such as viruses and bacteria, may trigger rheumatoid arthritis in people who have an inherited predisposition to the disease. Investigators are trying to discover which infectious agents may be responsible. More broadly, they are also working to understand the basic mechanisms by which these agents might trigger the development of rheumatoid arthritis. Identifying the agents and understanding how they work could lead to new therapies.

Scientists are searching for new drugs or combinations of drugs that can reduce inflammation, can slow or stop the progression of rheumatoid arthritis, and also have few side effects. Studies in humans have shown that a number of compounds have such potential. For example, some studies are breaking new ground in the area of "biopharmaceuticals," or "biologics." These new drugs are based on compounds occurring naturally in the body, and are designed to target specific aspects of the inflammatory process.

Investigators have also shown that treatment of rheumatoid arthritis with minocycline, a drug in the tetracycline family, has a modest benefit. The effects of a related tetracycline called doxycycline are under investigation. Other studies have shown that the omega-3 fatty acids in certain fish or plant seed oils also may reduce rheumatoid arthritis inflammation. However, many people are not able to tolerate the large amounts of oil necessary for any benefit.

Investigators are examining many issues related to quality of life for rheumatoid arthritis patients and quality, cost, and effectiveness of health care services for these patients. Scientists have found that even a small improvement in a patient's sense of physical and mental well-being can have an impact on his or her quality of life and use of health care services. Results from studies like these will help health care providers design integrated treatment strategies that cover all of a patient's needs—emotional as well as physical.

Hope for the Future

Scientists are making rapid progress in understanding the complexities of rheumatoid arthritis—how and why it develops, why some people get it and others do not, why some people get it more severely than others. Results from research are having an impact today, enabling people with rheumatoid arthritis to remain active in life, family, and work far longer than was possible 20 years ago. There is also hope for tomorrow, as researchers continue to explore ways of stopping the disease process early, before it becomes destructive, or even preventing rheumatoid arthritis altogether.

For More Information

National Arthritis and Musculoskeletal and Skin Diseases
Information Clearinghouse
NIAMS/National Institutes of Health
1 AMS Circle
Bethesda, MD 20892-3675

The text of this chapter is also available 24 hours a day by fax. Using the phone on a fax machine, call NIAMS Fast Facts at (301) 881-2731. Listen to the instructions and dial 01301; the text will print to the fax machine.

The National Arthritis and Musculoskeletal and Skin Diseases Information Clearinghouse (NAMSIC) is a public service sponsored by the NIAMS that provides health information and information sources. The Clearinghouse provides information on rheumatoid arthritis, including a fact sheet on arthritis and exercise. Fact sheets, additional information, and research updates can also be found on the NIAMS Web site at http://www.nih.gov/niams/.

Arthritis Foundation
1330 West Peachtree Street
Atlanta, GA 30309
(800) 283-7800
(404) 872-7100
or your local chapter, listed in the telephone directory
Web address: http://www.arthritis.org

The Arthritis Foundation is the major voluntary organization devoted to supporting arthritis research and providing educational and other services to individuals with arthritis. The foundation publishes a free pamphlet on rheumatoid arthritis and a magazine for members on all types of arthritis. It also provides up-to-date information on research and treatment, nutrition, alternative therapies, and self-management strategies. Chapters nationwide offer exercise programs, classes, support groups, physician referral services, and free literature.

Acknowledgments

The NIAMS gratefully acknowledges the assistance of the following people in the preparation and review of the material for this chapter:

John H. Klippel, M.D., NIAMS, NIH; Reva Lawrence, M.P.H., NIAMS, NIH; Amye L. Leong, San Pedro Peninsula, California; Michael D. Lockshin, M.D., Barbara Volcker Center for Women and Rheumatic Disease, Hospital for Special Surgery, New York, New York; Kate Lorig, R.N., Dr.P.H., Stanford University, Stanford, California; J. Lee Nelson, M.D., Fred Hutchinson Cancer Research Center, Seattle, Washington; Stanley R. Pillemer, M.D., NIH; Paul H. Plotz, M.D., NIAMS, NIH; Paul G. Rochmis, M.D., Fairfax Virginia; and Ronald L. Wilder, M.D., Ph.D., NIAMS, NIH. Special thanks also go to Cheryl Yarboro, R.N., B.S.P.A., NIAMS, NIH, and to the patients who reviewed this text and provided valuable input. This text for this chapter was written by Anne Brown Rodgers of Cygnus Corporation.

About NIAMS and NAMSIC

The National Arthritis and Musculoskeletal and Skin Diseases Information Clearinghouse (NAMSIC) is a public service sponsored by the NIAMS that provides health information and information sources. The NIAMS, a part of the National Institutes of Health (NIH), leads the Federal medical research effort in arthritis and musculoskeletal and skin diseases. The NIAMS supports research and research training throughout the United States as well as on the NIH campus in Bethesda, Maryland, and disseminates health and research information. Additional information and research updates can be found on the NIAMS Web site at http://www.nih.gov/niams/

Chapter 9

Gout

Say the word "gout" and some people will think of a bloated king surveying the remains of a sumptuous feast, wine glass in hand, swollen foot propped on a pillow—looking for all the world like the dismal product of a grossly overindulgent life.

There are a couple of flaws in that conventional image. We know, for example, that gout doesn't afflict only the privileged classes and that women, too, are susceptible, though a lot less than men.

But still there's a good deal right with that picture. It correctly reflects that:

- About 90 percent of people afflicted with gout are men over 40.

- Obesity in general, and in particular excessive weight gain in men between ages 20 and 40, has been shown to increase the risk of gout. In fact, about half of all gout sufferers are overweight.

- Alcohol abuse and so-called "binge" drinking are associated with gout, as is eating purine-rich foods such as brains, kidneys, liver, sardines, anchovies, and dried beans and peas.

In addition, careful scientific surveys have shown that occupational exposure to lead, the use of certain drugs to control high blood pressure, some surgical procedures, family history (possibly a genetic predisposition), and trauma are all linked to an increased risk of gout.

FDA Consumer, March 1995.

Indeed, the prevalence of gout—the number of gout sufferers for each 100,000 people—is rising rapidly in the United States and other developed countries. Some authorities believe the increase is related to higher living standards.

Our fanciful image of a gouty Henry VIII (or other bloated monarch) can't show, however, the one common denominator that ties together this mixed bag of risk factors: failure of the metabolic process that controls the amount of uric acid in the blood. For most people, the process works just fine. But in some one million Americans, uric acid metabolism has gone seriously haywire. As a result, they suffer from gout.

And suffer they do. An Englishman, Thomas Sydenham, writing in the 17th century, left this unfortunately all-too-accurate description of a typical attack of gout: *The victim goes to bed . . . in good health. About two o'clock in the morning, he is awakened by a severe pain in the great toe; more rarely in the heel, ankle, or instep. The pain is like that of a dislocation. [It] becomes more intense . . . . So exquisite and lively meanwhile is the feeling of the part affected, that it cannot bear the weight of the bedclothes nor the jar of a person walking in the room. The night is passed in torture . . .*

How Gout Gets Going

After several years of abnormal uric acid deposits, uric acid crystals can build up in joints and surrounding tissues. They form large lumpy deposits called tophi, which, if left untreated, can damage joints.

A Crystal Culprit

In spite of the agony and havoc it can cause, uric acid is a normal constituent of the human body. Ordinarily about one third of the uric acid in our system comes from food, especially foods like those noted earlier that are rich in purines. The rest we produce ourselves through ordinary metabolism.

The body converts purines to uric acid. The level of uric acid in the blood fluctuates in response to diet, fluid intake, overall health status, and other factors. Men normally have somewhat more uric acid than women do (although the difference begins to narrow after menopause), and in both sexes it tends to increase with advancing age.

Higher-than-normal amounts of uric acid in the blood, a condition called hyperuricemia, is quite common and only rarely warrants medical treatment. On the other hand, sustained hyperuricemia is the primary risk factor for gout. It's safe to say that, while not all people with hyperuricemia develop gout, virtually everyone with gout is hyperuricemic. It works this way:

At normal and even somewhat elevated levels, uric acid stays in solution in the blood. It moves through the circulation, gets filtered by the kidneys, and is excreted in the urine. When, however, blood uric acid levels rise above a certain concentration (which varies with temperature and blood acidity), it forms needle-like crystals that lodge in or around a joint.

In response to irritation caused by uric acid crystals, the skin covering the affected area rapidly becomes tight, inflamed, swollen, and red or purplish. These classical signs of inflammation, together with sudden and extreme pain (just as Thomas Sydenham described), strongly suggest an acute attack of gout. The diagnosis is confirmed by laboratory finding of uric acid crystals in fluid taken from the affected joint.

Why is the big toe the most common site for an initial gout attack? Perhaps because first, the extremities are a bit cooler than other parts of the body, and uric acid crystals form more readily at lower temperatures; and second, normal walking and standing subject the feet to considerable stress. Together, these factors might explain why the big toe, heel, instep, and Achilles tendon are among the places that gout attacks first. Other targets, especially in untreated patients who have recurrent attacks of gout, are the knee, elbow, wrist, fingers and, less often, the shoulder, pelvis, spine, and internal organs.

Gout is classified as a form of arthritis because it is initially and predominantly a disease of the joints. Other similar conditions exist; one called "pseudogout" is somewhat milder than true gout and is caused by calcium rather than uric acid crystals. Infection or trauma to the affected area can mimic gout and mislead both patients and health professionals. Accurate diagnosis is essential for appropriate treatment.

Without treatment, an initial acute attack of gout will run its painful course within several days or a few weeks, by which time all outward evidence of the disease disappears. The next acute attack—50 or more percent of gout sufferers will have a second attack—may not occur for months or years. Subsequent attacks, however, are likely to be more frequent, more severe, and more destructive to joints and other tissue unless the problem is treated. Over time, uric acid crystals accumulate in the body, causing gritty, chalky deposits called tophi that are sometimes visible under the skin, particularly around joints and in the edges of the ears. Tophi may also form inside bone near the joints, in the kidneys, and in other organs and tissues, causing permanent damage. Advances in treatment, fortunately, have made this kind of chronic gout extremely rare.

Treatment

As with most illnesses, effective treatment of gout depends on a correct diagnosis. Gout can be unequivocally diagnosed by telltale uric acid crystals in joint fluid. But appropriate treatment is often started after a "clinical" diagnosis based on painfully obvious signs and symptoms and other relevant factors, such as the patient's uric acid level, age, weight, gender, diet, and alcohol use. If this picture adds up to a strong suspicion of gout, treatment can be started with the immediate goal of arresting the acute attack.

Acute gout is treated with drugs that block the inflammatory reaction. One of the oldest agents known to be effective against acute gout is colchicine, which comes from a common European plant, the autumn crocus, and is marketed in this country primarily as a generic drug. An English clergyman, Sidney Smith, said a century and a half ago that he had only to go into his garden and hold out his gouty toe to the plant to obtain a prompt cure. This may have been an exaggeration, but a rapid response to colchicine suggests that the patient does indeed have gout.

This old, powerful remedy is now used less often than it once was because it can be quite toxic, causing nausea, vomiting, diarrhea, and stomach cramps when taken by mouth and severe (even fatal) blood disorders when taken intravenously. Moreover, modern agents, specifically nonsteroidal anti-inflammatory drugs (NSAIDs) are highly effective against acute gout and less toxic than colchicine. To treat an acute case of gout, the first choice of many physicians is the NSAID Indocin (and other brands of indomethacin). Naprosyn (naproxen) is another NSAID commonly used in acute gout.

Steroid drugs, such as Deltasone (and other brands of prednisone) and Acthar (and other brands of adrenocorticotropic hormone), may be used if NSAIDs fail to control an acute attack. Steroids may be taken by mouth or by injection into the bloodstream or muscle.

Drug treatment usually relieves the symptoms of acute gout within 48 hours. Subsequent treatment, which may well be lifelong, is aimed at preventing further attacks by controlling uric acid in the blood—keeping it below concentrations at which crystals can form. Two main treatment approaches are used, in some cases simultaneously.

One approach is to slow the rate at which the body produces uric acid. Zyloprim (allopurinol) has been approved for the treatment of gout and is frequently prescribed for gout patients who have uric acid kidney stones or other kidney problems. Side effects include skin rash and upset stomach, both of which usually subside as the body becomes used to the drug. Zyloprim makes some patients drowsy, so they need to be cautious about driving or using machinery.

The other approach to controlling gout following an initial acute attack is to increase the amount of uric acid excreted in urine. Two so-called uricosuric drugs commonly used for this are Benemid (probenecid) and Anturane (sulfinpyrazone), both approved by FDA for gout treatment. In addition to lowering blood uric acid levels, these drugs help dissolve deposits of uric acid crystals around joints and in other tissue. Zyloprim is also used to dissolve tophaceous gout in uric acid over-producers. Uricosurics can cause nausea, stomach upset, headache, and a potentially serious skin rash.

Drugs to control uric acid levels may, paradoxically, prolong an acute attack. For this reason, Benemid, Anturane and Zyloprim are not used during the acute stage of gout. They may, in fact, induce gout flare-ups during the early part of long-term use. Accordingly, colchicine in a dose low enough to avoid toxic side effects is some-times prescribed to prevent acute attacks during this phase of treatment.

Common-sense Measures

Better understanding of what gout is, what causes it, and how to treat it has perhaps dispelled some of the traditional myths about what has been erroneously called "the disease of kings." Then, too, folk wisdom about gout, coupled with good science and medicine, points to measures that prudent people can take to prevent or at least lessen the severity of the condition.

Many authorities and the Arthritis Foundation, which supports research and public service programs relating to gout, advocate weight control as a logical aid to gout prevention. They point out, however, that people who are overweight should get professional guidance in planning a weight reduction program, because fasting or severe diet-ing can actually increase uric acid levels.

Experts generally agree that people with gout can eat pretty much what they want, within limits. People who have kidney stones caused by uric acid may need to avoid purine-rich foods. But this problem can usually be handled effectively with drug treatment.

Curbing alcohol use and avoiding "binge" drinking can reduce the likelihood of acute attacks. So can drinking six or eight glasses of water a day, which dilutes uric acid and aids its removal by the kidneys. Some medicines—in particular the thiazide diuretics ("water pills") used to control high blood pressure—tend to increase uric acid levels. A gout patient taking one of these drugs may have to switch to another type of diuretic or blood pressure medicine.

Finally, although uncommon, it might be helpful to find out if an environmental or occupational exposure to lead is playing a role in a patient's problem with gout.

While a cure for gout—a treatment that gets rid of the condition once and for all—isn't on the horizon, reliable and effective ways of diagnosing gout and keeping it under control constitute one of the more impressive success stories of modern medical science.

There may be no sure-fire way to keep a person from having that first agonizing attack, but prompt treatment can minimize the risk of further attacks and virtually rule out the damaging and crippling effects of chronic gouty arthritis.

—by Ken Flieger

Ken Flieger is a writer in Washington, D.C.

Part Three

Other Forms of Arthritis and Related Disorders

Chapter 10

Spondyloarthropathies: A Family of Related Diseases

Introduction

In this chapter, you will learn about these five diseases:

- Ankylosing Spondylitis
- Reiter's Syndrome/Reactive Arthritis
- Psoriatic Arthritis and Psoriatic Spondylitis
- Spondylitis of Inflammatory Bowel Disease
- Undifferentiated Spondyloarthropathy

The following pages present the primary signs and symptoms of these diseases; what we think causes them; the risks of further complications; and various treatments and techniques to manage these conditions.

The information contained in this chapter cannot replace treatment provided by your doctor or other health care professionals. If you have questions as you read this chapter, you may want to consult further with your doctor.

The Five Spondyloarthropathies

The great numbers and types of rheumatic diseases present a challenge to patients and doctors alike. Among the 100 different rheumatic diseases (which affect the joints and muscles) is a group of five called the spondyloarthropathies. These include: ankylosing spondylitis, Reiter's syndrome/reactive arthritis, psoriatic arthritis or spondylitis, spondylitis of inflammatory bowel disease, and undifferentiated Spondyloarthropathy.

Like the other rheumatic diseases, the spondyloarthropathies display a variety of symptoms and signs. But they also share many common features, including:

- a tendency toward inflammatory arthritis of the spine, sacroiliac joints, and other joints of the body.

- a condition called enthesopathy, which is an inflammation where ligaments and tendons attach to bone.

- a tendency to occur in more than one family member.

- the absence of physical signs or testing markers found in other types of arthritis. For instance, other types of arthritis may be accompanied by subcutaneous nodules (or small lumps under the skin) and a blood test which is positive for the rheumatoid factor.

Who Is at Risk?

The complete medical term for this group of diseases is the "seronegative" spondyloarthropathies. ("Sero" refers to the blood and "negative" indicates that there is usually no rheumatoid factor present in the blood.) Most spondyloarthropathies begin around the ages of 20-30. Men are more likely to get the disease. Psoriatic arthritis, which affects men and women equally, is the exception to this. Those whose condition includes spinal involvement tend to have the gene that makes a protein called HLA-B27.

The Role of Genetics

For a long time, researchers suspected that these diseases had a hereditary component. They had noticed that family members of people with ankylosing spondylitis and psoriatic arthritis also frequently got these diseases. In 1973, scientists found an association between HLA-B27 and ankylosing spondylitis (AS) and other spondyloarthropathies. Since the discovery of HLA-B27, its link with spondyloarthropathies has been extensively documented: Over 95 percent of patients with ankylosing spondylitis; 90 percent of those with Reiter's syndrome/reactive arthritis; and about 70 percent of those with psoriatic spondylitis and the spondylitis of inflammatory bowel disease will have HLA-B27. On the other hand, those with psoriatic arthritis involving only the peripheral joints and not the spine only have a slightly increased frequency of HLA-B27 (25 percent) and those with peripheral arthritis and inflammatory bowel disease show no increased frequency of HLA-B27 above that of the healthy population, which shows a frequency of about 7 percent.

Should You Be Tested?

Although we now know that people with spondyloarthropathies most likely have HLA-B27, the marker does not predict who will get the disease. Most HLA-B27 positive people, in fact, do not have a spondyloarthropathy. Only about 1 to 2 percent of those who have HLA-B27 ever develop AS. For this reason, doctors do not advise family members of a person with a spondyloarthropathy to be tested, especially if they don't show any symptoms of the disease.

The Role of HLA-B27

While we still do not know exactly how HLA-B27 influences the development of spondyloarthropathy, studies conducted with rats seem to establish its role in causing the disease. When the human HLA-B27 gene was injected into rats, they developed the signs and symptoms of spondyloarthropathy. Recent studies have suggested that the presence of HLA-B27 may actually permit certain types of bacteria to enter and survive in certain tissues of the body, such as joints.

Types, Signs and Symptoms

Ankylosing Spondylitis (AS)

Ankylosing spondylitis (AS) is probably the best known of the spondyloarthropathies. This disease affects about two in every 1,000 Caucasians. It appears to be more common in men and is uncommon in African-Americans. AS can occur as early as the teenage years or as late as age 40-50, but usually begins in the person's 20s or 30s.

Early and Advanced Symptoms

Typically, people with AS first notice pain and stiffness in the lower back and buttocks, caused by arthritis in the sacroiliac joints. The symptoms are usually worse in the mornings, and the stiffness tends to improve with exercise. As the disease slowly progresses, the pain and stiffness may spread up the spine, sometimes even up to the neck. In severe cases, the spinal vertebrae may completely fuse. The joints where the ribs meet the spine may also fuse, making deep inhalation difficult. One way to adapt to this problem is to do breathing exercises using the abdominal muscles.

The spinal fusion in some patients with AS produces a column of bone which also causes the loss of the cushioning effect normally provided by intervertebral discs. As a result, the spine then becomes more prone to fracture. People with AS, particularly those with advanced disease, should take particular care to avoid situations that may cause spinal trauma.

Other Complications of AS

About one-fourth to one-half of patients with AS also have arthritis in the joints of the arms and legs. About a quarter of those with AS will get iritis or uveitis, an inflammation of the eye that requires treatment by an ophthalmologist to prevent permanent eye damage. Uncommon complications of AS include:

- involvement of the aortic valve of the heart, resulting in aortic insufficiency·caused by a leaky valve.

- blocks in the heart's electrical conduction system.

- fibrosis of the lungs, especially the upper segments.

Routine physical examinations by a physician can detect these complications before they become very serious.

Reiter's Syndrome/Reactive Arthritis

Originally described during WWI, Reiter's syndrome affects the following parts of the body:

- the joints (usually the knees, ankles and toes; occasionally those in the arms and hands; and less frequently the spine and sacroiliac).

- the skin, where rashes commonly appear as thickened red or brown spots, scaling rashes on the palms of the hands or the soles of the feet, or a red, scaling rash on the penis.

- the eyes, with frequent appearance of conjunctivitis, an inflammation of the eye's outer lining, or iritis or uveitis, an inflammation of the eye's inner parts.

- the bladder.

- the genitals.

- the mucus membranes.

People with Reiter's syndrome often have Achilles' tendinitis, a painful swelling behind the heel, or plantar fasciitis, pain and tenderness on the sole of the foot under the heel. Involved fingers and toes often swell, causing the so-called "sausage digit." Fingernails and toenails can also be affected, becoming thickened and crumbling as if infected by fungus.

Is Infection the Cause?

The term "reactive arthritis" is now considered synonymous with Reiter's syndrome, but usually refers to primary involvement of the joints without prominent skin or eye complications.

Reiter's syndrome and reactive arthritis usually result from one of two types of infection:

- a bacterium called Chlamydia, contracted during sexual activity and causing either burning on urination or a watery discharge from the penis or vagina.

- bacteria such as Salmonella, Shigella, Yersinia or Campylobacter that cause dysentery and are contracted by eating spoiled food, such as meat or dairy products sitting too long at room temperature, or handled without proper hygienic practices.

Genetics and Infection Combine

While anyone can get either of these bacterial infections, those who go on to develop Reiter's syndrome and reactive arthritis are those with the HLA-B27 gene. In fact, one out of every five HLA-B27-positive individuals who is infected with one of these bacteria will develop Reiter's syndrome or reactive arthritis.

Psoriatic Arthritis/Spondylitis

Psoriasis is a scaly rash that occurs most frequently on the elbows, knees and scalp, but can cover much of the body. In about 5 to 10 percent of those with this disease, arthritis also appears. In most cases, the psoriasis will precede the arthritis, sometimes by many years.

Conjunctivitis and iritis do occur, although much less frequently than in other spondyloarthropathies.

Types of Psoriatic Arthritis

The arthritis takes several different forms.

- The joints at the ends of the fingers are most commonly affected. This is usually accompanied by symptoms of the fingernails and toenails, ranging from small pits in the nails to nearly complete nail destruction and crumbling, as seen in Reiter's syndrome or fungal infections.

- About one-fifth of those with psoriatic arthritis will have involvement of the spine (spondylitis). The spinal disease can progress to complete spinal fusion (as in AS) or can skip areas, where, for example, only the lower back and neck are involved. Those with spinal involvement are most likely to be HLA-B27 positive.

- The least common type of psoriatic arthritis is also the most severe. Called psoriatic arthritis mutilans, it occurs in about one in 20 with psoriatic arthritis. As the name "mutilans" suggests, this disease results in widespread destruction of the joints.

Arthritis/Spondylitis Associated with Inflammatory Bowel Disease

This type of spondyloarthropathy involves inflammation of the intestinal wall. Abdominal pain and often bloody diarrhea are the primary symptoms of inflammatory bowel disease, the two best known types of which are ulcerative colitis and Crohn's disease.

About one in six patients with inflammatory bowel disease also has spinal inflammation, although the intensity of spinal inflammation is independent of the severity of the bowel disease. In many, this may just be arthritis in the sacroiliac joints, but in about 5 percent the entire spine can be involved, as it is in AS. Inflammation of the eye occurs less frequently than in AS.

Approximately one in five people with inflammatory bowel disease (especially Crohn's disease) will have arthritis in one of the joints of the arms or legs. In contrast to the spinal arthritis, the severity of arthritis in these joints follows that of the bowel disease when the diarrhea and abdominal pain are flaring, this arthritis tends to flare also.

Undifferentiated Spondyloarthropathy

Sometimes doctors see patients with signs and symptoms of spondyloarthropathy that don't quite fit into one of the categories outlined above. For example, a person may have iritis and heel pain and be HLA-B27 positive. In cases such as these the term "undifferentiated spondyloarthropathy" is often used. Some of these people may later develop symptoms of the so-called classic categories explained above. But many will continue to have chronic, but not severe symptoms, and remain undifferentiated.

Expectations for the Future

Most people with one of the spondyloarthropathies lead long and productive lives. Certain complications, however, can lead to disability. It is important to be on the lookout for signs and symptoms of the more serious complications. Fortunately, only a minority of those with AS, for instance, develop severe spinal deformities. And even then, several interventions are available. Likewise, chronic and severe eye inflammation can lead to visual impairment and even blindness. But with regular checkups, preferably with an ophthalmologist, a person with iritis or other eye problems can be effectively monitored for any sign of progressive eye damage.

Interventions and Treatments

A full range of interventions exist for those with the spondyloarthropathies. These range from exercise and postural controls, to analgesics (painkillers) and antibiotics, to surgical interventions in selected cases. These are all presented below.

Postural and Non-invasive Interventions

We do not know whether medical therapy can prevent spinal fusion in patients with a spondyloarthropathy. If it appears that fusion is occurring, therapy is aimed at trying to influence how the spine fuses. Therefore, early and aggressive intervention is recommended in someone just given a diagnosis of spondylitis. A spine that fuses in a straight and upright position allows a person to be much more functional than one that has fused in a bent forward position. If the neck fuses in a position so far forward that the chin is touching the chest, this can cause difficulties with forward gaze and even with chewing one's food.

Keeping the Spine Straight

Exercises designed at keeping the spine straight (and mobile, if possible) are very important. Just as important in keeping the spine straight are certain lifestyle changes, such as:

- Sleeping without a pillow. Up to one third of the day is spent in bed, and most people use at least one pillow. Using a pillow causes the head to be bent forward. For someone with a spondylo-arthropathy, maintaining that position for eight hours at a time can influence spinal fusion in the forward-flexed position.

- Sitting in an upright position, with the spine straight and erect. People with spondyloarthropathy must take certain measures to prevent slouching forward when seated at a desk or while watching television. They may prefer to watch TV while lying on the floor on their stomachs. If they work at a desk or computer terminal, periodic breaks for stretching can be helpful.

Other Helpful Measures

- Application of heat, ultrasound and massage, can provide at least temporary pain relief.

- Heel cups can be effective in relieving the heel pain and discomfort associated with planter fasciitis.

- Avoiding excess calories and obesity. However, dietary measures have not yet been found helpful in the management of the spondyloarthropathies.

- Maintaining physical fitness, which is so important in coping with the disease.

Exercise Is Important

Anyone with spondyloarthropathy, especially with spondylitis, should have a daily home exercise schedule. Excessive rest can actually put someone at greater risk for spinal fusion. Many exercise programs are possible, but any that are adopted should include the following elements:

- stretching; neck flexion (bending forward);
- neck extension (bending backward);
- neck rotation (bending around); side stretching; and
- spinal extension (bending the spine backward).

Many of these exercises are described in better detail in Straight Talk on Spondylitis, available from the Spondylitis Association.

Studies have shown that regular exercise in exercise groups led by a physiotherapist can give the best results. Keep in mind that if you are at higher risk for spinal fracture, you should avoid hard competitive sports, impact loading and heavy weight bearing exercises.

A Range of Medications

Many types of medications have been effective in managing the symptoms of spondyloarthropathy. The main types are summarized below.

Nonsteroidal Anti-inflammatory Drugs / NSAIDs

NSAIDs are the most commonly used medications for the spondyloarthropathies. NSAIDs can be quite effective in reducing the pain and stiffness associated with these diseases but often chronic, high doses of NSAIDs are required to maintain such relief. Indomethacin (Indocin) is the most widely used and probably one of the most effective. Phenylbutazone (Butazolidin) is also occasionally used, but the rare side effect of bone marrow toxicity has caused it to no longer be widely available in the U.S.

NSAIDs most frequently affect the gastrointestinal system. They prevent the production of gastric mucus and also cause some localized irritation. This can lead to heartburn, gastritis and even gastric or duodenal ulceration and bleeding. People can take drugs to neutralize or prevent the production of gastric acid (antacids or H2 blockers such as cimetidine) or coat the stomach (Carafate) or restore the lost gastric mucus (Cytotec). Other less common side effects of NSAIDs include fluid retention, headaches, dizziness and even confusion.

Sulfasalazine

Sulfasalazine can effectively control not only pain and joint swelling from arthritis of the extremities in patients with ankylosing spondylitis and other spondyloarthropathies, but also the intestinal lesions in inflammatory bowel disease. The usual dosage is between three and four grams of sulfasalazine per day. Side effects include headaches, abdominal bloating and nausea and oral ulcers. Rarely the patient can develop bone marrow suppression on this drug, thus requiring occasional monitoring of blood counts.

Methotrexate

Methotrexate is also effective in controlling the symptoms of arthritis in many patients with spondyloarthropathy, particularly psoriatic arthritis and Reiter's syndrome. It has the added benefit of improving the skin rash of psoriasis. It is given once a week, either in one dosage (if arthritis treatment is the major goal) or in three doses spaced at twelve hour intervals (if psoriasis treatment is most important). The weekly doses range between 7.5 and 25 mg. Side effects include bone marrow suppression, with lowering of the blood counts, oral ulcers, nausea, gastritis or peptic ulceration and liver toxicity. These require frequent monitoring of the blood counts and liver profile.

Antibiotics

Antibiotics, such as doxycycline, may be useful when administered for up to three months in patients in the early stages of Reiter's syndrome/reactive arthritis. Their usefulness in established disease or in other spondyloarthropathies is less clear, however.

Corticosteroids

Corticosteroids such as prednisone can be effective in relieving the inflammation associated with spondyloarthropathies, but their side effects (weight gain, osteoporosis, etc.) make the use of NSAIDs more desirable. The use of corticosteroid injections into inflamed joints can also provide temporary relief of the pain and swelling of arthritis or bursitis. Because of the concern of rupture of the Achilles' tendon, such injections are rarely, if ever, used to treat Achilles' tendinitis. Similarly, their usefulness in planter fasciitis is not clear.

Experimental Therapies

When the above medications fail to adequately control the symptoms of spondyloarthropathy, other more toxic or less well proven remedies are possible. Drugs that suppress the activity of the immune system, such as azathioprine (Imuran) or cyclophosphamide (Cytoxan) may be effective where others have failed. However, their higher side effect profile, including the increased frequency of cancers in patients receiving these medications, clearly limits their use.

Surgical Remedies

Occasionally the arthritis associated with the spondylo-arthropathies can be so severe as to cause destruction of the joint cartilage. In this case, particularly in the knees and hips, joint replacement can be effective in alleviating pain as well as in restoring function to severely damaged joints.

Ankylosing spondylitis can be associated with severe flexion deformities of the spine, particularly in the neck. Surgical correction of the flexion deformity is possible, although this procedure is risky (particularly with the concern of spinal cord injury and paralysis) and should only be attempted by surgeons who have extensive experience with this procedure.

Conclusion

Most people are able to manage these diseases well. They are able to continue to work, raise children, and lead a typically productive and active life. Some patients will need to change their recreational activities. Some will eventually need to modify or change their work. It is important to remember that there is much that can be done to help, and more importantly, much that people can do to help themselves.

Spondylitis Association of America

A national nonprofit organization founded in 1983, the Spondylitis Association of America is dedicated to providing information and support to patients and their families. Our mission includes educating physicians to recognize the early symptoms and initiate appropriate treatment, expanding public awareness and understanding of spondylitis, and advocating research to find the cure.

Publications include a quarterly newsletter called *Spondylitis Plus*, a comprehensive patient self-management book and exercise poster entitled *Straight Talk on Spondylitis*, *Fight Back* exercise videotape, *The Water Workout* exercise videotape, *A Guidebook for Patients*, an exercise audiotape, and a booklet on *Juvenile Ankylosing Spondylitis*.

For more information, please write or call:

Spondylitis Association of America
P. O. Box 5872
Sherman Oaks,
CA 91413
(800) 777-8189

Chapter 11

Psoriatic Arthritis

Psoriatic Arthritis: Advice, Information, and Guidance

What Is Psoriatic Arthritis?

Psoriatic (sore-ee-AA-tick) arthritis is a condition that causes pain and swelling in some joints and scaly skin patches on some areas of the body. Psoriatic arthritis is related to psoriasis (so-REYE-ah-sis), a chronic (long-lasting) skin condition that may affect up to 3 percent of the population. Psoriasis is characterized by a scaly, itchy skin rash, often on the elbows, knees and scalp. Psoriasis also causes lifting of the nails and pitting, a condition in which the nails become marked with several small depressions.

The joint pain caused by psoriatic arthritis often is associated with stiffness, especially in the morning. About a third of people with psoriatic arthritis also have neck and/or back pain and stiffness, which may further limit movement.

Psoriatic arthritis affects men and women of all races. It usually occurs between the ages of 20 and 50, but it can occur at any age. It

This chapter contains texts from two sources. ©1995 Excerpted from *Psoriatic Arthritis: Advice, Information, and Guidance*. Used by Permission of the Arthritis Foundation. For more information, please call the Arthritis Foundation's Information Line 1-800-283-7800. Reprinted with Permission. National Institute of Arthritis and Musculoskeletal and Skin Diseases. Office of Scientific and Health Communications web document, "Questions and Answers about Psoriasis." [http://www.nih.gov/niams/healthinfo/psoriafs.htm]

affects about 20 to 30 percent of people who have psoriasis. More than 80 percent of people with psoriatic arthritis have nail involvement. Nail lesions occur more commonly in people who have psoriatic arthritis and uncomplicated psoriasis. However, not everyone who has psoriasis develops psoriatic arthritis.

What Are the Patterns of Joint Involvement?

About 95 percent of those with psoriatic arthritis have swelling in joints outside the spine. In most of these people, more than five joints are affected. These joints often involve swollen fingers and toes.

Psoriatic arthritis may either occur in the same joints on both sides of the body at the same time or, more likely, in different joints on either side of the body at the same time. In some people there is just swelling in the outermost joints, such as in the tips of the fingers or in the toes.

About 5 percent of people with psoriatic arthritis just have spinal involvement. This form of psoriatic arthritis affects the sacroiliac joints and spine and usually involves pain and stiffness in the buttocks, lower back, neck or along the spine. Another 20 to 40 percent have both spinal involvement and joint involvement outside the spine.

What Are the Symptoms?

- Silver or gray scaly spots on the scalp, elbows, knees and/or the lower end of the backbone;

- Pitting, which is characterized by small depressions and/or detachment of fingernails and/or toenails;

- Pain and swelling in one or more joints, usually including the wrists, knees or ankles and/or joints at the ends of the fingers or toes; and

- Swelling of fingers and/or toes that gives them a "sausage" appearance.

The course of psoriatic arthritis varies. Most people do reasonably well and lead productive lives. However, in about 20 percent of the people the arthritis may become deforming and destructive. It is thought that this damage results from persistent inflammation within the affected joints. It is not yet known what factors lead to the development of the destructive rather than the mild form of the arthritis.

What Causes Psoriatic Arthritis?

The cause of psoriatic arthritis is not yet known. It may be partly inherited. Some people with psoriasis have a genetic background that makes them more likely to get psoriatic arthritis than the general population. The same is true of some people with psoriasis who later develop arthritis.

The body's immune system and the environment also may play a role in the disease. Some researchers believe that certain bacteria or fungal agents may cause chronic stimulation of the immune system, which in turn could cause arthritis.

How Is it Diagnosed?

To find out if you have psoriatic arthritis, your doctor will ask you about your symptoms and will perform a physical examination. Since the symptoms are similar to other forms of arthritis, such as gout, Reiter's syndrome and rheumatoid arthritis, your doctor also may perform:

- X-rays to look for changes in bones and joints;
- blood tests to rule out other diseases, such as rheumatoid arthritis; and/or
- joint fluid tests to rule out gout, which may resemble psoriatic arthritis.

It may take some time to determine if you have psoriatic arthritis. Usually, if your nails and skin are affected along with your joints, a firm diagnosis can be made.

Questions and Answers about Psoriasis

What Is Psoriasis?

Psoriasis is a chronic (long-lasting) skin disease characterized by scaling and inflammation. Scaling occurs when cells in the outer layer of skin reproduce faster than normal and pile up on the skin's surface.

Psoriasis affects 1.5 to 2 percent of the United States population, or almost five million people. It occurs in all age groups and about equally in men and women. People with psoriasis may suffer discomfort, restricted motion of joints, and emotional distress.

When psoriasis develops, patches of skin thicken, redden, and become covered with silvery scales. These patches are sometimes referred to as plaques. They may itch or burn. The skin at joints may crack. Psoriasis most often occurs on the elbows, knees, scalp, lower back, face, palms, and soles of the feet. The disease also may affect the fingernails, toenails, and the soft tissues inside the mouth and genitalia. About 10 percent of people with psoriasis have joint inflammation that produces symptoms of arthritis. This condition is called psoriatic arthritis.

What Causes Psoriasis?

Recent research indicates that psoriasis may be a disorder of the immune system. The immune system includes a type of white blood cell, called a T cell, that normally helps protect the body against infection and disease. Scientists now think that in psoriasis, an abnormal immune system produces too many T cells in the skin. These T cells trigger the inflammation and excessive skin cell reproduction seen in people with psoriasis.

In some cases, psoriasis is inherited. Researchers are studying large families affected by psoriasis to identify a gene or genes associated with the disease. (Genes govern every body function and determine inherited traits passed from parent to child.)

People with psoriasis may notice that there are times when their skin worsen, then improves. Conditions that may cause flare-ups include changes in climate, infections, stress, and dry skin. Also, certain medicines, such as the nonsteroidal anti-inflammatory drug indomethacin and medicines used to treat high blood pressure or depression, may trigger an outbreak or worsen the disease.

How Is Psoriasis Diagnosed?

Doctors usually diagnose psoriasis after a careful examination of the skin. However, diagnosis may be difficult because psoriasis often looks like other skin diseases. A pathologist may assist with diagnosis by examining a small skin sample under a microscope.

There are several forms of psoriasis. The most common form is plaque psoriasis (its scientific name is psoriasis vulgaris). In plaque psoriasis, lesions have a reddened base covered by silvery scales. Other forms of psoriasis include:

- **Guttate Psoriasis:** Drop-like lesions appear on the trunk, limbs, and scalp. Guttate psoriasis may be triggered by viral respiratory infections or certain bacterial (streptococcal) infections.

116

- **Pustular Psoriasis:** Blisters of noninfectious pus appear on the skin. Attacks of pustular psoriasis may be triggered by medications, sunlight, infections, pregnancy, perspiration, emotional stress, or exposure to certain chemicals.

- **Inverse Psoriasis:** Large, dry, smooth, vividly red plaques occur in the folds of skin near the genitals, under the breasts, or in the armpits. Inverse psoriasis is related to increased sensitivity to friction and sweating.

- **Erythrodermic Psoriasis:** Widespread reddening and scaling of the skin is often accompanied by itching or pain. Erythrodermic psoriasis may be precipitated by severe sunburn, use of oral steroids (such as cortisone), or a drug-related rash.

What Treatments Are Available for Psoriasis?

Doctors generally treat psoriasis in steps according to the severity of the disease or responsiveness to initial treatments. This is sometimes called the "1-2-3" approach. In step 1, medicines are applied to the skin (topical treatment). Step 2 involves treatments with light (phototherapy). Step 3 involves taking medicines internally, usually by mouth (systemic treatment).

Over time, affected skin tends to resist some treatments. Also, a treatment that works like magic in one person may have little effect in another. Thus, doctors commonly use a trial and error approach to find a treatment that works, then switch treatments every 12 to 24 months to reduce resistance and adverse reactions. Selection of treatment depends on the location of lesions, their size, the amount of the skin affected, previous response to treatment, and a patient's perceptions about their skin condition and patient preferences for treatment. In addition, treatment is often tailored to the specific form of the disorder.

Topical Treatment

Treatments applied directly to the skin are sometimes effective in clearing psoriasis. Doctors find that some patients respond well to sunlight, steroid ointments, medicines made from vitamin D, coal tar, or anthralin. Other topical measures, such as bath solutions and moisturizers, may be soothing but are seldom strong enough to clear lesions for a sustained length of time and may need to be combined with more potent remedies.

Sunlight. Daily, regular, short doses of sunlight without burning clears psoriasis in many people with the disease. However, exposure to sunlight is not recommended for those undergoing ultraviolet light treatments or using certain topical treatments, such as coal tar, which make the skin extra sensitive to the sun's effects.

Corticosteroids. Available in different strengths, corticosteroids (cortisone) are usually applied twice each day. Short-term treatment is often effective. If less than 10 percent of the body's skin is involved, some doctors will begin treatment with a high-potency corticosteroid ointment (for example, Diprolene, Temovate, Ultravate, or Psorcon). High-potency steroids may also be used for treatment-resistant plaques, particularly those on the hands or feet. Long-term use or overuse of high-potency steroids can lead to thinning of skin, internal side effects, resistance to the treatment's benefits, and worsening of the psoriasis. Medium-potency corticosteroids may be used on the torso or limbs; low-potency preparations are used on delicate skin areas.

Calcipotriene. This drug is a synthetic form of vitamin D. (This is not the same as vitamin D supplements.) Application of calcipotriene ointment (for example, Dovonex) twice daily controls the excessive production of skin cells in psoriasis. Because calcipotriene can irritate the skin, it is not recommended for the face or genitals. After four months of treatment, about 60 percent of patients have a good to excellent response to calcipotriene. The safety of using the drug for psoriasis affecting more than 20 percent of the body's skin is unknown; use on widespread areas of skin may raise the amount of calcium in the body to unhealthy levels.

Coal tar. Coal tar may be applied directly to the skin, used in a bath solution, or used as a shampoo for the scalp. It is available in different strengths, but the most potent form may be irritating. Because coal tar makes skin more sensitive to ultraviolet (UV) light, it is sometimes combined with ultraviolet B (UVB) phototherapy. Compared with steroids, coal tar has fewer side effects but is messy and less effective and thus is not popular with many patients. Other drawbacks include its failure to provide long-term help for most patients, its strong odor, and its tendency to stain skin or clothing.

Anthralin. Doctors sometimes use a 15- to 30-minute application of anthralin ointment, cream, or paste to treat chronic psoriasis lesions. However, this treatment often fails to adequately clear lesions, it irritates the skin, and it stains skin and clothing brown or purple. In addition, anthralin is unsuitable for acute or actively inflamed eruptions.

Salicylic acid. Used to remove scales, salicylic acid is usually more effective when combined with topical steroids, anthralin, or coal tar.

Bath solutions. People with psoriasis may find that bathing in water with an oil added, then applying a moisturizer, can soothe the skin. Scales can be removed and itching reduced by soaking 15 minutes in water containing a tar solution, oiled oatmeal, Epsom salts, or Dead Sea salts.

Moisturizers. When applied regularly over a long period, moisturizers have a cosmetic and soothing effect. Preparations that are thick and greasy usually work best because they lock water into the skin.

Phototherapy

UV light from the sun stimulates production of vitamin D by the skin, which slows the over-production of skin cells that causes scaling. Daily, short, non-burning exposure to sunlight clears or improves psoriasis in some people. Therefore, sunlight may be included among initial treatments for the disease. A more controlled artificial light treatment may be used in mild psoriasis (UVB phototherapy) or in more severe or extensive psoriasis (psoralen and ultraviolet A (PUVA therapy).

UVB Phototherapy. Artificial sources of UVB light are similar to sunlight. Some physicians will start with UVB treatments instead of topical agents. UVB phototherapy also is used to treat widespread psoriasis and lesions that resist topical treatment. This type of phototherapy is normally administered in a doctor's office by using a light panel or light box, although with a doctor's guidance, some patients can use UVB light boxes at home. UVB phototherapy also may be combined with other treatments. One combined therapy program, referred to as the Ingram regime, involves a coal tar bath, UVB phototherapy, and application of an anthralin-salicylic acid paste, which is left on the skin for 6 to 24 hours. A similar regime, the Goeckerman treatment, involves application of coal tar ointment and UVB phototherapy.

PUVA. This treatment combines oral or topical administration of a medicine called psoralen with exposure to ultraviolet A (UVA) light. Psoralen makes the body more sensitive to UVA light. PUVA is normally used when more than 10 percent of the body's skin is affected or when rapid clearing is required because the disease interferes with a person's occupation (for example, when a model's face or a carpenter's hands are affected by psoriasis). Compared with daily UVB treatment, PUVA treatment taken two to three times per week clears psoriasis more consistently but less quickly. However, it is associated with more side effects, including nausea, headache, fatigue, burning, and itching. Long-term treatment is associated with irregular skin pigmentation. Researchers have found that PUVA is effective and relatively safe when combined with some oral medications (retinoids and hydroxyurea) but appears to be associated with skin cancer when combined with other oral medications (for example, methotrexate or cyclosporine). In rare cases, patients who must travel long distances for PUVA treatments may, with a physician's close supervision, be taught to administer this treatment at home.

Systemic Treatment

Doctors sometimes prescribe medicines that are taken internally for more severe forms of psoriasis, particularly when more than 10 percent of the body is involved.

Retinoids. These drugs are derived from vitamin A and include etretinate (Tegison) and isotretinoin (Accutane). Etretinate is most effective against pustular and erythrodermic psoriasis. Isotretinoin is also helpful against pustular psoriasis. Both drugs can cause birth defects and are not recommended for women of childbearing age. At high doses, etretinate can affect liver function. Therefore it is often combined with UVB phototherapy or PUVA so that a lower, less toxic, dose can be taken.

Methotrexate. This treatment, which can be taken by pill or injection, slows down cell production and suppresses the immune system. Patients taking methotrexate must be closely monitored because this drug can cause liver damage or decrease the production of oxygen-carrying red blood cells, infection-fighting white blood cells, and clot-enhancing platelets. As a precaution, doctors do not prescribe the drug for people with long-term liver disease or anemia. Also, methotrexate should not be used by pregnant women, by women who are planning to get pregnant, or by their male partners.

Hydroxyurea (Hydrea). Compared with methotrexate, hydroxyurea is less toxic but also less effective. Hydroxyurea is sometimes combined with PUVA or retinoids. Possible side effects include anemia and a decrease in white blood cells and platelets. Like methotrexate, hydroxyurea must be avoided by pregnant women or those who are planning to get pregnant.

Antibiotics. Although seldom used in routine treatment, antibiotics may be employed when an infection such as streptococcus has triggered the outbreak of psoriasis, as in certain cases of guttate psoriasis.

What Are Some Promising Areas of Psoriasis Research?

Researchers continue to search for genes that contribute to the inheritance and causes of psoriasis. Scientists are also working to improve our understanding of what happens in the body to trigger this disease. In addition, much research is focused on developing new and better psoriasis treatments. Some of these experimental treatments, such as cyclosporine and agents that are directed at T cells, work by suppressing the immune system.

How Can I Contribute to Psoriasis Research?

The National Psoriasis Tissue Bank, which is supported by the National Psoriasis Foundation, is helping researchers worldwide to study the inherited tendency toward psoriasis by collecting white blood cells from over 250 families affected by the disease. Tissue specimens may also be collected from some patients. There is particular interest in large families in which psoriasis is both common and spans two or more generations. More recently, the tissue bank has begun research involving families that have at least two siblings with psoriasis. A living parent also must be available for examination. People seeking more information or families interested in participating in a study should contact:

National Psoriasis Tissue Bank
Baylor University Medical Center
Suite 656, Wadley Tower
3600 Gaston Ave.
Dallas, TX 75246
PHONE: (214) 820-2635
FAX: (214) 820-1296

Where Can I Get More Information about Psoriasis?

The National Psoriasis Foundation provides physician referrals and publishes pamphlets and a newsletter that includes information on support groups, research, and new drugs and other treatments. The foundation also promotes community awareness of psoriasis. For information, contact:

National Psoriasis Foundation
6600 S.W. 92nd Ave.
Portland, OR 97223
Phone: (503) 244-7404, or
(800) 723-9166

The NIAMS gratefully acknowledges the assistance of Gerald G. Krueger, M.D., of the University of Utah and Laurence H. Miller, M.D., in the preparation and review of the NIAMS' portion of this chapter.

Chapter 12

Arthritis and Inflammatory Bowel Disease

Introduction

Arthritis means inflammation of joints. Inflammation is a body process that can result in pain, swelling, warmth, redness, and stiffness. Sometimes inflammation can also affect the bowel. When it does, that process is called inflammatory bowel disease (IBD). IBD is actually two separate diseases: Crohn's (krons) disease and ulcerative colitis (UL-ser-a-tiv ko-LI-tis). With proper treatment, most people who have these diseases can lead full, active lives.

What causes these conditions?

The cause of inflammatory bowel disease is not known. Research suggests that the immune system, the body's natural defense against foreign invaders, is somehow altered in people with these conditions. Researchers believe that the chronic (long-lasting) inflammation present in the intestines of persons with both forms of IBD damages the bowel. This may permit bacteria to enter the damaged bowel wall and circulate through the bloodstream. The body's reaction to this bacteria may then cause problems in other areas of the body. The most common is inflammation of the joints. Other problems include skin sores, inflammation of the eyes, and certain types of liver disease.

Who gets IBD with arthritis?

Symptoms of arthritis (such as pain and swelling of joints) occur in about one-fourth of all people with IBD. Both men and women are affected equally. The arthritis of IBD can appear at any age, but is most common between the ages of 25 and 45. Joint inflammation begins most often when the colon (the large intestine) is involved in the disease process. In adults, the arthritis is usually most active when the bowel disease is active. Indeed, the amount of bowel disease usually influences the severity of the arthritis. In children, the arthritis is not as often associated with increased bowel disease activity.

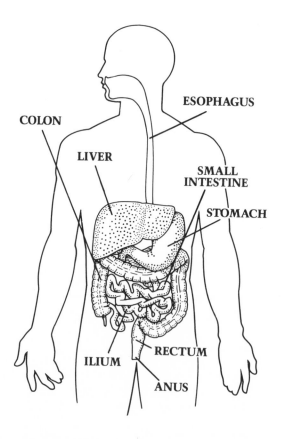

Figure 12.1. *Digestive Tract*

What are the symptoms of ulcerative colitis?

Ulcerative colitis produces inflammation and breakdown along the lining of the colon. Inflammation usually begins in the rectum and extends up the colon (see Figure 12.1). Symptoms may include rectal bleeding, abdominal cramping, weight loss, and fever.

The bowel symptoms often occur before the symptoms of arthritis. When ulcerative colitis is present, the arthritis is most likely to occur if there is severe bleeding or if the area around the anus is inflamed. When only the rectum is involved, the chance of getting arthritis is less.

Most of the time, the arthritis flares (becomes worse) when the bowel symptoms flare. An exception is during the first episode of arthritis, which can come at any time. One or more joints may be affected, and the symptoms often move from joint to joint. The hips, knees, and ankles are involved most often, although any joint may be affected. The joints may be very painful, red, and hot, but these symptoms usually do not result in permanent damage.

About one-fourth of people with IBD who develop arthritis have a skin rash on the lower legs, frequently seen when the arthritis flares. One characteristic rash usually consists of small, reddish lumps which are very painful to the touch. This skin condition is called erythema nodosum (AIR-uh-THE-mah no-DOH-sum).

People with ulcerative colitis can develop another form of arthritis called ankylosing spondylitis (ANG-ki-lo-sing SPON-di-LI-tis), which involves inflammation of the spine. It usually begins around the sacroiliac (SA-kro-IL-e-ak) joints, at the bottom of the back (see Figure 12.2). Symptoms of spondylitis generally do not accompany bowel symptoms in ulcerative colitis. If just the sacroiliac joints are inflamed, the symptoms are fairly mild. When the spine is affected, however, it may be quite painful and even disabling. This can result in stiffness or rigidity.

What are the symptoms of crohn's disease?

Crohn's disease usually involves either the colon or the ileum (IL-e-um), the lower small intestine. It may affect both, or any part of the digestive tract, from the mouth to the rectum. The inflammation involves all layers of the intestinal wall, and may lead to scarring and narrowing of the bowel. Fever, weight loss, and loss of appetite are common symptoms of Crohn's disease.

The arthritis of Crohn's disease can occur before, after, or at the same time as the bowel symptoms. As with ulcerative colitis, the large joints such as the knees and ankles are generally affected, though not necessarily on both sides of the body, and back pain can result from ankylosing spondylitis.

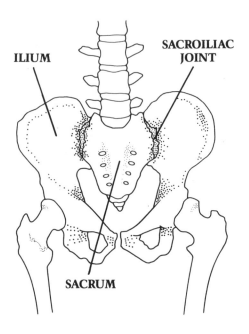

Figure 12.2. The Pelvis

How are these conditions diagnosed?

The history taken by the doctor is the most important part of the diagnosis. Certain information such as the way the arthritis began, the specific joints involved, and the relationship between joint and bowel symptoms is very helpful for diagnosis. The appearance of the joints, their range of motion, and pain or tenderness during the physical examination are also important.

Usually, x-rays of the joints are normal, unless the joints of the spine are affected. Then damage is visible in x-rays. A blood test for the presence of a substance called HLA-B27 in the blood cells is sometimes helpful in diagnosing ankylosing spondylitis. This substance is an inherited factor present in a much higher frequency among people who have IBD and spondylitis than in the normal population.

Chapter 13

Ankylosing Spondylitis

What is spondylitis?

Spondylitis is a chronic, inflammatory condition that involves primarily the spine and the joints of the extremities (such as shoulders, hips, and knees). Spondylitis is the shortened name for the medical term Ankylosing Spondylitis.

Is Spondylitis related to any other diseases?

Spondylitis is one in a group of diseases called spondyloarthropathies, which include Reiter's syndrome, psoriatic arthritis, and arthritis associated with inflammatory bowel disease (Crohn's disease and ulcerative colitis).

What are the early symptoms?

Symptoms usually begin in late adolescence or early adulthood (before age 40) Common symptoms are low back pain that starts gradually and lasts more than three months, and back stiffness that is worse in the morning and eased by mild physical activity or a hot shower. The inflammation may cause a general feeling of physical illness and fatigue.

How is spondylitis diagnosed?

The diagnosis depends on the history of your symptoms, physical examination, and x-ray findings. X-rays are taken of the sacroiliac joints to note changes in tissues caused by inflammation. However, tissue changes do not always appear on x-rays in the early stages of the disease. Since it is critical to initiate treatment early to minimize years of uncontrolled inflammation and pain, experienced physicians will often diagnose the disease and start treatment even before x-ray findings are conclusive.

What is the HLA-B27 gene?

HLA-B27 is a perfectly normal gene found in 8 percent of the general population. Generally speaking, no more than 2 percent of people born with this gene will eventually get spondylitis. It has to be emphasized, however, that more than 95 percent of HLA-B27 positive people never develop the disease. The gene itself does not cause spondylitis, but people with HLA-B27 are more susceptible to getting spondylitis. Researchers believe that an intestinal infection from one or more unknown bacteria may trigger spondylitis in susceptible people. Researchers are trying to identify which bacteria are involved.

If a parent, brother or sister has spondylitis, and I test positive for HLA-B27, what is my chance of getting the disease?

Since the gene runs in families, we sometimes see more than one family member with spondylitis or a related disease. If a family member had spondylitis and you test positive for the HLA-B27 gene, your chance of getting the disease increases to 20 percent, if you are under age 40. Many of these patients will have mild disease. If you are over 40, your chance of developing spondylitis is almost nonexistent.

Is HLA-B27 helpful in diagnosis?

Since the majority of persons with HLA-B27 never get spondylitis, it has limited help in diagnosis. However, when x-rays aren't clear, the doctor may want to know if you are HLA-B27 positive to better assess the likelihood of the diagnosis.

Is there a cure?

No. While medical science has not yet discovered the trigger mechanism or developed a cure, new research brings greater knowledge and increased hope each year. However, there is much that can be done to help.

How is it treated?

Treatment consists of medicines, regular exercise, good posture habits, and learning habits, and learning how to incorporate relaxation into your daily schedule.

What types of medicines are used?

Non steroidal anti-inflammatory drugs (NSAIDs) are the most common used medications. Other medications are sometimes prescribed such as Sulfasalazine or Methotrexate. However, these drugs can cause serious side effects and require careful monitoring by your doctor.

What is the best NSAID to use?

Each person may respond differently to each of the many NSAIDs available. Patients will most likely go through a period of trial and error until the doctor finds the drug that works best for them with the least number of side effects. To minimize the risk stomach upset or ulcers, medications are taken with a meal or after a snack and with a full glass of water. Sometimes it may be necessary to take antacids or H2 blockers such as Cimetidine or Carafate which coats the stomach in order to prevent heartburn, gastritis and even ulceration caused by taking NSAIDS.

Are any new drugs being tested?

New exciting arthritis drugs called COX-2 blockers are being developed and tested by major drug companies. These new medications promise to produce the potential benefits of current NSAIDs such as decreasing inflammation and relieving pain but without causing stomach problems and other side effects. Drug companies hope to apply for FDA approval within three years.

What kind of exercise is best?

It is important to remain physically fit with an all around exercise program. Additionally, there are important specific stretching and strengthening exercises for this disease. We recommend that patients be evaluated by a physical therapist and be given a program of exercise to meet their individual needs. Staying physically active is also important (swimming, hiking, etc), The Spondylitis Association of America (SAA) publishes books and videotapes with comprehensive information on exercise and sports that are appropriate for spondylitis.

Why is good posture important?

As the disease slowly progresses, the upper back tends to gradually stoop forward; sometimes quite severely. The good news is that with NSAIDs, exercise and attention to maintaining erect posture, this forward stooping posture is usually preventable. People who have a more mild condition won't have to deal with this problem, but it's hard to predict early on who is at risk.

Will I become disabled?

Most people are able to manage the disease well. They are able to continue to work, raise children, etc. While some patients will eventually need to modify or change their work, the vast majority remain employed full-time (a recent study showed that less than 15 percent of patients end up unemployed.)

What kind of doctor treats spondylitis?

A rheumatologist is an arthritis specialist and most familiar with the disease. There are no additional credentials that determine which rheumatologists are more knowledgeable or experienced in diagnosing and treating spondylitis. Before deciding upon a rheumatologist, you may want to ask how many spondylitis patients he or she currently treats. Ask whether it would be possible for you to speak with one or two of them. Your regular doctor may also be knowledgeable about spondylitis and able to treat you

How can I find a rheumatologist?

Ask your doctor for a referral to a rheumatologist or contact a rheumatology clinic at a large medical center. Also, SAA lists members of the SAA Professional Membership Network.

Where can I learn more?

The Spondylitis Association of America, a nonprofit foundation established in 1983, is the leading information source for patients and physicians in the United States, and the only organization that devotes all of its efforts and all of its funds to helping persons with spondylitis and related conditions. Our mission includes helping people affected by these diseases to lead more productive lives, to familiarize health care professionals with early symptoms and appropriate treatment, and support the advancement of research.

Table13.1. Differentiating between Mechanical Back Pain and Spondylitis Back Pain.

Factors for Comparison	Mechanical Back Pain	Spondylitis Back Pain
Onset	Sudden at any age	Gradual 20s-40s
History	Pain caused by injury or strain	Not caused by trauma; pain due to inflammation
Localization	Across lower back	Widespread pain from lower back often into buttocks
Morning stiffness	Usually not present	Often dominant throughout the spine
Prolonged rest (more than 1-2 hours)	Tends to relieve pain	Aggravates pain
Exercise	Often worsens pain	Often relieves pain

Chapter 14

Systemic Lupus Erythematosus

This chapter is for people who have systemic lupus erythematosus, commonly called SLE or lupus, as well as for their family and friends and others who want to better understand the disease. The chapter describes the disease and its symptoms and contains information about diagnosis and treatment as well as current research efforts supported by the National Institute of Arthritis and Musculoskeletal and Skin Diseases (NIAMS) and other components of the National Institutes of Health (NIH). It also discusses issues such as health care, pregnancy, and quality of life for people with lupus. If you have further questions after reading this chapter, you may wish to discuss them with your doctor.

Defining Lupus

Lupus is a type of immune system disorder known as an autoimmune disease. In autoimmune diseases, the body harms its own healthy cells and tissues. This leads to inflammation and damage of

NIH Web Publication. Systemic Lupus Erythematosus. This is a publication of the National Institutes of Health, National Institute of Arthritis and Musculoskeletal and Skin Diseases. This material is not copyrighted. Readers are encouraged to duplicate and distribute as many copies as needed. Printed copies of this chapter are available from the National Arthritis and Musculoskeletal and Skin Diseases Information Clearinghouse, National Institutes of Health (NAMSIC/NIH), 1 AMS Circle, Bethesda, Maryland 20892-3675. Phone: (301) 495-4484 Fax: (301) 587-4352. Web site [http://www.nih.gov/niams/healthinfo/slehandout/menu.html]

various body tissues. Lupus can affect many parts of the body, including the joints, skin, kidneys, heart, lungs, blood vessels, and brain. Although people with the disease may have many different symptoms, some of the most common ones include extreme fatigue, painful or swollen joints (arthritis), unexplained fever, skin rashes, and kidney problems.

Lupus is also known as a rheumatic disease. The rheumatic diseases are a group of disorders that cause aches, pain, and stiffness in the joints, muscles, and bones.

At present, there is no cure for lupus. However, the symptoms of lupus can be controlled with appropriate treatment, and most people with the disease can lead active, healthy lives. Lupus is characterized by periods of illness, called flares, and periods of wellness, or remission. Understanding how to prevent flares and how to treat them when they do occur helps people with lupus maintain better health. Intense research is underway and scientists funded by the NIH are continuing to make great strides in understanding the disease, which ultimately may lead to a cure.

Two of the questions researchers are studying are who gets lupus and why. We know that many more women than men have lupus. Lupus is three times more common in black women than in white women and is also more common in women of Hispanic, Asian, and Native American descent. In addition, lupus can run in families, but the risk that a child or a brother or sister of a patient also will have lupus is still quite low. It is difficult to estimate how many people in the United States have the disease because its symptoms vary widely and its onset is often hard to pinpoint.

Although "lupus" is used as a broad term, there actually are several kinds of lupus:

- **Systemic lupus erythematosus (SLE)**, which is the form of the disease that most people are referring to when they say "lupus." The word "systemic" means the disease can affect many parts of the body. The symptoms of SLE may be mild or serious. Although SLE usually first affects people between the ages of 15 and 45 years, it can occur in childhood or later in life as well. This chapter focuses on SLE.

- **Discoid lupus erythematosus** primarily affects the skin. A red, raised rash may appear on the face, scalp, or elsewhere. The raised areas may become thick and scaly. The rash may last for days or years and may recur. A small percentage of people with discoid lupus later develop SLE.

- **Drug-induced lupus** refers to a form of lupus caused by medication. It causes some symptoms similar to those of SLE (arthritis, rash, fever, and chest pain, but not kidney disease) that go away when the drug is stopped. Common medications that may cause drug-induced lupus include hydralazine (Apresoline), procainamide (Procan, Pronestyl), methyldopa (Aldomet), quinidine (Quinaglute), isoniazid (INH), and some anti-seizure medications such as phenytoin (Dilantin) or carbamazepine (Tegretol).

- **Neonatal lupus** can affect some newborn babies of women with SLE or certain other immune system disorders. Babies with neonatal lupus may have a serious heart defect. Other affected babies may have a skin rash, liver abnormalities, or low blood counts. Physicians can now identify most at-risk SLE patients, allowing for prompt treatment of the infant at birth. Neonatal lupus is very rare, and most infants of mothers with SLE are entirely healthy.

Understanding What Causes Lupus

Lupus is a complex disease whose cause is unknown. It is likely that there is no single cause but rather a combination of genetic, environmental, and possibly hormonal factors that work together to cause the disease. The exact cause may differ from one person to another. Scientists are making progress in understanding the causes of lupus, as described here and in the Current Research section of this chapter. Research suggests that genetics plays an important role; however, no specific "lupus gene" has been identified. Instead, it appears that several genes may increase a person's susceptibility to the disease.

The fact that lupus can run in families indicates that development of this disease has a genetic basis. In addition, studies of identical twins have shown that lupus is much more likely to affect both members of a pair of identical twins, who share the exact same set of genes, than two nonidentical twins or other siblings. Because the risk for identical twins is far less than 100 percent, however, scientists think that genes alone cannot account for who gets lupus. Other factors must also play a role.

Some of the factors that scientists are studying include sunlight, stress, certain drugs, and infectious agents such as viruses. Even though a virus might trigger the disease in susceptible individuals, a person cannot "catch" lupus from someone else.

In lupus, the body's immune system doesn't work as it should. A healthy immune system produces antibodies, which are special proteins that help fight and destroy viruses, bacteria, and other foreign substances that invade the body. In lupus, the immune system produces antibodies against the body's healthy cells and tissues. These antibodies, called autoantibodies ("auto"means self), contribute to the inflammation of various parts of the body, causing swelling, redness, heat, and pain. In addition, some autoantibodies join with substances from the body's own cells or tissues to form molecules called immune complexes. A buildup of these immune complexes in the body also contributes to inflammation and tissue injury in people with lupus. Researchers do not yet understand all of the factors that cause inflammation and tissue damage in lupus, and this is an active area of research.

Symptoms of Lupus

Each person's experience with lupus is different. Symptoms can range from mild to severe and may come and go over time. Common symptoms of lupus include extreme fatigue, painful or swollen joints, unexplained fever, and skin rashes. A characteristic skin rash may appear across the nose and cheeks—the so-called butterfly or malar rash. Other rashes occur elsewhere on the face and ears, upper arms, shoulders, chest, and hands.

Other symptoms of lupus include chest pain, hair loss, sensitivity to the sun, anemia (a decrease in red blood cells), and pale or purple fingers and toes from cold and stress. Some people also experience headaches, dizziness, depression, or seizures. New symptoms may continue to appear years after the initial diagnosis, and different symptoms can occur at different times.

Common Symptoms of Lupus

- Painful or swollen joints and muscle pain
- Unexplained fever
- Extreme fatigue
- Red rash or color change on the face
- Chest pain upon deep breathing
- Unusual loss of hair
- Pale or purple fingers or toes from cold or stress (Raynaud's phenomenon)
- Sensitivity to the sun
- Swelling (edema) in legs or around eyes
- Swollen glands

In some people with lupus, only one system of the body such as the skin or joints is affected. Other people experience symptoms in many parts of their body. Just how seriously a body system is affected also varies from person to person. Most commonly, joints and muscles are affected, causing arthritis and muscle pain. Skin rashes also are quite common. The following systems in the body also can be affected by lupus:

Kidneys. Inflammation of the kidneys (nephritis) can impair their ability to effectively get rid of waste products and other toxins from the body. Because the kidneys are so important to overall health, lupus in the kidneys generally requires intensive drug treatment to prevent permanent damage. There is usually no pain associated with kidney involvement, although some patients may notice that their ankles swell. Most often the only indication of kidney disease is an abnormal urine test.

Central nervous system. In some patients, lupus affects the brain or central nervous system. This can cause headaches, dizziness, memory disturbances, vision problems, stroke, or changes in behavior. Some of these symptoms, however, also can be caused by some treatments of lupus or by the emotional stress of dealing with the disease.

Blood vessels. Blood vessels may become inflamed (vasculitis), affecting the way blood circulates through the body. The inflammation may be mild, and may not require treatment.

Blood. People with lupus may develop anemia or leukopenia (a decreased number of white blood cells). Lupus also may cause thrombocytopenia, a decreased number of platelets in the blood that contributes to an increased chance of bleeding. Some people with lupus may have an increased risk for blood clots.

Lungs. Some people with lupus develop pleuritis, an inflammation of the lining of the chest cavity that causes chest pain, particularly with breathing. Patients with lupus also may get pneumonia.

Heart. In some people with lupus, inflammation can occur in the arteries that supply blood to the heart (coronary vasculitis), the heart itself (myocarditis and endocarditis), or the membrane that surrounds it (pericarditis), causing chest pains or other symptoms.

Diagnosing Lupus

Diagnosing lupus can be difficult. It may take months or even years for doctors to piece together the symptoms to accurately diagnose this complex disease. Making a correct diagnosis of lupus requires knowledge and awareness on the part of the doctor and good communication on the part of the patient. Telling the doctor a complete, accurate medical history (for example, what health problems you have had and for how long) is critical to the process of diagnosis. This information, along with a physical examination and the results of laboratory tests, helps the doctor consider other diseases that may mimic lupus, or determine if the patient truly has the disease. Reaching a diagnosis may take time and occur gradually as new symptoms appear.

No single test can determine whether a person has lupus, but several laboratory tests may help the doctor to make a diagnosis. The most useful tests identify certain blood autoantibodies often present in people with lupus. For example, the antinuclear antibody (ANA) test is commonly used to look for autoantibodies that react against components of the nucleus, or "command center," of the patient's own cells. Many people with lupus test positive for ANA; however, some drugs, infections, and other diseases also can cause a positive result. The ANA test simply provides another clue for the doctor to consider in making a diagnosis. There are also blood tests for individual types of autoantibodies that are more specific to people with lupus, although not all people with lupus test positive for these. These antibodies include anti-DNA, anti-Sm, anti-RNP, anti-Ro (SSA), and anti-La (SSB). The doctor may use these antibody tests to help make a diagnosis of lupus.

Some tests are used less frequently but may be helpful if the cause of a person's symptoms remains unclear. The doctor may order a biopsy of the skin or kidneys if those body systems are affected. Some doctors may order a syphilis test because some lupus antibodies in the blood may cause the test to be falsely positive. A positive test does not mean that a patient has syphilis. Again, all these tests merely serve as tools to give the doctor clues and information in making a diagnosis. The doctor will look at the entire picture—medical history, symptoms, and test results—to determine if a person has lupus.

Other laboratory tests are used to monitor the progress of the disease once it has been diagnosed. A complete blood count (CBC), urinalysis, blood chemistries, and erythrocyte sedimentation rate (ESR) test can provide valuable information. (The ESR is a measure of inflammation in the body. It tests how quickly red blood cells drop to the bottom of a tube of unclotted blood.) Another common test measures the blood level of a group of proteins called complement. People with lupus often have low complement levels, especially during flares of the disease.

Diagnostic Tools for Lupus

- Medical history

- Complete physical examination

- Laboratory tests:
  - Complete blood count
  - Erythrocyte sedimentation rate (ESR)—an elevated ESR indicates inflammation in the body
  - Urinalysis
  - Blood chemistries
  - Complement levels—often low in people with lupus, especially during a flare
  - Antinuclear antibody test (ANA)—positive in most lupus patients, but a positive ANA test can have other causes
  - Other autoantibody tests (anti-DNA, anti-Sm, anti-RNP, anti-Ro [SSA], anti-La [SSB]): One or more of these tests may be positive in some people with lupus
  - Syphilis test—may be falsely positive in people with lupus

- Skin or kidney biopsy

Treating Lupus

Diagnosing and treating lupus is often a team effort between the patient and several types of health care professionals. A person can go to his or her family doctor or internist, or can visit a rheumatologist. A rheumatologist is a doctor who specializes in arthritis and other diseases of the joints, bones, and muscles. Clinical immunologists (doctors specializing in immune system disorders) may also treat people with lupus. As treatment progresses, other professionals often help. These may include nurses, psychologists, social workers, and specialists such as nephrologists (doctors who treat kidney disease), hematologists (doctors specializing in blood disorders), dermatologists (doctors who treat skin disease), and neurologists (doctors specializing in disorders of the nervous system).

The range and effectiveness of treatments for lupus have increased dramatically, giving doctors more choices in how to treat the disease.

It is important for the patient to work closely with the doctor and take an active role in treatment. Once lupus has been diagnosed, the doctor will develop a treatment plan based on the patient's age, gender, health, symptoms, and lifestyle. Treatment plans are tailored to the individual's needs and may change over time. In developing a treatment plan, the doctor has several goals: to prevent flares, to treat them when they do occur, and to minimize complications. The doctor and patient should reevaluate the plan regularly to ensure that it is as effective as possible.

Several types of drugs are used to treat lupus. The treatment the doctor chooses is based on the patient's individual symptoms and needs. For people with joint pain, fever, and swelling, drugs that decrease inflammation, referred to as nonsteroidal anti-inflammatory drugs (NSAIDs), are often used. While some NSAIDs are available over the counter, a doctor's prescription is necessary for others. NSAIDs may be used alone or in combination with other types of drugs to control pain, swelling, and fever. Even though some NSAIDs may be purchased without a prescription, it is important that they be taken under a doctor's direction because the dose for people with lupus may differ from the dose recommendations on the bottle. Common side effects of NSAIDs, including those available over the counter, can include stomach upset, heartburn, diarrhea, and fluid retention. Some lupus patients also develop liver and kidney inflammation while taking NSAIDs, making it especially important to stay in close contact with the doctor while taking these medications:

NSAIDs Used to Treat Lupus*

Generic Name	Brand Name
Ibuprofen	Motrin, Advil
Naproxen	Naprosyn, Aleve
Sulindac	Clinoril
Diclofenac	Voltaren
Piroxicam	Feldene
Ketoprofen	Orudis
Diflunisal	Dolobid
Nabumetone	Relafen
Etodolac	Lodine
Oxaprozin	Daypro
Indomethacin	Indocin

* Brand names included in this fact sheet are provided as examples only and their inclusion does not mean that these products are endorsed by the National Institutes of Health or any other Government agency or by Omnigraphics Inc. Also, if a particular brand name is not mentioned, this does not mean or imply that the product is unsatisfactory.

Antimalarials are another type of drug commonly used to treat lupus. These drugs were originally used to treat the symptoms of malaria, but doctors have found that they also are useful treatments for lupus. Exactly how antimalarials work in lupus is unclear, but scientists think that they may work by suppressing parts of the immune response. Specific antimalarials used to treat lupus include hydrochloroquine (Plaquenil), chloroquine (Aralen), and quinacrine (Atabrine). They may be used alone or in combination with other drugs and generally are used to treat fatigue, joint pain, skin rashes, and inflammation of the lungs. Research doctors have found that continuous treatment with antimalarials may prevent flares from recurring. Side effects of antimalarials can include stomach upset and, extremely rarely, damage to the retina of the eye.

The mainstay of lupus treatment involves the use of corticosteroid hormones, such as prednisone (Deltasone), hydrocortisone, methylprednisolone (Medrol), and dexamethasone (Decadron, Hexadrol). Corticosteroids are related to cortisol, which is a natural anti-inflammatory hormone. They work by rapidly suppressing inflammation. Corticosteroids can be given by mouth, in creams applied to the skin, or by injection. Because they are potent drugs, the doctor will seek the lowest dose with the greatest benefit.

Short-term side effects of corticosteroids include swelling, increased appetite, weight gain, and emotional ups and downs. These side effects generally stop when the drug is stopped. It can be dangerous to stop taking corticosteroids suddenly, so it is very important that the doctor and patient work together in changing the corticosteroid dose. Sometimes doctors give very large amounts of corticosteroid by vein ("bolus" or "pulse" therapy). With this treatment, the typical side effects are less likely and slow withdrawal is unnecessary.

Long-term side effects of corticosteroids can include stretch marks on the skin, excessive hair growth, weakened or damaged bones, high blood pressure, damage to the arteries, high blood sugar, infections, and cataracts. Typically, the higher the dose of corticosteroids, the more severe the side effects. Also, the longer they are taken, the greater the risk of side effects. Researchers are working to develop alternative strategies to limit or offset the use of corticosteroids. For example, corticosteroids may be used in combination with other, less potent drugs, or the doctor may try to slowly decrease the dose once the disease is under control. People with lupus who are using corticosteroids should talk to their doctors about taking supplemental calcium and vitamin D to reduce the risk of osteoporosis (weakened, fragile bones).

For patients whose kidneys or central nervous systems are affected by lupus, a type of drug called an immunosuppressive may be used. Immunosuppressives, such as azathioprine (Imuran) and cyclophosphamide (Cytoxan), restrain the overactive immune system by blocking the production of some immune cells and curbing the action of others. These drugs may be given by mouth or by infusion (dripping the drug into the vein through a small tube). Side effects may include nausea, vomiting, hair loss, bladder problems, decreased fertility, and increased risk of cancer and infection. The risk for side effects increases with the length of treatment. As with other treatments for lupus, there is a risk of relapse after the immunosuppressives have been stopped.

In special circumstances, patients may require stronger drugs to combat the symptoms of lupus. For patients who cannot take corticosteroids, a type of immunosuppressive drug called methotrexate (Folex, Mexate, Rheumatrex) may be used to help control the disease. Patients who have many body systems affected by the disease may receive intravenous gamma globulin (Gammagard, Gammar, Gamine), a blood protein that increases immunity and helps fight infection. Gamma globulin also may be used to control acute bleeding in patients with thrombocytopenia or to prepare a person with lupus for surgery.

Working closely with the doctor helps ensure that treatments for lupus are as successful as possible. Because some treatments may cause harmful side effects, it is important to promptly report any new symptoms to the doctor. It is also important not to stop or change treatments without talking to the doctor first.

Because of the nature and cost of the medications used to treat lupus, their potentially serious side effects, and the lack of a cure, many patients seek other ways of treating the disease. Some alternative approaches that have been suggested include special diets, nutritional supplements, fish oils, ointments and creams, chiropractic treatment, and homeopathy. Although these methods may not be harmful in and of themselves, no research to date shows that they help. Some alternative or complementary approaches may help the patient cope or reduce some of the stress associated with living with a chronic illness. If the doctor feels the approach has value and will not be harmful, it can be incorporated into the patient's treatment plan. However, it is important not to neglect regular health care or treatment of serious symptoms.

Lupus and Quality of Life

Despite the symptoms of lupus and the potential side effects of treatment, people with lupus can maintain a high quality of life overall. One key to managing lupus is to understand the disease and its impact. Learning to recognize the warning signs of a flare can help the patient take steps to ward it off or reduce its intensity. Many people with lupus experience increased fatigue, pain, a rash, fever, stomach discomfort, headache, or dizziness just before a flare. Developing strategies to prevent flares can also be helpful, such as limiting exposure to the sun (intense sun exposure triggers flares in some patients) and scheduling adequate rest and quiet times.

It is also important for people with lupus to receive regular health care, instead of seeking help only when symptoms worsen. Having a medical exam and lab work on a regular basis allows the doctor to note any changes and may help predict flares. The treatment plan, which is tailored to the individual's specific needs and circumstances, can be adjusted accordingly. If new symptoms are identified early, treatments may be more effective. Other concerns also can be addressed at regular checkups. The doctor can provide guidance about such issues as the use of sunscreens, stress reduction, and the importance of structured exercise and rest, as well as birth control and family planning. Because people with lupus can be more susceptible to infections, the doctor may recommend yearly influenza vaccinations for some patients.

Warning Signs of a Flare

- Increased fatigue
- Pain
- Rash
- Fever
- Stomach discomfort
- Headache
- Dizziness

Preventing a Flare

- Learn to recognize warning signals
- Maintain good communication with your doctor
- Set realistic goals and priorities
- Limit exposure to the sun
- Maintain a healthy, balanced diet
- Try to limit stress
- Schedule adequate rest and quiet times
- Participate in moderate exercise when possible
- Develop a support system

People with lupus should receive regular preventive health care, such as gynecological and breast examinations. Regular dental care will help avoid potentially dangerous infections. If a person is taking corticosteroids or antimalarial medications, a yearly eye exam should be done to screen for and treat eye problems.

Staying healthy requires extra effort and care for people with lupus, so it becomes especially important to develop strategies for maintaining wellness. Wellness involves close attention to the body, mind, and spirit. One of the primary goals of wellness for people with lupus is coping with the stress of having a chronic disorder. Effective stress management varies from person to person. Some approaches that may help include exercise, relaxation techniques such as meditation, and setting priorities for spending time and energy.

Developing and maintaining a good support system is also important. A support system may include family, friends, medical professionals, community organizations, and organized support groups. Participating in a support group can provide emotional help, boost self-esteem and morale, and help develop or improve coping skills. (For more information on support groups, see the Additional Resources section at the end of this chapter).

Learning more about lupus may also help. Studies have shown that patients who are well informed and participate actively in their own care experience less pain, make fewer visits to the doctor, build self confidence, and remain more active.

Tips for Working with Your Doctor

- Find a doctor who will listen to and address your concerns.
- Provide complete, accurate medical information.
- Make a list of your questions and concerns in advance.

- Be honest and share your point of view with the doctor.
- Ask for clarification or further explanation if you need it.
- Talk to other members of the health care team, such as nurses, therapists, or pharmacists.
- Don't hesitate to discuss sensitive subjects (for example, birth control, sex) with your doctor.
- Discuss any treatment changes with your doctor before making them.

Pregnancy for Women with Lupus

Twenty years ago, women with lupus were counseled not to become pregnant because of the risk of a flare of the disease and an increased risk of miscarriage. Thanks to research and careful treatment, more and more women with lupus can have successful pregnancies. Although a lupus pregnancy is still considered high risk, most women with lupus carry their babies safely to the end of their pregnancy. Experts disagree on the exact numbers, but 20 to 25 percent of lupus pregnancies end in miscarriage, compared to 10 to 15 percent of pregnancies in women without the disease. Pregnancy counseling and planning before pregnancy is important. Ideally, a woman should have no signs or symptoms of lupus and be taking no medications for at least six months before she becomes pregnant.

Some women may experience a mild to moderate flare during or after their pregnancy; others do not. Pregnant women with lupus, especially those taking corticosteroids, also are more likely to develop high blood pressure, diabetes, hyperglycemia (high blood sugar), and kidney complications, so regular care and good nutrition during pregnancy are essential. It is also advisable to have access to a neonatal (newborn) intensive care unit at the time of delivery in case the baby requires special medical attention. About 25 percent (one in four) of babies of women with lupus are born prematurely, but do not suffer from birth defects.

It is important to consider treatment options during pregnancy. The woman and her doctor must weigh the potential risks and benefits of each option to both mother and baby. Some drugs used to treat lupus should not be used at all during pregnancy because they may harm the baby or cause a miscarriage. A woman with lupus who becomes pregnant needs to work closely with both her obstetrician and her lupus doctor. They can work together to evaluate her individual needs and circumstances.

The fear of miscarriage is very real for many pregnant women with lupus. Researchers have now identified two closely related lupus autoantibodies, anticardiolipin antibody and lupus anticoagulant (together called the antiphospholipid antibodies), that are associated with risk of miscarriage. One-third to one-half of women with lupus have these antibodies, which can be detected by blood tests. Identifying women with these antibodies early in the pregnancy may help doctors take steps to reduce the risk of miscarriage. Pregnant women who test positive for these antibodies and who have had previous miscarriages are generally treated with baby aspirin or the drug heparin throughout their pregnancy. In a small percentage of cases, babies of women who have specific antibodies called anti-Ro (SSA) and anti-La (SSB) have symptoms of lupus such as a rash or low blood count. This is not the same as systemic lupus erythematosus and is almost always temporary. Most babies with symptoms of neonatal lupus need no treatment at all.

Current Research

Lupus is the focus of much research as scientists try to determine what causes the disease and how it can best be treated. Some of the questions they are working to answer include: Exactly who gets lupus, and why? Why are women more likely than men to have the disease? Why are there more cases of lupus in some racial and ethnic groups?

What goes wrong in the immune system, and why? How can we correct the way the immune system functions once something goes wrong? What treatment approaches will work best to lessen or cure symptoms of lupus?

To help answer these questions, scientists are developing new and better ways to study the disease. They are doing laboratory studies that compare various aspects of the immune systems of people with lupus with those of other people both with and without lupus. They also use mice with disorders resembling lupus to explore how the immune system functions in the disease and to identify possible new therapies.

The National Institute of Arthritis and Musculoskeletal and Skin Diseases (NIAMS), a component of the National Institutes of Health (NIH), funds many individual researchers across the United States who are studying lupus. To help scientists gain new knowledge, NIAMS also has established Specialized Centers of Research devoted specifically to lupus research. In addition, NIAMS is funding several lupus registries that will gather medical information as well as blood and tissue samples from patients and their relatives. This will give researchers across the country access to information and materials they can use to help identify genes that determine susceptibility to the disease.

Identifying genes that play a role in the development of lupus is an active area of research. For example, researchers suspect a genetic defect in a cellular process called apoptosis, or "programmed cell death" in people with lupus. Apoptosis allows the body to safely get rid of damaged or potentially harmful cells. If there is a problem in the apoptosis process, harmful cells may stay around and do damage to the body's own tissues. For example, in a mutant mouse strain that develops a lupus-like illness, one of the genes that controls apoptosis, called the fas gene, is defective. When it is replaced with a normal fas gene, the mice no longer develop signs of the disease. Scientists are studying what role genes involved in apoptosis may play in human disease development.

Studying genes for complement, a series of proteins in the blood that play an important part in the immune system, is another active area of lupus research. Complement acts as a backup for antibodies, helping them destroy foreign substances that invade the body. If there is a decrease in complement, the body is less able to fight or destroy foreign substances. If these substances are not removed from the body, the immune system may become overactive and begin to make autoantibodies.

Research to identify genes that predispose some people to the more serious complications of lupus, such as kidney disease, is producing significant findings. NIAMS-supported researchers have identified a gene associated with an increased risk of lupus kidney disease in African Americans. Variations in this gene affect the immune system's ability to remove potentially harmful immune complexes from the body. Researchers are also making progress in identifying other genes that play a role in lupus.

Researchers also are studying other factors that may affect a person's susceptibility to lupus. For example, because lupus is more common in women than in men some researchers are investigating the role of hormones and other male-female differences in the development and course of the disease.

Promising Areas of Research

- Identifying lupus susceptibility genes
- Searching for environmental agents that cause lupus
- Developing drugs or biologic agents that cure lupus

A current study funded by the NIH is focusing on the safety and effectiveness of oral contraceptives (birth-control pills) and hormone replacement therapy in women with lupus. Doctors have worried about the wisdom of prescribing oral contraceptives or estrogen replacement therapy for women with lupus because of a widely held view that estrogens can make the disease worse. However, recent limited data suggest these drugs may be safe for some women with lupus. Researchers hope this study will yield options for safe, effective methods of birth control for young women with lupus and enable postmenopausal women with lupus to benefit from estrogen replacement therapy.

Researchers are also focusing on finding better treatments for lupus. A primary goal of this research is to develop treatments that can effectively minimize the use of corticosteroids. Scientists are trying to identify combination therapies that may be more effective than single-treatment approaches. Researchers are also interested in using male hormones, called androgens, as a possible treatment for the disease. Another goal is to improve the treatment and management of lupus in the kidneys and central nervous system. For example, a 20-year study supported by NIAMS and NIH found that combining cyclophosphamide with prednisone helped delay or prevent kidney failure, a serious complication of lupus.

On the basis of new information about the disease process, scientists are using novel "biologic agents" to selectively block parts of the immune system. Development and testing of these new drugs, which are based on compounds that occur naturally in the body, is an exciting and promising new area of lupus research. The hope is that these treatments not only will be effective but also will have fewer side effects. Other treatment options currently being explored include reconstructing the immune system by bone marrow transplantation. In the future, gene therapy also may play an important role in lupus treatment.

Hope for the Future

With research advances and a better understanding of lupus, the prognosis for people with lupus today is far brighter than it was even 20 years ago. It is possible to have lupus and remain active and involved with life, family, and work. As current research efforts unfold, there is continued hope for new treatments; improvements in quality of life; and ultimately, a way to prevent or cure the disease. The research efforts of today may yield the answers of tomorrow, as scientists continue to unravel the mysteries of lupus.

Additional Resources

Lupus Foundation of America (LFA), Inc.
1300 Piccard Drive, Suite 200
Rockville, MD 20850
(301) 670-9292
(800) 558-0121
or your local chapter, listed in the telephone directory
Web address: http://www.lupus.org/lupus

This is the main voluntary organization devoted to lupus. The LFA assists local chapters in providing services to people with lupus, works to educate the public about lupus, and supports lupus research. Through a network of more than 500 branches and support groups, the chapters provide education through information and referral services, health fairs, newsletters, publications, and seminars. Chapters provide support to people with lupus, their families, and friends through support group meetings, hospital visits, and telephone help lines.

Acknowledgments

The NIAMS gratefully acknowledges the assistance of Patricia A. Fraser, M.D., Brigham and Women's Hospital, Boston, Massachusetts; John H. Klippel, M.D., NIAMS, NIH; Michael D. Lockshin, M.D., Barbara Volcker Center for Women and Rheumatic Disease, Hospital for Special Surgery, New York, New York; and Rosalind Ramsey-Goldman, M.D., Dr.P.H., Northwestern University Medical School, Chicago, Illinois, in the preparation and review of this publication. Special thanks also go to Cheryl Yarboro, R.N., B.S.P.A., NIAMS, NIH, and to the many patients who reviewed this publication and provided valuable input. This text for this chapter was written by Debbie Novak of Johnson, Bassin and Shaw, Inc. About NIAMS and NAMSIC

The National Arthritis and Musculoskeletal and Skin Diseases Information Clearinghouse (NAMSIC) is a public service sponsored by the NIAMS that provides health information and information sources. The NIAMS, a part of the National Institutes of Health (NIH), leads the Federal medical research effort in arthritis and musculoskeletal and skin diseases. The NIAMS supports research and research training throughout the United States as well as on the NIH campus in Bethesda, Maryland, and disseminates health and research information. Additional information and research updates can be found on the NIAMS Web site at //www.nih.gov/niams

Chapter 15

Chronic Lyme Disease

Important Information

- Ticks that Most Commonly transmit *B. burgdorferi* in the U.S.
- Most Common Symptoms of Lyme Disease
- Tips for Personal Protection
- How to Remove a Tick

Introduction

In the early 1970s, a mysterious clustering of arthritis occurred among children in Lyme, Connecticut, and surrounding towns. Medical researchers soon recognized the illness as a distinct disease, which they called Lyme disease. They subsequently described the clinical features of Lyme disease, established the usefulness of antibiotic therapy in its treatment, identified the deer tick as the key to its spread, and isolated the bacterium that caused it.

Lyme disease is still mistaken for other ailments, and it continues to pose many other challenges: it can be difficult to diagnose because of the inadequacies of today's laboratory tests; it can be

NIH Publication No. 92-3193, April 1992. Lyme Disease—The Facts, The Challenge. Prepared by the Office of Communications, NIAID and the Office of Scientific and Health Communications, NIAMSD. This text is not copyrighted and users are encouraged to reproduce and distribute as many free copies as needed. Single copies are available by writing to: Lyme Disease Booklet, NIAMS/ NIH, 1 AMS Circle, Bethesda, Maryland 20892 or from the NIH website at http://www.nih.gov/niams/healthinfo/lyme.

troublesome to treat in its later phases; and its prevention through the development of an effective vaccine is hampered by the elusive nature of the bacterium.

The National Institutes of Health (NIH), a part of the U.S. Public Health Service, conducts and supports biomedical research aimed at meeting the challenges of Lyme disease. This chapter presents the most recently available information on the diagnosis, treatment, and prevention of Lyme disease.

How Lyme Disease Became Known

Lyme disease was first recognized in 1975 after researchers investigated why unusually large numbers of children were being diagnosed with juvenile rheumatoid arthritis in Lyme and two neighboring towns. The investigators discovered that most of the affected children lived near wooded areas likely to harbor ticks. They also found that the children's first symptoms typically started in the summer months coinciding with the height of the tick season. Several of the patients interviewed reported having a skin rash just before developing their arthritis, and many also recalled being bitten by a tick at the rash site.

Further investigations resulted in the discovery that tiny deer ticks infected with a spiral-shaped bacterium or spirochete (which was later named *Borrelia burgdorferi*) were responsible for the outbreak of arthritis in Lyme.

In Europe, a skin rash similar to that of Lyme disease had been described in medical literature dating back to the turn of the century. Lyme disease may have spread from Europe to the United States in the early 1900s but only recently became common enough to be detected.

The ticks most commonly infected with *B. burgdorferi* usually feed and mate on deer during part of their life cycle. The recent resurgence of the deer population in the northeast and the influx of suburban developments into rural areas where deer ticks are commonly found have probably contributed to the disease's rising prevalence.

The number of reported cases of Lyme disease, as well as the number of geographic areas in which it is found, has been increasing. Lyme disease has been reported in nearly all states in this country, although most cases are concentrated in the coastal northeast, mid-Atlantic states, Wisconsin and Minnesota, and northern California. Lyme disease is endemic in large areas of Asia and Europe. Recent reports suggest that it is present in South America, too.

Ticks That Most Commonly Transmit B. Burgdorferi *in the United States*

(These ticks are all quite similar in appearance.)

* Ixodes dammini—most common in the Northeast and Midwest
* Ixodes scapularis—found in south and southeast
* Ixodes pacificus—found on west coast

Symptoms of Lyme Disease

Erythema Migrans

In most people, the first symptom of Lyme disease is a red rash known as *erythema migrans*. The telltale rash starts as a small red spot that expands over a period of days or weeks, forming a circular, triangular, or oval-shaped rash. Sometimes the rash resembles a bull's eye because it appears as a red ring surrounding a central clear area. The rash, which can range in size from that of a dime to the entire width of a person's back, appears within a few weeks of a tick bite and usually occurs at the site of a bite. As infection spreads, several rashes can appear at different sites on the body.

Erythema migrans is often accompanied by symptoms such as fever, headache, stiff neck, body aches, and fatigue. Although these flu-like symptoms may resemble those of common viral infections, Lyme disease symptoms tend to persist or may occur intermittently.

Arthritis

After several months of being infected by *B. burgdorferi*, slightly more than half of those people not treated with antibiotics develop recurrent attacks of painful and swollen joints that last a few days to a few months. The arthritis can shift from one joint to another; the knee is most commonly affected. About 10 to 20 percent of untreated patients will go on to develop chronic arthritis.

Neurological Symptoms

Lyme disease can also affect the nervous system, causing symptoms such as stiff neck and severe headache (meningitis), temporary paralysis of facial muscles (Bell's palsy), numbness, pain or weakness in the limbs, or poor motor coordination. More subtle changes such as memory loss, difficulty with concentration, and a change in mood or sleeping habits have also been associated with Lyme disease.

153

Nervous system abnormalities usually develop several weeks, months, or even years following an untreated infection. These symptoms often last for weeks or months and may recur.

Heart Problems

Fewer than one out of ten Lyme disease patients develops heart problems, such as an irregular heartbeat, which can be signalled by dizziness or shortness of breath. These symptoms rarely last more than a few days or weeks. Such heart abnormalities generally surface several weeks after infection.

Other Symptoms

Less commonly, Lyme disease can result in eye inflammation, hepatitis, and severe fatigue, although none of these problems is likely to appear without other Lyme disease symptoms being present.

How Lyme Disease Is Diagnosed

Lyme disease may be difficult to diagnose because many of its symptoms mimic those of other disorders. In addition, the only distinctive hallmark unique to Lyme disease—the *erythema migrans* rash—is absent in at least one-fourth of the people who become infected. Although a tick bite is an important clue for diagnosis, many patients cannot recall having been bitten recently by a tick. This is not surprising because the tick is tiny, and a tick bite is usually painless.

When a patient with possible Lyme disease symptoms does not develop the distinctive rash, a physician will rely on a detailed medical history and a careful physical examination for essential clues to diagnosis, with laboratory tests playing a supportive role.

Blood Tests

Unfortunately, the Lyme disease microbe itself is difficult to isolate or culture from body tissues or fluids. Most physicians look for evidence of antibodies against *B. burgdorferi* in the blood to confirm the bacterium's role as the cause of a patient's symptoms. Antibodies are molecules or small substances tailor-made by the immune system to lock onto and destroy specific microbial invaders.

Some patients experiencing nervous system symptoms may also undergo a spinal tap. Through this procedure doctors can detect brain and spinal cord inflammation and can look for antibodies in the spinal fluid.

The inadequacies of the currently available antibody tests may prevent them from firmly establishing whether the Lyme disease bacterium is causing a patient's symptoms. In the first few weeks following infection, antibody tests are not reliable because a patient's immune system has not produced enough antibodies to be detected. Antibiotics given to a patient early during infection may also prevent antibodies from reaching detectable levels, even though the Lyme disease bacterium is the cause of the patient's symptoms.

Because some tests cannot distinguish Lyme disease antibodies from antibodies to similar organisms, patients may test positive for Lyme disease when their symptoms actually stem from other bacterial infections. A lack of standardization of antibody tests and poor quality control also contribute to inaccuracies in test results.

Due to these pitfalls, physicians must rely on their clinical judgement in diagnosing someone with Lyme disease even though the patient does not have the distinctive *erythema migrans* rash. Such a diagnosis would be based on the history of a tick bite, the patient's symptoms, a thorough ruling out of other diseases that might cause those symptoms, and other implicating evidence. This evidence could include such factors as an initial appearance of symptoms during the summer months when tick bites are most likely to occur, outdoor exposure in an area where Lyme disease is common, and a clustering of Lyme disease symptoms among family members.

New Tests under Development

To improve the accuracy of Lyme disease diagnosis, NIH-supported researchers are developing a number of new tests that promise to be more reliable than currently available procedures. Some of these detect distinctive protein fragments of the Lyme disease bacterium in fluid samples.

NIH scientists are developing tests that use the highly sensitive genetic engineering technique, known as polymerase chain reaction (PCR), to detect extremely small quantities of the genetic material of the Lyme disease bacterium in body tissues and fluids.

Several new methods to detect infection are under development in NIH laboratories. Scientists have isolated a protein of *B. burgdorferi*, called p39, that reacts strongly on blood tests. The presence of antibodies to this protein was found to be a strong indicator of the presence of *B. burgdorferi*. Although further research will be needed to determine how soon after infection it can detect the bacterium, p39 may prove to be an ideal test for Lyme disease.

A somewhat different approach is the use of an assay based on two closely related spirochetal proteins that are not found in other species of bacterial spirochetes. This assay differs from blood tests now in use because it detects products of the spirochete itself rather than detecting human antibodies to the bacterium.

Most Common Symptoms of Lyme Disease

(One or more may be present at different times during infection)

Early Infection

- Rash (*erythema migrans*)
- Muscle and joint aches
- Headache
- Stiff neck
- Significant fatigue
- Fever
- Facial paralysis (Bell's palsy)
- Meningitis
- Brief episodes of joint pain and swelling

- **Less common:**

    Eye problems such as conjunctivitis
    Heart abnormalities such as heart block and myocarditis

Late Infection

- Arthritis, intermittent or chronic

- **Less common:**

    Neurologic conditions such as encephalitis or confusion

How Lyme Disease Is Treated

Nearly all Lyme disease patients can be effectively treated with an appropriate course of antibiotic therapy. In general, the sooner such therapy is begun following infection, the quicker and more complete the recovery.

Antibiotics, such as doxycycline or amoxicillin taken orally for a few weeks, can speed the healing of the *erythema migrans* rash and usually prevent subsequent symptoms such as arthritis or neurological problems.

Patients younger than nine years or pregnant or lactating women with Lyme disease are treated with amoxicillin or penicillin because doxycycline can stain the permanent teeth developing in young children or unborn babies. Patients allergic to penicillin are given erythromycin.

Lyme disease patients with neurological symptoms are usually treated with the antibiotic ceftriaxone given intravenously once a day for a month or less. Most patients experience full recovery.

Lyme arthritis may be treated with oral antibiotics. Patients with severe arthritis may be treated with ceftriaxone or penicillin given intravenously. To ease these patients' discomfort and further their healing, the physician might also give anti-inflammatory drugs, draw fluid from affected joints, or surgically remove the inflamed lining of the joints.

Lyme arthritis resolves in most patients within a few weeks or months following antibiotic therapy, although it can take years to disappear completely in some people. Some Lyme disease patients who are untreated for several years may be cured of their arthritis with the proper antibiotic regimen. If the disease has persisted long enough, however, it may irreversibly damage the structure of the joints.

Physicians prefer to treat Lyme disease patients experiencing heart symptoms with antibiotics such as ceftriaxone or penicillin given intravenously for about two weeks. If these symptoms persist or are severe enough, patients may also be treated with corticosteroids or given a temporary internal cardiac pacemaker. People with Lyme disease rarely experience long-term heart damage.

Following treatment for Lyme disease, some people still have persistent fatigue and achiness. This general malaise can take months to subside, although it generally does so spontaneously without requiring additional antibiotic therapy.

Researchers are currently conducting studies to assess the optimal duration of antibiotic therapy for the various manifestations of Lyme disease. Investigators are also testing newly developed antibiotics for their effectiveness in countering the Lyme disease bacterium.

Unfortunately, a bout with Lyme disease is no guarantee that the illness will be prevented in the future. The disease can strike more than once in the same individual if he or she is reinfected with the Lyme disease bacterium.

Lyme Disease Prevention

Avoidance of Ticks

At present, the best way to avoid Lyme disease is to avoid deer ticks. Although generally only about 1 percent of all deer ticks are infected with the Lyme disease bacterium, in some areas more than half of them harbor the microbe.

Most people with Lyme disease become infected during the summer, when immature ticks are most prevalent. Except in warm climates, few people are bitten by deer ticks during winter months.

Deer ticks are most often found in wooded areas and nearby grasslands, and are especially common where the two areas merge. Because the adult ticks feed on deer, areas where deer are frequently seen are likely to harbor sizable numbers of deer ticks.

To help prevent tick bites, people entering tick-infested areas should walk in the center of trails to avoid picking up ticks from overhanging grass and brush.

To minimize skin exposure to both ticks and insect repellents, people outdoors in tick-infested areas should wear long pants and long-sleeved shirts that fit tightly at the ankles and wrists. As a further safeguard, people should wear a hat, tuck pant legs into socks, and wear shoes that leave no part of the feet exposed. To make it easy to detect ticks, people should wear light-colored clothing.

To repel ticks, people can spray their clothing with the insecticide permethrin, which is commonly found in lawn and garden stores. Insect repellents that contain a chemical called DEET (N,NdiethylM-toluamide) can also be applied to clothing or directly onto skin. Although highly effective, these repellents can cause some serious side effects, particularly when high concentrations are used repeatedly on the skin. Infants and children may be especially at risk for adverse reactions to DEET.

Pregnant women should be especially careful to avoid ticks in Lyme disease areas because the infection can be transferred to the unborn child. Such a prenatal infection can make the woman more likely to miscarry or deliver a stillborn baby.

Checking for Ticks

Once indoors, people should check themselves and their children for ticks, particularly in the hairy regions of the body. The immature deer ticks that are most likely to cause Lyme disease are only about the size of a poppy seed, so they are easily mistaken for a freckle or a speck of dirt. All clothing should be washed. Pets should be checked for ticks before entering the house, because they, too, can develop symptoms of Lyme disease. In addition, a pet can carry ticks into the house. These ticks could fall off without biting the animal and subsequently attach to and bite people inside the house.

If a tick is discovered attached to the skin, it should be pulled out gently with tweezers, taking care not to squeeze the tick's body. An antiseptic should then be applied to the bite. Studies by NIH-supported researchers suggest that a tick must be attached for many hours to transmit the Lyme disease bacterium, so prompt tick removal could prevent the disease.

The risk of developing Lyme disease from a tick bite is small, even in heavily infested areas, and most physicians prefer not to treat patients bitten by ticks with antibiotics unless they develop symptoms of Lyme disease.

Vaccine Development

Because Lyme disease is difficult to diagnose and sometimes does not respond to treatment, researchers are trying to create a vaccine that will protect people from the disorder. Vaccines work in part by prompting the body to generate antibodies. These custom-shaped molecules lock onto specific proteins made by a virus or bacterium— often those proteins lodged in the microbe's outer coat. Once antibodies attach to an invading microbe, other immune defenses are evoked to destroy it.

Development of an effective vaccine for Lyme disease has been difficult to create for a number of reasons. Scientists need to find out how the immune system protects against the bacterium because people who have been infected once can acquire the infection again. In addition, there are several different strains of the bacterium, each with its own distinct set of proteins, and bacteria within an individual strain may change the shape of their proteins over time so that antibodies can no longer identify and lock onto them.

Tick Eradication

In the meantime, researchers are trying to develop an effective strategy for ridding areas of deer ticks. Studies show that a single fall spraying of pesticide in wooded areas can substantially reduce the number of adult deer ticks residing there for as long as a year. Spraying on a large scale, however, may not be economically feasible and may prompt environmental or health concerns.

Scientists are also pursuing biological control of deer ticks by introducing tiny stingerless wasps, which feed on immature ticks, into tick-infested areas. Researchers are currently assessing the effectiveness of this technique.

Successful control of deer ticks will probably depend on a combination of tactics. More studies are needed before wide-scale tick control strategies can be implemented.

Tips for Personal Protection

- Avoid tick-infested areas, especially in May, June, and July.*
- Wear light-colored clothing so that ticks can be easily spotted.
- Wear long-sleeved shirts and closed shoes and socks.
- Tuck pant legs into socks or boots and tuck shirt into pants.
- Apply insect repellent containing permethrin to pants, socks, and shoes, and compounds containing DEET on exposed skin. Do not overuse these products.
- Walk in the center of trails to avoid overgrown grass and brush.
- After being outdoors in a tick-infested area, remove, wash, and dry clothing.
- Inspect the body thoroughly and remove carefully any attached ticks.
- Check pets for ticks.

*Local health departments and park or agricultural extension services may have information on the seasonal and geographic distribution of ticks in your area.

How to Remove a Tick

- Tug gently but firmly with blunt tweezers near the head of the tick until it releases its hold on the skin.
- To lessen the chance of contact with the bacterium, try not to crush the tick's body or handle the tick with bare fingers.
- Swab the bite area thoroughly with an antiseptic to prevent bacterial infection.

Research—the Key to Progress

Although Lyme disease poses many challenges, they are challenges the medical research community is well equipped to meet.

New information on Lyme disease is accumulating at a rapid pace, thanks to the scientific research being conducted around the world.

This chapter is not copyrighted and users are encouraged to reproduce and distribute as many free copies as needed. Single copies are available by writing to:

Lyme Disease Booklet
NIAMS/NIH
1 AMS Circle
Bethesda, Maryland 0892

For more information about Lyme disease, you may want to contact your State or local Department of Health (check the government listings in your phone book). This agency may be able to tell you whether Lyme disease is common in your area. Also, staff of the Department may suggest nearby hospitals or clinics where you can be tested for Lyme disease. They may also know local places where ticks can be tested for the bacterium.

Chapter 16

Arthritis in Children

What Kinds of Arthritis Affect Children?

The word arthritis refers to inflammation (that is, swelling, heat, and pain) involving the joints. Arthritis is frequently a chronic illness, meaning that it may last for months or years. About 200,000 children or 2.9 in every 1,000 in the United States have some form of arthritis.

The most common form of arthritis in children is Juvenile Rheumatoid Arthritis. However, children may also be affected by arthritis as a feature of other diseases including:

Systemic lupus erythematosus. (ee-RI-them-a-TOE-sus)—a chronic inflammatory disease characterized by fever and rash that may attack organs such as joints, kidneys, the brain, lungs, and heart.

Juvenile dermatomyositis. (der-MA-toe-MY-o-SY-tis)—a disease that causes a skin rash and weak muscles in children, and may be accompanied by swollen joints.

The spondyloarthropathies of childhood. (SPON-dill-o-arth-ROP-a-thees)—diseases in children that involve the spine. In some but not all children with these diseases, a protein called HLA-B27 is found on the white blood cells. The spondyloarthropathies of child-hood include:

— **Ankylosing spondylitis.** (an-ki-LOW-sing spon-dill-EYE-tis)— a type of arthritis which primarily affects the spine and hips. It usually occurs in males.

— **Reiter's Disease**—a form of arthritis that may cause inflam-mation of the urinary tract, inflammation of the eyelids, mouth ulcers, and/or skin rash.

— **B-27 Arthritis**—a form of arthritis that occurs more often in older boys and affects only a few joints—usually the back, and large joints of the legs such as hips, knees, and ankles. It occurs more often in children who inherit the HLA-B27 protein. If par-ticular changes are seen in X-rays, B-27 arthritis may be reclas-sified as Ankylosing Spondylitis.

— **Psoriatic Arthritis**. (sore-ee-A-tick)—a type of arthritis that may occur with the skin condition, psoriasis. It affects both boys and girls.

— **Scleroderma**—a disease that can affect the skin, joints, blood vessels, and internal organs.

— **Inflammatory Bowel (Crohn's) Disease**—a disease that can affect the intestines, causing diarrhea and abdominal pain. It can be associated with arthritis and fever; these sometimes ap-pear before the digestive symptoms.

Chapter 17

Juvenile Ankylosing Spondylitis

What is it?

Ankylosing Spondylitis (AS) is a kind of arthritis. It especially affects the joints of the spine (backbone) and the sacroiliac joints, which join the pelvis (hip bones) to the spine. The disease also often affects other joints as well, such as the knees, ankles, toes, hips, and rib cage. When it begins before age seventeen, it is called Juvenile Ankylosing Spondylitis (JAS).

JAS and diseases related to it are uncommon but account for a significant proportion of all young people with arthritis. JAS may occur in 1 in 1,000 children, and it occurs much more commonly in boys than in girls. It usually begins in the preteen or teen years.

The cause of JAS is not known. Nevertheless, we do know that children who inherit a gene called HLA B27 from one or both parents are more likely to develop the illness than other children. On the other hand, JAS is still rare in the 8 percent or so of Caucasian children who have the HLA B27 gene. Moreover, HLA B27 does not in itself cause disease. Many physicians believe that a common infection of the intestinal or genito-urinary tract may actually trigger the onset of ankylosing spondylitis.

What are the symptoms?

In children, ankylosing spondylitis usually starts in an ankle, knee, or hip. Months or years later, other joints may be affected, particularly joints of the spine or the sacroiliac joints. In each person the disease behaves somewhat differently.

The first symptom of JAS may be enthesitis, a painful inflammation in ligaments and tendons where they attach to the bone, often near or around the joints. The pain is usually not in the joint (as it is in rheumatoid arthritis) but next to the joint. In children this type of pain occurs most commonly under or behind the heel, under the toes, or around the knee cap.

About one fifth of JAS patients develop an inflammation of the inner eye called iridocyclitis or uveitis. It can occur in one or both eyes and is usually accompanied by acute eye redness, sensitivity to sunlight, and pain. Other complications (which may affect the heart, kidneys, or spinal cord) are very rare.

How is JAS diagnosed?

The diagnosis of JAS is made on the basis of:

- the clinical history
- physical characteristics of the joint and tissue inflammation
- the results of certain laboratory tests

Physicians experienced in the care of children with JAS will carefully evaluate for arthritis; ask careful questions about enthesitis and examine for it; and test for good spinal mobility, sacroiliac tenderness, and good chest movement with breathing.

There is no specific laboratory test for JAS, but laboratory testing can still be very helpful. Blood tests show that children with JAS do not have rheumatoid factor or antinuclear antibodies common in other types of chronic childhood arthritis. The HLA B27 genetic marker is not in itself an abnormality, but its presence correlates with the presence of JAS in a child with arthritis. More than 90 percent of Caucasian children with JAS test positive for the HLA B27 gene, but no more than 40 percent of blacks. This means the test for HLA B27 is an important, but not diagnostic, test for JAS.

X-rays of the sacroiliac joints, which must show changes for a clear diagnosis of ankylosing spondylitis in adults, are seldom useful. These X-ray changes are rarely present in children with JAS, and they may never develop. Moreover, sacroiliac films are often difficult to interpret in teenagers because the bones are growing along the joint.

JAS can look like many other diseases, and physicians must take care to make a proper diagnosis. Many physicians think of JAS as one of many joint diseases under the umbrella called juvenile arthritis.

Younger children with juvenile rheumatoid arthritis can have pauci-articular arthritis (arthritis in a few joints). But, unlike children with JAS, most children with pauciarticular Juvenile rheumatoid arthritis are girls, often have a positive antibody test; only rarely have enthesitis, and may develop chronic, as opposed to acute, eye inflammation.

There are several diseases related to ankylosing spondylitis which have other problems in addition to arthritis. These include: Crohn's disease and ulcerative colitis (inflammation of the intestine) Reiter's syndrome (inflammation of the eyes and urinary tract), and psoriasis (severe skin rash). All these may occur in children.

How is JAS treated?

The treatment of a child with JAS is individualized according to how severe the disease is and whether there are complications. In general, however, a three-part approach is used:

1. **Education and Counseling.** Children with JAS and their families must understand that JAS is likely to last many months, probably years. Furthermore, the disease may seem to greatly improve or even go away altogether, and then the child may have an unpredictable relapse. This characteristic makes evaluating the effectiveness of treatment very difficult. In addition, the child with JAS and the parents must understand the risks of complications and of treatment.

    Finally, the psychological effects of the illness on the child and the family need to be anticipated and evaluated. Families may overprotect children with JAS and treat them as more ill than necessary.

2. **Physical and Occupational Therapy.** The child with JAS must strive to maintain range of motion in affected joints and strengthen weakened muscles in the back, abdomen, and limbs. The well-designed therapy program will involve daily activities designed to promote normal function.

    The three areas of emphasis are stretching exercises, posture, and regular daily exercise. Simple stretching exercises for range of motion in the chest, back, and other joints may be prescribed depending upon the specific joints and ligaments affected. Children with JAS tend to slouch, with the head thrust forward. Attention to posture will keep the head, shoulders, and back well aligned and reduce pain and fatigue.

167

Children with JAS should normally be encouraged to participate in physical activities appropriate to their age, and general exercise should be accomplished in the regular course of
the child's day (such as walking, riding a bicycle, swimming).
Any deviations from this principle should be made by the pediatric rheumatologist or physical therapist.

Children with JAS can also benefit from custom-made equipment that can help control the effects of their arthritis. Specifically, they may benefit from splinting affected joints at
night to prevent and help treat joint contractures. Custom-
fitted insoles may help relieve heel or foot pain.

3. **Medication.** Several anti-inflammatory drugs are effective in
the treatment of JAS. The major class of drugs is called nonsteroidal anti-inflammatory drugs (NSAIDS). These drugs include aspirin, tolmetin (Tolectin), naproxen (Naprosyn), and
in the adolescent, indomethacin (Indocin) or diclofenac
(Voltaren).

Although aspirin is still used for treatment of the rare, very
young child with JAS, aspirin is not the most potent drug for
this condition. In addition, parents are often concerned about
the side effects of aspirin and worry particularly about the
very small risk of Reye's syndrome.

Accordingly, many physicians are now treating JAS with
other, apparently more effective, NSAIDS—Tolectin and
Naprosyn. Naprosyn is particularly useful in children because
it is available both as a liquid and a tablet and requires a dose
only twice a day.

Most pediatric rheumatologists agree that indomethacin is
the most potent NSAID for JAS. Unfortunately, its possible
side effects include severe headaches, dizziness, nightmares,
and other nervous system effects, and it therefore may not be
given to young children. Indocin is approved, however, for
children age 14 and older.

All NSAIDS may cause gastrointestinal distress (discomfort
or pain in the stomach or intestines) or even ulcers. Children
seem less susceptible to these problems than adults, but still
should be closely watched by routine blood tests. These medications should not be taken on an empty stomach but taken

with food in order to minimize stomach distress. Medications (such as ranitidine or sucralfate) can be prescribed if required to control gastrointestinal symptoms.

Other medications are sometimes used in treating JAS. A drug called salazopyrine is rapidly gaining regard as an important treatment. The drug has been used for many years to treat children with certain kinds of bowel disease that may be complicated by an arthritis that mimics JAS, and its side effects are well known. Oral corticosteroids like prednisone are rarely used in JAS, although they may be needed to control eye inflammation. Topical steroids are used to treat the eye disease of JAS. Injection of steroid into an inflamed joint that has not responded to NSAID therapy may be highly effective.

Surgery

Surgery for joint disease is usually not required for the child with JAS. In some very uncommon cases, however, removal of some fluid from a joint is performed by the pediatric rheumatologist or orthopedic surgeon to test the possibility that the arthritis might be infectious. In very rare cases, children with JAS may have such bad joint destruction in a knee or hip joint that they need a joint replacement to improve very poor function or severe pain.

Who can help?

Care of children with JAS is best accomplished by a team of health care professionals. They will assist the pediatrician or family doctor in the evaluation and management of the disease. Members of that team may include:

Pediatric Rheumatologist. The pediatric rheumatologist is a physician with highly specialized training and experience in the care of children with rheumatic diseases like JAS. In the United States, most pediatric rheumatologists are employed by university medical centers.

Nurse. In most medical centers, the health care team includes a nurse with special experience in the care of children with arthritis. The nurse generally has a central role in educating the child, the family, and often the child's school about JAS.

Physical Therapist. The physical therapist will evaluate joint motion and strength. The therapist also has the responsibility to develop exercise programs for the child to be carried out at home or with a local therapist.

Most physical therapists also maintain contact with physical education teachers in the school system, so that the most appropriate program will be undertaken in school for the child with JAS.

Occupational Therapist. People generally don't think of children as needing an occupational therapist; certainly, eight-year-olds don't have formal jobs. Yet, children really do have a lob: they go to school. A major focus of the occupational therapist, then, is to be certain that the child can perform well physically in school and that any needed adaptive equipment (like special chairs, for example) are available. In addition, the occupational therapist will teach the child and the family about activities of daily living so that the child with severe joint disease can still function as well as possible independently.

Social Worker or Psychologist. The potential for psychological stress of JAS on a child and the family should never be taken lightly. Children may perceive themselves as different from their peers even if their disease is not severe. They may be even more upset if JAS limits their activities significantly. Therefore, children and families should be routinely followed by psychological experts, such as social workers and child psychologists who have experience in the evaluation and care of chronically ill children.

Nutritionist. Good nutrition is critically important for any child with a chronic illness. Children with JAS are particularly at risk for becoming overweight because of decreased physical activity. Unfortunately, extra weight can also worsen the symptoms of the illness by producing more stress on affected joints.

Other Physicians. During the course of care of JAS, children may require the services of a number of other physicians. This group might include the Ophthalmologist, who would generally see the child for acute eye pain and redness. The Orthopaedic Surgeon might become involved to evaluate and treat a very severely affected joint, particularly the hip. The Physiatrist, a specialist in physical and rehabilitative medicine, can help design a complicated physical therapy program.

What about school?

Children with JAS and their families should be aware that the disease may affect school life. Parents and teachers can help plan appropriate educational goals and activities with a goal of maintaining as normal a routine as possible.

One potential problem area to watch for is side effects of medication. In some children, some medications may create a feeling of "fuzziness" that might interfere with the child's ability to concentrate. The physician must watch for such problems and work to come up with medication that will not impair the child's school performance.

Children with JAS may experience some difficulty in dealing with other children. They may need help in learning how to handle being different, how to handle the stress of the special things they may need to do (such as getting up to stretch during class or taking medication during the school day).

Special preparation for physical education classes may be required. For example, the child with JAS who has been sitting all day may need to do stretches before participating in Physical Education.

Finally, fatigue may be a factor for the child with JAS. In particular, fatigue may influence the child's ability to do homework. Careful attention to a balanced schedule of school, exercise, and rest can help manage fatigue.

What's in the future?

JAS is usually a chronic disorder. It can last months or years with periods of remission (when the patient seems "cured"). It may persist into adulthood, and children with enthesitis may develop back problems as adults. Treatment is aimed at preventing loss of function and preserving healthy joints. With therapy, most persons with JAS are not significantly disabled and can continue to lead productive lives.

Recommended Reading

From the Ankylosing Spondylitis Association:

- "A Guidebook for Patients"
- "ASA Newsletter"
- "Straight Talk on Ankylosing Spondylitis"

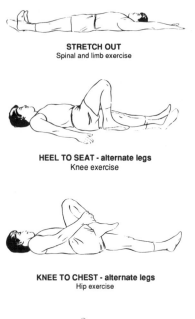

STRETCH OUT
Spinal and limb exercise

HEEL TO SEAT - alternate legs
Knee exercise

KNEE TO CHEST - alternate legs
Hip exercise

CHIN TO KNEE - alternate legs
Spinal mobility, hip/knee mobility

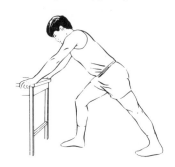

HIP & KNEE ROLLS
Spinal mobility (rotation)

ANKLE STRETCH

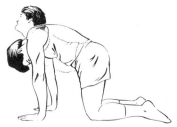

BACK HUMP & HOLLOW
Spinal mobility

Figure 17.1. Exercises

From the Arthritis Foundation:

- "Ankylosing Spondylitis"—Pamphlet
- "When Your Student Has Arthritis" Pamphlet
- "We Can: A Guide for Parents of Children With Arthritis"

About the ASA

The Ankylosing Spondylitis Association is a national volunteer health organization, established in 1983, to work exclusively toward meeting the needs and addressing the concerns of people with AS. We are an organization of people with AS, their families, friends therapists, and doctors, as well as researchers working on the problems of the disease.

Our mission is to provide information, education, and support for people affected by AS, to educate the medical community and public in the unique needs of people with the disease, and to stimulate interest in and support for research.

A tax-deductible membership contribution entitles you to the ASA Newsletter(published quarterly). Guidebook for Patients and Pharmacy Service. Make cheque payable to ASA. Write for membership application form to **ASA, P.O. Box 5872, Sherman Oaks. California 91413.**

Chapter 18

Juvenile Rheumatoid Arthritis

Juvenile Rheumatoid Arthritis (JRA) affects about 71,000 children in the United States. It is a disease of the joints that may also affect other organs. JRA is often a mild condition which causes few problems, but in severe cases it can produce serious complications. Its signs and symptoms may change from day to day, even from morning to afternoon. Joint stiffness and pain may be mild one day but become so severe the next that the child cannot move without great difficulty.

Periods when the arthritis is particularly active are called flares. There are at least three forms of JRA. Each form begins in a different way and has different signs and symptoms. The three forms are:

- Polyarticular JRA ("poly" means several or many and "articular" means joint): this type affects five or more joints

- Pauciarticular JRA ("pauci" means few): this type affects four or fewer joints

- Systemic JRA ("systemic" means internal organs and other body parts are involved): this type affects both the joints and the internal organs

No one knows the cause of JRA, but we know that it involves abnormalities of the immune system.

©1995 Excerpted from brochure "Arthritis in Children." Used by permission of the Arthritis Foundation. For more information, please call the Arthritis Foundation's information line, 1-800-283-7800. Reprinted with permission.

Some research suggests that in autoimmune diseases such as JRA, one type of white blood cells called lymphocytes loses the ability to tell parts of one's body, such as cartilage, from harmful agents like bacteria or viruses. This results in the release of chemicals that can damage the body's own tissues, in a process called inflammation.

The painful joint swelling children with JRA experience is one example of inflammation; another is iridocyclitis, an inflammation in the front of the eye, near the iris.

JRA is not contagious, so your child didn't "catch" it from anyone and can't give it to anyone. We also know that heredity plays some part in the development of several forms of arthritis. However, the inherited trait alone does not cause the illness. We think that this trait along with some other unknown factors triggers the disease. It is unusual for more than one child in a family to have arthritis.

The most common features of JRA are:

• joint inflammation
• joint contracture
• joint damage
• altered growth

Other symptoms:

• joint stiffness following decreased activity, and
• muscle and other soft-tissue weakness.

Joint Inflammation

Joint inflammation is the most common symptom of JRA. It causes heat, pain, swelling, and stiffness in joints. The lining of the joint, called the synovium (si-NO-vee-um), becomes swollen and overgrown and produces too much fluid. This causes swelling, stiffness, pain, warmth, and sometimes redness of the skin over the affected joints.

Contracture

Since it usually hurts to move an inflamed joint, the child will often hold it still in a bent position. If she holds a sore joint in a fixed position for a long time, the muscles around the joint will become stiff and weak.

After a while, the tendons (tissues which connect the muscles to the bone) may tighten up and shorten, causing a deformity called a joint contracture.

Joint Damage

In some children with severe disease, long-lasting inflammation damages the joint surfaces. This is called joint erosion, and can cause pain and limitation of motion.

Altered Growth

Sometimes joint inflammation either speeds up or slows down the growth centers in bones. This can make the affected bones longer, shorter, or bigger than normal. If the growth centers in many bones have been damaged by inflammation, a child may stop growing entirely. If no damage has occurred, however, the child will usually continue to grow once the JRA is under control.

Polyarticular JRA

Polyarticular means "many joints." In this form of JRA, five or more joints are affected. Girls get polyarticular arthritis more often than boys. Because it can be severe, the most powerful medications are recommended for this type of JRA.

Most Common Features

- usually affects the small joints of the fingers and hands
- can also affect weight-bearing and other joints, especially the knees, as well as hips, ankles and feet, neck, and jaw
- often affects the same joint on both sides of the body

Other Possible Features

- low fever
- a positive blood test for rheumatoid factor
- rheumatoid nodules, or lumps, on an elbow or other point of the body that receives a lot of pressure from chairs, shoes, etc.

Pauciarticular JRA

Pauciarticular (PAW-see-ar-TICK-u-lar) means "few joints." In this form of JRA, four or fewer joints are affected.

Most Common Features

- usually affects the large joints (knees, ankles or elbows)

- often affects a particular joint on only one side of the body
- may cause iridocyclitis, an eye inflammation

Systemic JRA

"Systemic" means "affecting the body generally." Systemic JRA affects a child's internal organs as well as the joints. It may take months to diagnose. This is the least common form of JRA. Boys and girls are equally likely to get this kind of JRA. In some, the systemic symptoms of the disease and the fever may go away completely, although the joint-related symptoms of arthritis may remain.

Most Common Features

- **high fevers usually starting in the late afternoon or evening.** The child's temperature may go up to 103 degrees or higher and then return to normal within a few hours. Chills and shaking often go along with the fever and the child may feel very sick. Periods of fever can last for weeks or even months but rarely go on for more than six months.

- **a rash along with the fever.** Pale red spots often appear on the child's chest and thighs and sometimes on other parts of the body. This rash comes and goes for many days in a row.

- **inflammation in many joints.** Joint problems may begin with the fever or may not start until weeks or even months later. Some children have severe pain in their joints when they have a fever and then feel much better when their temperature goes down. Joint problems can also go on after the period of fever ends and can be a major long-term difficulty for children with this kind of arthritis.

Other Possible Features

- inflammation of the outer lining of the heart (pericarditis: PARE-i-car-DE-tis), the heart itself, or the lungs (pleuritis: plur-EYE-tis)
- anemia (low red blood count)
- a high level of white cells in the blood
- enlarged lymph nodes, liver, and spleen

Regular visits to your doctor are important so these problems can be checked and treated from the beginning.

How Is JRA Diagnosed?

The signs and symptoms of JRA vary from child to child. There is no single test that makes the diagnosis of JRA. Therefore, your doctor may go though many steps to find out if your child really does have JRA. The main steps involved in diagnosis are:

The Child's Health History

To make a correct diagnosis, the doctor will ask questions about your child's recent symptoms, medications she is taking, and any previous medical problems.

In order to make a diagnosis of JRA, the arthritis must have been constantly present for six or more consecutive weeks.

The doctor may also wish to rule out other possible causes of arthritis through various tests. Many viral infections can lead to temporary joint problems in children, but in these cases the arthritis usually goes away rapidly. Other diseases can cause arthritis. Sometimes a bacterial infection of bone or cartilage can cause joint swelling or pain. Prompt diagnosis is important to allow proper antibiotic treatment.

The doctor may also want to know if other members of the family have had any other form of arthritis, since some forms may be inherited.

Physical Examination

During the physical examination, the doctor will look for:

- joint inflammation
- rash
- nodules
- eye problems

The doctor must be able to find evidence of joint inflammation to be sure the problem is JRA. A child who complains of aches and pains, but who shows no joint changes, may not have JRA. In a few cases, a physically healthy child experiencing acute emotional stress may complain of sore joints.

An ophthalmologist may also need to examine your child's eyes to check for signs of iridocyclitis.

179

Laboratory Tests

Although there are several laboratory tests that may support a diagnosis of JRA, there is no single test that provides positive proof one way or another. The most common tests are:

- erythrocyte sedimentation rate ("sed" rate)
- rheumatoid factor test
- antinuclear antibody test (ANA)
- HLA-B27 typing
- hemoglobin test
- urinalysis

If the diagnosis is particularly hard to make, the doctor may do additional tests to rule out other diseases. The diagnosis of JRA is made by excluding other diseases.

X-ray Examinations

X-ray examinations of joints may be helpful early in the course of the illness to find out if another condition such as a bone infection, tumor, or fracture is causing the problem. Later on, x-rays may be used to check on joint damage, or changes in bones. X-rays of the spine help the doctor tell if ankylosing spondylitis is present.

Your child's physician may also suggest Magnetic Resonance Imaging (MRI), a new technology that uses magnetic waves to provide images of the inside of the body without harmful radiation.

Joint Fluid and Tissue Tests

A sample of fluid from one or more joints may be withdrawn by a needle and examined to find out if there is an infection in the joint.

Sometimes the doctor will take a small bit of tissue from a joint or a nodule for examination in the laboratory. This is called a biopsy.

Does JRA Have Long-term Effects?

JRA is a chronic disease one that may last for many years. Eventually, there are good chances that your child will get well and experience no serious, permanent disability. Children with JRA can usually keep up with school and many social activities. Some changes may need to be made when the child is in a flare or if there has been joint damage.

Sometimes, the signs and symptoms of JRA may go away. When this happens, it is called a remission. A remission may last for months, or years, or even forever. But no one can be sure this will happen in your child.

While most children with JRA do well in the long run, parents should be aware of possible long-term consequences. Children with pauciarticular JRA have a higher risk of chronic eye inflammation. Some children with polyarticular or systemic JRA may have serious joint problems or develop other long-term complications, such as decreased growth.

There is no fast and simple solution to JRA.

How JRA Is Treated

Your child's treatment program will be based on the kind of arthritis she has and on her specific symptoms. The goals of any treatment program for juvenile rheumatoid arthritis are to:

- control inflammation
- relieve pain
- prevent or control joint damage
- maximize functional abilities

To reach these goals, the treatment program usually includes:

- medications
- exercise
- eye care
- dental care
- healthy eating practices

Each of these treatments is discussed Part VI: Arthritis Treatments later in this Sourcebook.

Other types of treatment, such as surgery, may be necessary for special long-term problems.

Some physicians have also found that pain can be lessened by combining medical treatment with techniques such as progressive muscle relaxation, meditative breathing, and guided imagery.

Because so many techniques are used to treat children with JRA, the ideal type of care is sometimes called "team care" or "coordinated care." Your child's health care team will include many different specialists who work together to offer your child a complete treatment program. Pediatric rheumatology centers found in many major medical centers offer this care in one location. If you do not live near a pediatric rheumatology center, your child's physician will refer you to the specialists she needs.

Note: Because there is no cure for JRA, you may be tempted to try an unproven remedy. Some unproven remedies are harmless, but others are dangerous. Bring any questions to your doctor.

Exercise

Exercise is a very important part of the treatment for JRA. For children with arthritis, the purpose of regular exercise is to:

- keep joints mobile
- keep muscles strong
- regain lost motion or strength in a joint or muscle
- make everyday activities like walking or dressing easier
- improve general fitness and endurance

Your child might do therapeutic exercise with physical therapists or occupational therapists or sports and recreational activities

Morning Stiffness Relief

Many children experience a period of stiffness upon getting up each day. Morning stiffness can be one of the best measures of disease activity; the longer the morning stiffness lasts, the more active the disease. Morning stiffness can be relieved by these methods:

- a hot bath or shower
- sleeping in a sleeping bag
- range of motion exercises
- a paraffin bath (a tub of warmed wax which coats the small joints of the hands)
- a cold pack: though most children do better with warmth, there are a few who respond to cold (a plastic bag filled with ice or frozen vegetables works well)

Diet

Children with JRA sometimes have nutritional problems associated with their illness such as:

- lack of appetite leading to weight loss and poor growth in height
- excessive weight gain

Although there is no special diet for children with arthritis, and no special foods that will cure the disease, proper nutrition can improve your child's overall health and promote normal growth. A registered dietitian can help you make sure your child eats properly by teaching you ways of improving your child's diet.

Poor Appetite

Loss of appetite often occurs when a child is in a flare. Some children with JRA might feel too sick or too tired to eat. To help your child:

- Encourage her to eat a well-balanced diet at regular meal intervals and include planned snacks even when she may not feel much like eating.

- Try to reduce the amount of food she needs to eat by increasing the nutrient content of each bite of food or drink she eats. For example, add melted cheese, gravies, margarine, dips, and offer whole milk. This can help prevent weight loss and poor growth.

Weight Gain

Children with JRA may limit their physical activity if their joints are stiff and painful. As a result, the child may gain too much weight. Corticosteroids can also cause a child to gain weight. Excess weight is unhealthy because it puts more stress on joints such as knees, hips, and ankles. Appropriate exercise combined with eating a well-balanced diet which includes planned snacks based on the basic four food groups can help your child keep a normal body weight.

Note: Taking medicines, particularly NSAIDs, with food helps prevent damage to the stomach and upper part of the intestine.

Dental Care

The most important aspect of dental care for everyone is the prevention of dental disease. Some children with JRA may have difficulty brushing and flossing. Your dentist may suggest various toothbrush handles, electric toothbrushes, floss holders, toothpicks, and rinses that will help your child maintain healthy teeth and gums.

Eye Care

An eye inflammation called iridocyclitis (EER-i-doe-sy-ELLY-tis), or closely-related forms called anterior uveitis and iritis, are sometimes associated with JRA, especially the pauciarticular type. Iridocyclitis occurs more often in young girls with pauciarticular JRA whose blood contains a kind of protein known as an Antinuclear Antibody (ANA). In iridocyclitis, certain tissues in the eyes become inflamed. But this inflammation may not cause any obvious eye symptoms until it has gone on for a long time. The symptoms of iridocyclitis which might appear after a while include red eyes, eye pain, and failing vision.

It is important for all children with JRA to have their eyes checked by an ophthalmologist as soon as they are diagnosed. The ophthalmologist can detect the problem early and start treatment to avoid any serious problems.

Children should continue to get periodic eye exams even when the arthritis is inactive and they have no joint swelling, because iridocyclitis may still be present.

Your child should visit the ophthalmologist for a complete medical eye evaluation, including a slit lamp test. This is a simple and painless procedure that can spot problems before you can tell anything is wrong. The eye examination may need to be repeated from time to time, depending on your child's risk for developing the eye problem. Your doctor will tell you how often your child should be examined. If iridocyclitis is found early and treated properly, it is unlikely to cause any trouble. If it is allowed to go on, it can result in impaired vision or even blindness.

If your child has iridocyclitis, eye drops will be prescribed. One type of eye drops is used to dilate the pupil (make the black spot in the center of the eye bigger). This will keep scars from forming on the pupil. Another kind of eye drop contains a corticosteroid drug which will decrease the inflammation in the eye tissues. When corticosteroids are taken in this form, the side effects are not as serious as when the drug is taken by mouth. If the drops cannot control the iridocyclitis, your child may need to take an anti-inflammatory medication in pill form.

Surgery

Surgery is rarely used to treat JRA early in the course of the disease. However, surgery can be used to:

- relieve pain
- release joint contractures
- replace a damaged joint

If surgery is necessary, your doctor may consider joint replacement or soft tissue release as treatment.

What about Emotions?

Your child may feel angry or sad about having arthritis. But be aware that you as parents, siblings, and other family members may also have troubling feelings about the disease and its effect on the family. However, acceptance and settling into a routine will benefit everyone in the family.

When you are first told your child has arthritis, you might feel shocked, numbed, or disbelieving. You might also feel guilty, and ask yourself if something you did or didn't do caused your child's arthritis. While these thoughts are common to all parents whose children are ill, work hard to put such thinking into perspective. Remember: you are not the reason for your child's arthritis.

The child with arthritis may feel many different emotions. Children can feel "hurt" by an illness that isn't their fault, blame parents for the illness, adopt a "why me?" attitude, engage in self-pity or become angry because of restrictions on activities. They may also resent other children who are well, including brothers and sisters.

Other children in the family may feel left out and resentful because of the amount of time and attention the child with arthritis requires. Or they may feel guilty, as if their normal "bad thoughts" towards their brother or sister had somehow caused the illness.

Children may over-identify with the brother or sister with special needs. Some feel a pressure to achieve or make up for what their brother or sister can no longer do. Others want to involve themselves in care giving to the point where they give up their own normal activities. In these cases, try to help siblings find other ways to deal with their feelings. Whenever possible, let brothers and sisters settle their own differences. Encourage non-disabled siblings to talk with peers who live in homes with similar concerns.

The key to dealing with all these emotions is to talk about them with one another.

Talk to your child about how she feels about the illness. Allow your child to express her anger about arthritis from time to time.

Encourage your child to develop her special talents.

Expect your child to behave as well as other children do not give her special privileges, like avoiding light household chores that she is physically able to do, just because she has arthritis.

Encourage your child to learn as much as she can about arthritis and about her treatment program. Older children can be responsible for taking medications on time, reporting any medication side effects to you, and following an exercise program. Prepare them for the change to adult health-care.

Remember: Your attitude toward arthritis will affect the way your child feels about arthritis.

Talk to your child's brothers and sisters about arthritis let them express their feelings about the disease. Encourage the family to treat the child with JRA as they did before she became ill but at the same time, do remember that she will need some special attention.

Try not to overprotect your child. Your child might become too dependent if you do everything for her or if you keep her from tasks which she is capable of doing. Don't be manipulated into allowing activities that shouldn't be done, but compromise when you can. Being as consistent as possible will help your child learn what is expected. Plan special time to spend alone with your spouse, or with the entire family. When your child first becomes ill, you may set aside relationships with other family members. It is important, however, to continue to talk and spend time with all family members.

Chapter 19

Sjögren's Syndrome

What is Sjögren's Syndrome?

Sjögren's (SHOW-grens) syndrome is an autoimmune disease that causes dry eyes and a dry mouth. An autoimmune disease is a disease in which the immune system turns against itself. Your immune system is your body's natural defense against antigens, which are substances that your body regards as foreign. Bacteria and viruses are examples of antigens. The immune system fights off antigens by activating certain white blood cells and producing antibodies, which are special types of blood protein. These cells and antibodies then attack antigens and render them harmless.

Occasionally, the immune system does not function properly and loses the ability to distinguish between its own body cells and antigens. Instead of fighting antigens, the immune system mistakenly fights the body's own cells. This is referred to as an autoimmune response (auto means self, and this is a response directed against the body's own cells).

Sjögren's syndrome can occur in two forms: primary and secondary. Primary Sjögren's syndrome occurs by itself and is not associated with other diseases. Secondary Sjögren's syndrome occurs with rheumatic diseases such as rheumatoid arthritis, systemic lupus erythematosus (lupus), polymyositis and some forms of scleroderma.

Rheumatic diseases are conditions that affect joints, bones, muscles, skin and sometimes other organs.

Sjögren's syndrome can affect people of any race and any age, although it is relatively rare in people under age 20. Ninety percent of the people affected are women. The tendency to develop Sjögren's syndrome increases if someone in your family has had the condition. It is estimated that Sjögren's syndrome affects more than one million people in the United States.

What happens in Sjögren's Syndrome?

In Sjögren's syndrome, a type of white blood cell called a lymphocyte invades moisture-producing glands, such as tear and salivary glands in the head and Bartholin's glands in the vagina. Lymphocytes can damage these glands and prevent them from producing moisture.

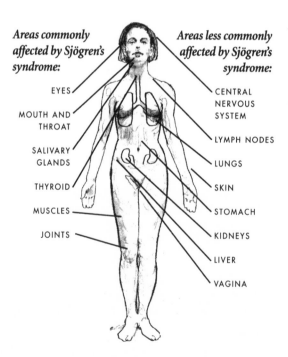

Figure 19.1.

Sjögren's syndrome also can cause problems in other parts of the body. These problems can include joint inflammation as well as inflammation in parts of the lungs, kidneys, liver, nerves, thyroid gland and brain.

What are the symptoms?

Sjögren's syndrome affects everyone differently. You may not have every symptom listed in this section. The symptoms may very from mild at times to severe at others. Symptoms include:

- Dry mouth
- Dry eyes
- Swollen salivary glands
- Dental caries (cavities)
- Oral yeast infection (candidiasis—can-di-DYE-ah-sis)
- Dry Nose, Throat and Lungs
- Dryness of the Vagina
- Fatigue
- Other problems can include inflamed, achy joints; muscle weakness; dry skin; rashes; constipation; inflamed nerves; feelings of numbness and tingling; and swollen lymph nodes. (In rare situations, lymph gland swelling can result in a type of cancer called lymphoma.) These are reasons why medical exams and continued follow-up are important.

How is Sjögren's Syndrome diagnosed?

Your doctor's diagnosis may be based on several sources of information. These include:

- Your medical history
- Your Physical Examination
- Chest X-rays
- Laboratory Tests. These include:
  - Blood Tests for specific blood markers.
  - Schirmer Test to determine how dry your eyes are.
  - Slit-Lamp examination as a more accurate way to find out if your eyes are dry.
  - Lip Biopsy in which the doctor removes a few minor salivary glands from inside your lip and examines them under a microscope.
  - Salivary Function Tests measure the actual amount of saliva you produce.
  - Urine tests may be done to check your kidney function.

How is Sjögren's Syndrome treated?

As yet, there is no cure for Sjögren's syndrome. But proper treatment can help relieve symptoms so that you can live a comfortable and productive life.

One of the main goals of treatment is to relieve discomfort and lessen or prevent the effects of the dryness. Since Sjögren's syndrome affects everyone differently, your treatment plan needs to be based upon your specific needs. Following are some things that can help you cope with the symptoms.

For Systemic Problems.

- Since Sjögren's syndrome is a systemic disorder, which means that it can affect various internal organs and body parts, several different medications can be used to treat it. Aspirin and nonsteroidal anti-inflammatory drugs (NSAIDs) can help reduce joint pain and stiffness, as well as muscle aches. Recent studies have shown that hydroxychloroquine (Plaquenil) can help relieve joint pain, rashes and fatigue in some people. If you have serious complications, your doctor may recommend stronger medicines, such as steroids (cortisone) or medications that may alter or modify your immune system response.

- Exercise also can help treat systemic problems by keeping joints and muscles flexible. Walking, swimming and range-of-motion exercises are well suited for people with Sjögren's syndrome.

For Dry mouth.

- Sip water throughout the day as needed.

- Use sugar-free gum or candies to stimulate saliva production.

- Seek treatment for oral yeast infection (candidiasis) from your dentist or physician. Your mouth will feel better afterward. However, candidiasis is a condition that can reoccur, which means you may need additional treatment.

- Try saliva substitutes or mouth-coating gels. They are particularly useful at night and are available without a prescription.

To Prevent Dental Caries (cavities).

- Have frequent dental checkups.

- Ask your dentist to recommend fluoride-containing products, particularly for dry mouth.

- Brush and floss your teeth effectively and regularly, especially after meals.

- Eliminate sugary foods and drinks between meals.

For Dry Eyes.

- Use artificial tears to help relieve the discomfort of dry eyes. You may wish to use preservative-free products if you apply the drops more than four times per day.

- Try lubricating eye ointments at night and small, long-acting pellets during the day.

- Your doctor may recommend a procedure called punctal occlusion. This is a simple operation that prevents tears from draining out of your eyes and into your nose. This procedure helps retain tears so your eyes can benefit from natural moisture.

For Dry Skin.

- Use moisturizing lotions for sensitive skin.

- Avoid drafts from air conditioners, heaters and radiators whenever possible.

- Avoid detergents, deodorant soaps and excessively hot water.

- Use a humidifier whenever possible.

For Vaginal Dryness.

- Use lubricants made specifically to help vaginal dryness. Don't use petroleum jelly.

The Future

Sjögren's syndrome is generally not life-threatening. The outlook for people with this condition is usually good. Dryness, however, may last for the rest of your life. By using artificial moisture and preventing dental caries (cavities), you can help prevent serious problems.

If you have Sjögren's Syndrome and a rheumatic disease, make sure you follow your doctor's complete treatment program.

191

Chapter 20

Polymyalgia Rheumatica and Giant Cell Arteritis

Questions and Answers

What are Polymyalgia Rheumatica and giant cell arteritis?

Polymyalgia Rheumatica is a rheumatic disorder that is associated with moderate to severe muscle pain and stiffness in the neck, shoulder, and hip area. Stiffness is most noticeable in the morning. This disorder may develop rapidly—in some patients overnight. In other people, Polymyalgia Rheumatica develops more gradually. The cause of Polymyalgia Rheumatica is not known; however, possibilities include immune system abnormalities and genetic factors. The fact that Polymyalgia Rheumatica is rare in people under the age of 50 suggests it may be linked to the aging process.

Polymyalgia Rheumatica may go away without treatment in one to several years. But with treatment the symptoms of Polymyalgia Rheumatica disappear quickly.

Giant cell arteritis, also known as temporal arteritis and cranial arteritis, is a disorder that results in swelling of in the head (most often the temporal arteries), neck, and arms. This swelling causes the arteries to narrow, reducing blood flow. Giant cell arteritis should be treated as soon as it is detected to prevent blindness.

NIH, NIAMS Web Document http://www.nih.gov/niams/healthinfo/pmrgcafs.htm.

How are Polymyalgia Rheumatica and giant cell arteritis related?

It is unclear how or why Polymyalgia Rheumatica and giant cell arteritis are related, but an estimated 15 percent of people in the United States with Polymyalgia Rheumatica also develop giant cell arteritis. Patients can develop giant cell arteritis either at the same time as Polymyalgia Rheumatica, or after the symptoms disappear. About half of the people suffering from giant cell arteritis also have Polymyalgia Rheumatica.

When a person is diagnosed with Polymyalgia Rheumatica, the doctor also should look for symptoms of giant cell arteritis because of the risk of blindness. With proper treatment, the disease is not threatening. Untreated, however, giant cell arteritis can lead to serious complications including permanent vision loss and stroke. Patients must learn to recognize the signs of giant cell arteritis, because they can develop even after the symptoms of Polymyalgia Rheumatica disappear. Patients should report any symptoms to the doctor immediately.

Who is at risk?

White women over the age of 50 are most at risk of developing Polymyalgia Rheumatica and giant cell arteritis. Women are twice as likely as men to develop the conditions. Both conditions almost exclusively affect people over the age of 50. The average age of onset is 70 years. Polymyalgia Rheumatica and giant cell arteritis are quite common. In the United States, it is estimated that 500 per 100,000 people in the general population over 50 years of age develop Polymyalgia Rheumatica.

What are the symptoms?

The primary symptoms of Polymyalgia Rheumatica are moderate to severe stiffness and muscle pain near the neck, shoulders, or hips. The stiffness is more severe upon waking or after a period of inactivity, and typically lasts longer than 30 minutes. People with this condition also may have flu-like symptoms, including fever, weakness, and weight loss.

Early symptoms of giant cell arteritis also may resemble the flu. As the condition progresses, people are likely to experience headaches, pain in the temples, and blurred or double vision. Pain may also affect the jaw and tongue. Doctors suspect giant cell arteritis in people with these symptoms who previously were diagnosed with Polymyalgia Rheumatica.

How are Polymyalgia Rheumatica and giant cell arteritis diagnosed?

No single test is available to definitively diagnose Polymyalgia Rheumatica. To diagnose the condition, a physician considers the patient's medical history, including symptoms that the patient reports; and results of laboratory tests that can rule out other possible diagnoses.

The most typical laboratory finding in people with Polymyalgia Rheumatica is an elevated erythrocyte sedimentation rate, commonly referred to as the sed rate. This test measures how quickly red blood cells fall to the bottom of a test tube of unclotted blood. Rapidly descending cells (an elevated sed rate) indicate inflammation in the body. While the sed rate measurement is a helpful diagnostic tool, it alone does not confirm Polymyalgia Rheumatica. An abnormal result indicates only that tissue is inflamed, which also is a symptom of many other types of arthritis. Before making a diagnosis of Polymyalgia Rheumatica, the doctor may perform additional tests to rule out other conditions including rheumatoid arthritis, because symptoms of Polymyalgia Rheumatica and rheumatoid arthritis are very similar.

The doctor may recommend a test for rheumatoid factor (RF). RF is an antibody sometimes found in the blood. (An antibody is a special protein made by the immune system.) People with rheumatoid arthritis are likely to have RF in their blood, but most people with Polymyalgia Rheumatica do not. If the diagnosis still is unclear, a physician may conduct additional tests to rule out other disorders.

Doctors and patients both need to be aware of the risk of giant cell arteritis in people with Polymyalgia Rheumatica, and should be on the lookout for symptoms of the disorder. Severe headaches, jaw pain, and vision problems are typical symptoms of giant cell arteritis. In addition, physical examination may reveal an abnormal temporal artery (located on the temples on each side of the head)—tender to the touch, inflamed, and with reduced pulse. Because of the possibility of permanent blindness, a temporal artery biopsy is recommended if there is any doubt about the diagnosis. In a person with giant cell arteritis, the biopsy will show abnormal cells in the artery walls. Some patients showing symptoms of giant cell arteritis will have negative biopsy results. In such cases the doctor may suggest a second biopsy.

What are the treatments?

Polymyalgia Rheumatica usually disappears without treatment in one to several years. With treatment, however, symptoms disappear quickly, usually in 24 to 48 hours. If there is no improvement the doctor is likely to consider other possible diagnoses.

The treatment of choice is corticosteroid medication, usually prednisone. Polymyalgia Rheumatica responds to a low daily dose of prednisone. The dose is increased as needed until symptoms disappear. Once symptoms disappear, the doctor may gradually reduce the dosage to determine the lowest amount needed to alleviate symptoms. The amount of time that treatment is needed is different for each patient. Most patients can discontinue medication after six months to two years. If symptoms recur, prednisone treatment is required again.

Nonsteroidal anti-inflammatory drugs (NSAIDs)such as aspirin and ibuprofen also may be used to treat Polymyalgia Rheumatica. The medication must be taken daily and long-term use may cause stomach irritation. For most patients, NSAIDs alone are not enough to relieve symptoms.

Giant cell arteritis carries a small but definite risk of blindness. The blindness is permanent once it happens. A high dose of prednisone is needed to prevent blindness and should be started as soon as possible, perhaps even before the diagnosis is confirmed with a temporal artery biopsy. When treated, symptoms quickly disappear. Typically, people with giant cell arteritis must continue taking a high dose of prednisone for one month. Once symptoms disappear and the sed rate is normal and there is no longer a risk of blindness, the doctor can begin to gradually reduce the dose. When treated properly, giant cell arteritis rarely recurs.

People taking low doses of prednisone rarely experience side effects. Side effects are more common among people taking higher doses. But all patients should be aware of potential effects, which include:

- fluid retention and weight gain
- rounding of the face
- delayed wound healing
- bruising easily
- diabetes
- glaucoma
- increase in blood pressure
- decreased calcium absorption in the bones, which can lead to osteoporosis
- irritation of the stomach

People taking corticosteroids may have some side effects or none at all. A patient should report any side effects to the doctor. When the medication is stopped, the side effects disappear. Because prednisone and other corticosteroid drugs change the body's natural production of corticosteroid hormones, the patient should not stop taking the medication unless instructed by the doctor. The patient and doctor must work together to gradually reduce the medication.

What is the outlook?

Most people with Polymyalgia Rheumatica and giant cell arteritis lead normal, active lives. The duration of drug treatment differs by patient. Once treatment is discontinued, Polymyalgia may recur; but once again, symptoms respond rapidly to prednisone. When properly treated, giant cell arteritis rarely recurs.

What research is being conducted to help people who have Polymyalgia Rheumatica and giant cell arteritis?

Researchers studying possible causes of Polymyalgia Rheumatica and giant cell arteritis are investigating the role of genetic predisposition, immune system abnormalities, and environmental factors.

Scientists also are studying why the two disorders often occur together and are exploring other treatments. Preliminary findings suggest that low doses of methotrexate, a drug used to treat some other rheumatic disorders, controls Polymyalgia Rheumatica and may be an effective treatment for giant cell arteritis.

Where can people get more information about Polymyalgia Rheumatica and giant cell arteritis?

Arthritis Foundation
1314 Spring Street, N.W.
Atlanta, Georgia
30309
(404) 872-7100
(800) 283-7800 (or your local chapter of the Arthritis Foundation listed in your local telephone directory)
World Wide Web address: www.arthritis.org

Chapter 21

Chronic Arthropathy: Parvovirus B19

Human parvovirus B19, discovered by serendipity and subsequently implicated in a wide variety of clinical conditions, has been linked to yet another illness in a new population. A 2-year study conducted by Dr. Stanley J. Naides and his colleagues at the University of Iowa in Iowa City shows that this tiny human virus can persist in otherwise healthy adults who have a type of chronic joint disease that may be mistakenly diagnosed as rheumatoid arthritis. Called chronic arthropathy to distinguish it from true arthritis, this condition joins an expanding repertoire of clinical consequences of B19 infection, ranging from a mild, short-lived illness in children—somewhat more severe when contracted by adults—to more serious effects in fetuses and in people with certain types of anemia or suppressed immune systems.

Almost 100 years separate the description of a distinctive, "slapped-cheek" childhood facial rash and flu-like illness (erythema infectiosum) from the incidental discovery of its cause by Dr. Y. E. Cossart and her colleagues in 1975. This British team was developing diagnostic tests for hepatitis B when they happened upon an antigen in normal donor sera that was eventually identified as parvovirus B19, the first human parvovirus to be described. Subsequent experimental infection of normal adult volunteers with the virus proved it to be the cause of erythema infectiosum. Parvovirus B19 infection occurs throughout

"Recently Discovered Human Virus Causes Joint Disease, Many Other Conditions," *Research Resources Reporter*, August 1991.

the world and is so common, says Dr. Naides, that 40 to 60 percent of adults have antibodies in their blood that indicate a past encounter with the virus. The risk of infection can be higher for people in certain occupations such as nursing, teaching, and day-care, Dr. Naides adds.

Dr. Naides and his associates tested 21 adults who visited the University of Iowa Hospitals and Clinics rheumatology service over a 2-year period. All had a type of antibody to parvovirus B19 in their blood that indicated a recent, rather than past, infection. Nine of the twenty-one had erythema infectiosum, which is typically characterized by muscle and joint pain in adults. Eight of these nine patients showed varying degrees of pain, stiffness, or swelling in several joints, but these symptoms lasted only 2 to 21 days. In contrast, the other 12 patients came to the hospital with acute pain, stiffness, and inflammation in their joints that lasted an average of 14 months.

Ordinarily those 12 patients would have been diagnosed with rheumatoid arthritis rather than chronic parvovirus arthropathy. "Four of seven criteria are required for a diagnosis of rheumatoid arthritis," says Dr. Naides, assistant professor of rheumatology in the University of Iowa's department of internal medicine. "Most of the patients with parvovirus arthropathy meet three if not four of those criteria."

None of the 12 patients in the Iowa study developed nodules under the skin or erosion of bone at the affected joints, both common findings in rheumatoid arthritis. The blood of one patient did show a low to moderate level of rheumatoid factor, a protein associated with rheumatoid arthritis; however, he says, "rheumatoid factor can be elevated in any number of infectious or inflammatory diseases. It is an antibody made against other antibodies and so is not specific for any one disease."

The precise way in which parvovirus B19 arthropathy develops remains elusive, as does the reason it strikes disproportionately more women than men. The natural history of the virus and the other clinical conditions it may induce are better understood. Besides arthropathy and erythema infectiosum, says Dr. Naides, B19 infection causes a critical shortage of oxygen-carrying red blood cells—aplastic crisis—in people with chronic anemias. The virus can also be transmitted from mother to fetus and cause anemia and subsequent cardiac failure when the heart can no longer meet the demands of oxygen-starved tissues. Finally, persistent infection with B19 may result in episodic or chronic bone marrow suppression in people whose immune systems are compromised, either hereditarily or through chemotherapy or acquired disorders such as AIDS.

These three clinical phenomena—aplastic crisis, fetal anemia and heart failure, and bone marrow suppression—all stem from the virus's preference for replicating in rapidly dividing cells, explains Dr. Naides. In children and adults the B19 virus targets the bone marrow, specifically the precursors of erythrocytes, or red blood cells. In fetuses, which have a higher rate of cell turnover overall, the virus may also infect other tissues, including heart muscle, he says.

Once entrenched in the nucleus, the replicating parvovirus stops the host cell from maturing into an erythrocyte, causing production of new red blood cells to cease for approximately 7 to 10 days. According to Dr. Naides, other investigators have shown that healthy people infected with the B19 virus can survive a shortage of this duration because their existing erythrocytes stay in circulation for 120 days. However, he adds, in people with conditions such as sickle cell anemia even a week's worth of lost new erythrocytes "becomes critical because these people need a brisk production of red cells to keep up with the equally brisk destruction caused by the anemia."

A similar problem confronts the fetus infected with B19. "In many respects the fetus is like a child with sickle cell anemia," notes Dr. Naides. "Its red cells survive only about 45 to 70 days, which is normal for a fetus, and because it is growing it has an increased pool of red cell precursors, providing an excellent milieu for the virus."

For people with compromised immune systems, "the virus can do long-term what it does short-term in immunocompetent people," says Dr. Naides. "Some immunocompromised individuals fail to make neutralizing antibodies against the virus and therefore become persistently infected." Persistent arrest of red cell maturation translates into chronic bone marrow suppression, Dr. Naides explains.

Returning to the question of how B19 causes chronic arthropathy, two possibilities present themselves, says Dr. Naides. The virus may persist after its acute phase, alternately replicating or remaining latent for periods. Alternatively, the virus may do its damage—perhaps to the immune system—during the acute infection, after which it might be cleared from the body, with the arthropathy a consequence of the damage.

The former possibility seems more likely so far. "We have identified B19 DNA in bone marrow aspirated from individuals who have had chronic arthropathy for at least two years, but not in normal volunteer bone marrow donors both with and without evidence of past infection with B19," Dr. Naides says. The Iowa researchers are now looking for B19 DNA in synovia—the membranes that secrete the viscous fluid found in joint cavities—of both the arthropathy patients and patients who have had joint trauma or joint replacements for other reasons. "The next questions will be how much of the viral genome is present and whether it represents persistent or latent infection," Dr. Naides notes.

Early and accurate diagnosis can improve the outcome of several of the conditions caused by parvovirus B19. For example, in the fetus an accumulation of fluid in the abdominal cavity—fetal hydrops—signals the clinician that something is wrong. From this point it takes only six hours to detect viral particles in the fluid by electron microscopy, after which the fetus can receive a blood transfusion in utero, "with very good results," says Dr. Naides. Similarly, he adds, immunocompromised patients who are infected with B19 benefit from administration of gamma-globulin, which contains normal donors' neutralizing antibodies against B19.

For both fetuses and immunocompromised patients, prevention is equally important. Dr. Naides recommends that closer attention be paid to pregnant women who have been exposed to children or adults with erythema infectiosum. He also cautions that although the probability is low, B19 virus can be transmitted in factor VIII and prothrombin preparations, blood products that are given to people with certain coagulation disorders who in some cases may be immunocompromised.

In the case of chronic arthropathy, the serologic testing for B19 infection must be done when the patient is first seen, say the Iowa investigators, because the particular type of antibody that reveals recent infection is no longer detectable after about three months. Furthermore, because the courses of the two diseases differ, knowing whether a patient has chronic parvovirus arthropathy or rheumatoid arthritis may affect the choice of therapy.

"Some rheumatologists would like to use cytotoxic agents such as methotrexate earlier in treatment to prevent the erosions of rheumatoid arthritis. My concern is that if we don't make the diagnosis of parvovirus arthropathy, we'll pat ourselves on the back when these patients don't develop erosions, never knowing that they would not have developed erosions anyway. Also, we do not know what effects cytotoxic agents might have on an individual in whose bone marrow the virus may be persisting," he says.

Until recently, says Dr. Naides, B19 virus has been too difficult to obtain and to culture for routine diagnostic purposes. He and others currently are using whole virus in antibody detection. However, he expects several groups that are now using recombinant DNA technology to produce viral proteins that should be as useful in testing as is whole virus.

Additional Reading:

1. Naides, S. J., Scharosch, L. L., Foto, F., and Howard, E. J., Rheumatologic manifestations of human parvovirus B19 infection in adults. *Arthritis s Rheumatism* 33:1297-1309, 1990.

2. Graeve, J. L. A., de Alarcon, P. A., and Naides, S. J., Parvovirus B19 infection in patients receiving cancer chemotherapy: The expanding spectrum of disease. *American Journal of Pediatric Hematology/Oncology* 11:441-444, 1989.

3. Naides, S. J. and Weiner, C. P., Antenatal diagnosis and palliative treatment of non-immune hydrops fetalis secondary to fetal parvovirus B19 infection. *Prenatal Diagnosis* 9:105-114, 1989.

4. Anderson, M. J., Higgins, P. G., Davis, L. R., et al., Experimental parvoviral infection in humans. *Journal of Infectious Diseases* 152:257-265,1985.

The research described in this article was supported by the General Clinical Research Centers Program of the National Center for Research Resources; the National Heart, Lung, and Blood Institute; the Arthritis Foundation; the American Philosophical Society; the Veterans Affairs Disease Fund, Iowa City; and the March of Dimes Birth Defects Foundation.

Chapter 22

Myositis

What Is Myositis?

Myositis refers to inflammation of the muscles (*myo* means muscle and *itis* means inflammation). Myositis is a term that describes several different illnesses, including polymyositis, dermatomyositis and inclusion body myositis.

Myositis is a rare disease. In the United States, it is estimated that each year five to 10 out of every one million people get one of the forms of myositis.

Although myositis can affect people of any age, most children who get the disease are between five and 15 years of age and most adults are between 30 and 60. Like many other inflammatory diseases, most forms of myositis attack more women than men. The exception is inclusion body myositis, a form of myositis in which holes, called inclusion bodies, develop in the muscle fibers. This form affects more men than women.

All forms of myositis involve chronic, or persistent, muscle inflammation. This muscle inflammation almost always results in weakness, and less often in heat, swelling and pain of the muscles. Myositis can affect many parts of the body. Sometimes the joints, heart, lungs, intestines and skin can become inflamed.

Some forms of myositis, like dermatomyositis (*dermato* refers to the skin), result in particular rashes over the knuckles, around the eyes or sometimes in other parts of the body. Other forms or myositis occur in children. Some forms are seen with other connective tissue diseases, like lupus or rheumatoid arthritis. Still other forms may occur in people with tumors. Rarely, myositis can occur in a single part of the body such as one arm, one leg or just the muscles that move the eye.

What Causes Myositis?

We do not know what causes myositis. But because myositis has many forms, it probably has many causes. Some scientists think that myositis results when a person with a certain genetic background is exposed to particular chemicals, viruses or other infectious agents.

Whatever triggers these diseases also results in abnormalities in the immune system. The immune system consists of groups of cells called lymphocytes that circulate throughout the body. In healthy people, these lymphocytes act as a defense force that produces substances that attack viruses, bacteria and other agents of disease. But in many people with myositis, there is an abnormality in the immune system that results in the production of proteins called autoantibodies. Autoantibodies and some of the lymphocytes turn against the body's own tissues and may cause damage.

What Happens in Myositis?

The many forms of myositis begin and progress in different ways. In most people the illness develops slowly over a period of months or even years, but in some people problems can occur suddenly. The disease often appears to come and go for no apparent reason, and sometimes its form changes over time.

Muscle Weakness

The major symptom of myositis is muscle weakness. Hip and shoulder muscles are most likely to be involved. This often results in difficulty combing hair; putting on heavy clothes; getting out of a bathtub, bed, chair or car; and climbing stairs. Other muscles sometimes affected are those in the front of the neck, making it difficult to raise your head when lying down. Occasionally, other neck and throat muscles may be affected, making it hard to swallow, sing or even speak clearly. If your chest muscles or lungs are affected, you may have trouble breathing. Many people with myositis learn ways of compensating, however, and adjust so well that even they are not aware of the slow, gradual, progression of their disease.

Skin Changes

Symptoms of dermatomyositis include a bumpy, patchy, reddish or purplish skin rash on the face; around the eyes (called heliotrope rash); on the knuckles, elbows, or knees (called Gottron's papules); or over the chest or back. Some people have puffy eyelids, wrists or hands as a result of myositis. If you have myositis you also may develop a rash around the base of your fingernails; overgrown cuticles; or cracked and bleeding skin on the sides and tips of your fingers.

Other Symptoms

Other possible symptoms of myositis include fever, weight loss, pain, tenderness in the muscles and arthritis. It sometimes is very difficult to tell whether the joints or the muscles between the joints are causing pain and other problems.

Sometimes Raynaud's phenomenon develops. This is an extreme sensitivity and reaction to cold that is most often felt in the fingers. Raynaud's phenomenon is caused by a narrowing of the blood vessels in the fingers, which reduces blood flow and turns the fingers white and then gradually blue.

Occasionally the heart can become damaged by myositis. This damage can result in irregular heartbeat. Occasionally, myositis can cause the heart to become enlarged and result in swelling of the lower legs.

Course of the Disease

How myositis begins and progresses is quite variable and differs from person to person. Some people first experience rashes, some shortness of breath and some arthritis. As time goes on, new symptoms may develop or existing symptoms may go away. Children with myositis are more likely than adults to develop a condition called calcinosis in which small lumps of calcium are deposited in the skin and muscle fibers.

A small minority of people with myositis have tumors that seem to be related to their myositis. Scientists have found that tumors occur more in people past the age of 50 and in persons with dermatomyositis. Sometimes the removal of the tumor results in the disappearance of the myositis.

How Is Myositis Diagnosed?

Because myositis closely resembles many other diseases and differs from person to person, it can be difficult to diagnose. Your doctor may have to perform many tests and see you many times before deciding on a diagnosis of myositis.

During the process of reaching a diagnosis, your doctor will ask a series of questions about the problems you are experiencing and will perform a physical examination. There are blood tests that may be done, including some for autoantibodies and muscle enzymes. One of the most useful is a blood test for a muscle enzyme called creatine kinase, or CK. In most people with active myositis, the CK level in the blood is abnormally high. The CK level tends to go up with increasing myositis disease activity and tends to go down as the myositis improves.

Another procedure that is very useful in diagnosing myositis is an electromyogram (EMG). An EMG measures the electrical pattern of the muscles, just as an electrocardiogram (EKG) measures the electrical pattern of the heart.

Your doctor will probably also request that a muscle biopsy be done. This is the removal of a small piece of muscle for staining and examination with a microscope. The muscle biopsy shows your doctor whether and how the muscle fibers are damaged.

Chapter 23

Fibromyalgia

Questions and Answers

What is fibromyalgia?

Fibromyalgia is a chronic disorder characterized by widespread musculoskeletal pain, fatigue, and multiple tender points. "Tender points" refers to tenderness that occurs in precise, localized areas, particularly in the neck, spine, shoulders, and hips. People with this syndrome may also experience sleep disturbances, morning stiffness, irritable bowel syndrome, anxiety, and other symptoms.

How many people have fibromyalgia?

According to the American College of Rheumatology, fibromyalgia affects three to six million Americans. It primarily occurs in women of childbearing age, but children, the elderly, and men can also be affected.

What causes fibromyalgia?

Although the cause of fibromyalgia is unknown, researchers have several theories about causes or triggers of the disease. Some scientists believe that the syndrome may be caused by an injury or trauma.

NIAMS Web Document. 10/95 Updated 1/98 National Institute of Arthritis and Musculoskeletal and Skin Diseases.

This injury may affect the central nervous system. Fibromyalgia may be associated with changes in muscle metabolism, such as decreased blood flow, causing fatigue and decreased strength. Others believe the syndrome may be triggered by an infectious agent such as a virus in susceptible people, but no such agent has been identified.

How is fibromyalgia diagnosed?

Fibromyalgia is difficult to diagnose because many of the symptoms mimic those of other diseases. The physician reviews the patient's medical history and makes a diagnosis of fibromyalgia based on a history of chronic widespread pain that persists for more than three months. The American College of Rheumatology (ACR) has developed criteria for fibromyalgia that physicians can use in diagnosing the disease. According to ACR criteria, a person is considered to have fibromyalgia if he or she has widespread pain in combination with tenderness in at least 11 of 18 specific tender point sites.

How is fibromyalgia treated?

Treatment of fibromyalgia requires a comprehensive approach. The physician, physical therapist, and patient may all play an active role in the management of fibromyalgia. Studies have shown that aerobic exercise, such as swimming and walking, improves muscle fitness and reduces muscle pain and tenderness. Heat and massage may also give short-term relief. Antidepressant medications may help elevate mood, improve quality of sleep, and relax muscles. Fibromyalgia patients may benefit from a combination of exercise, medication, physical therapy, and relaxation.

What research is being conducted on fibromyalgia?

The NIAMS is sponsoring research that will increase understanding of the specific abnormalities that cause and accompany fibromyalgia with the hope of developing better ways to diagnose, treat, and prevent this disorder.

Recent NIAMS studies show that abnormally low levels of the hormone cortisol may be associated with fibromyalgia. At Brigham and Women's Hospital in Boston, Massachusetts, and at the University of Michigan Medical Center in Ann Arbor, researchers are studying regulation of the function of the adrenal gland (which makes cortisol) in fibromyalgia. People whose bodies make inadequate amounts of cortisol experience many of the same symptoms as people with fibromyalgia. It is hoped that these studies will increase understanding about fibromyalgia and may suggest new ways to treat the disorder.

Other NIAMS research studies are looking at different aspects of the disease. At the University of Alabama in Birmingham, researchers are concentrating on how specific brain structures are involved in the painful symptoms of fibromyalgia. Researchers at Vanderbilt University in Nashville, Tennessee, are using magnetic resonance imaging (MRI) and magnetic resonance spectroscopy (MRS) techniques to study patients with fibromyalgia. MRI and MRS are powerful tools that have been shown to be useful in evaluating muscle disorders and muscle performance. At the New York Medical College in Valhalla, scientists are investigating the causes of a post-Lyme disease syndrome as a model for fibromyalgia. Some patients develop a fibromyalgia-like condition following Lyme disease, an infectious disorder associated with arthritis and other symptoms.

NIAMS-supported research on fibromyalgia also includes several projects in the Institute's Multipurpose Arthritis and Musculoskeletal Diseases Centers. Researchers at these centers are studying individuals who do not seek medical care, but who meet the criteria for fibromyalgia. (Potential subjects are located through advertisements in local newspapers asking for volunteers with widespread pain or aching.) Other studies at the Centers are attempting to uncover better ways to manage the pain associated with the disease through behavioral interventions such as relaxation training.

The NIAMS supports and encourages outstanding basic and clinical research that increases the understanding of fibromyalgia. However, much more research needs to be done before fibromyalgia can be successfully treated or prevented.

The Federal Government, in collaboration with researchers, physicians, and private voluntary health organizations, is committed to research efforts that are directed to significantly improving the health of all Americans afflicted with fibromyalgia.

Where can people get more information about fibromyalgia?

Arthritis Foundation
1330 West Peachtree Street
Atlanta, GA 30309
404/872-7100
800/283-7800 or call your local chapter (listed in the telephone directory)
World Wide Web address: http://www.arthritis.org

This is the main voluntary organization devoted to all forms of arthritis. The Foundation publishes a pamphlet on fibrositis. Single copies are free with a self-addresses stamped envelope. The Foundation also can provide physician referrals.

Fibromyalgia Alliance of America
P.O. Box 21990
Columbus, OH 43221-0990
614/457-4222
Contact: Mary Anne Saathoff, R.N.

Fibromyalgia Association of Texas
3810 Keele Drive
Garland, TX 75041
972/271-5085
Contact: Ms. Faye Wright

Fibromyalgia Network
P.O. Box 31750
Tucson, AZ 85751-1750
800/853-2929
Contact: Ms. Kristin Thorson

Fibromyalgia Association of Greater Washington (FMAGW)
13203 Valley Drive
Woodbridge, VA 22191-1531
Phone: 703/790-2324
Fax: 703/494-4103
Web: www.fmagw.org
Contact person: Tamara Liller

These are the main organizations devoted to fibromyalgia. They publish newsletters and provide pamphlets on the disease.

The National Arthritis and Musculoskeletal and Skin Diseases Information Clearinghouse (NAMSIC) is a public service sponsored by the NIAMS that provides health information and information sources. The NIAMS, a component of the National Institutes of Health, leads and coordinates the Federal medical effort in arthritis, musculoskeletal, bone, muscle, and skin diseases by conducting and supporting research projects, research training, clinical trials, and epidemiological studies, and by disseminating information on research initiatives and research results.

Chapter 24

Paget's Disease

Help for People with Paget's Disease

Something weighs heavily on Jan Brown's head every day. Something called Paget's disease of bone, and it affects her skull. She feels the effects constantly, like 5 pounds of pressure, she says.

"It's always there," the 57-year-old Rockville, Md., woman says. "I can feel it right now as I speak."

Sometimes she takes Tylenol (acetaminophen) for the pain.

Seventy-two-year-old Kenneth Halstead, of Raleigh, N.C., also has Paget's disease. It affects his skull, as well as his spine, hips, pelvis, and right leg. It's evident from his right leg, which is bowed. On his right foot, he wears a "built-up" shoe to compensate for the half an inch his leg has shrunk. He also wears a hearing aid.

A 78-year-old woman from Washington, D.C., who asked that her name not be used, also has the disease. She, too, wears a hearing aid, and her head is pushed forward and down, preventing her from tilting her head back to look up.

Paget's disease is the second most common bone disease in the United States. Osteoporosis is No. 1. Paget's disease can cause pain, deformities, hearing loss, and limits on activity. The disease, which affects people in different ways, also can cause arthritis and other serious consequences.

This chapter contains two documents: "Help for People with Paget's Disease," *FDA Consumer*, October 1996, and *Research Developments: Paget's Disease of Bone*, NIH Publication No. 92-3414. June 1992.

213

Many people may dismiss these disabilities as a natural part of aging. The average age of diagnosis is 58 (although the disease actually may begin much earlier). But the disease is treatable, and with newer drugs on the market—including two approved by the Food and Drug Administration in 1991 and 1995—there is greater opportunity for patients with Paget's disease to find pain relief, limit the progression of their disease, and, in some cases, reverse bone damage.

The challenge now, experts say, is to identify patients early and, if feasible, start treatment promptly. It's estimated that 3 percent of the American population over 40 is affected. The problem is that many people with Paget's disease don't know they have it because often it develops without symptoms.

Bone Gone Awry

Paget's disease gets its name from Sir James Paget, an English doctor who served as surgeon to Queen Victoria. He first described the disease's characteristics in 1876.

Many years later, scientists realized Paget's disease is a disruption in the normal activity of bone tissue.

Bone is constantly being broken down by cells called osteoclasts and rebuilt by cells called osteoblasts. This is called bone turnover, and throughout the entire skeleton, this process is normally in precise balance.

In Paget's disease, the process goes awry. In discrete portions of bone, overly large osteoclasts dissolve bone too quickly—as much as 50 times faster than normal. Osteoblasts try to compensate for the increased pace by rapidly depositing new bone. But, in the hurried process, the newly deposited bone is loose and bulky in structure, rather than strong, compact, and neatly arranged.

Over time, pagetic bone becomes weak and soft and can easily bend, actually shortening the part of the body affected: for example, a leg or the spine. The bone may enlarge in diameter, though, and it can become painful and break easily.

Any bone can be affected, but the most common sites are the spine, skull, pelvis, and legs. Some patients may have only one affected bone, while others may have two or more. The disease usually does not spread to unaffected bones.

Common deformities include bowed legs, an enlarged head or pelvis, and a curved back. Pagetic bone can affect other parts of the body, causing added problems. For example, it can change bones around joints, causing arthritis. If in the skull and the temporal bone (the bone surrounding the inner ear), Paget's disease can affect hearing. When it affects the facial bones, it can cause dental problems.

Because of changes to the bone, pagetic bones often contain more blood vessels than normal, increasing blood flow to affected bones. Because the heart has to work harder to pump the extra blood, Paget's patients with heart disease may be at even greater risk for heart failure.

Paget's disease is rarely fatal. However, fewer than 1 percent of patients may develop osteosarcoma, a form of bone cancer, and other sarcomas. Most Paget's patients die from causes unrelated to Paget's disease.

Causes

No one knows what causes Paget's disease, although genetics may play a role. Several studies indicate that 15 to 30 percent of Paget's patients have family members with the disease. Those with a first-degree relative—parent, sibling or child—with Paget's disease are seven times more likely to develop the disease than those without an affected first-degree relative.

"It clearly runs in families," says Ethel Siris, M.D., an endocrinologist at Columbia University College of Physicians and Surgeons in New York City. She says the risk increases if the first-degree relative has more severe disease and an early age at diagnosis. Paget's disease is rarely diagnosed in people under 40, although there have been cases. Siris says she's treated patients in their late 20s and early 30s.

The family history related by several patients seems to bear out Siris' conclusions: Evelyn Nef, 83, of Washington, D.C., who was diagnosed with Paget's disease in 1962, says her brother and sister also suffer from the disease. Halstead, who was diagnosed in his 30s, says his two brothers have the disease and his mother, who is 102, was diagnosed three years ago.

The role of genetics also is supported by observations that certain ethnic groups have higher rates of Paget's disease. According to the Paget Foundation, Paget's disease is most common in Caucasian people of Anglo-Saxon and European descent, but it also occurs in African Americans. It is rare in people of Asian descent.

Research by Frederick Singer, M.D., an endocrinologist with the John Wayne Cancer Institute at Saint John's Hospital and Health Center in Santa Monica, Calif., may eventually yield proof of a genetic role. Studying an Iowa family with a history of Paget's disease, Singer and his colleagues traced a genetic abnormality to chromosome

18. The precise gene has yet to be identified, Singer says, but when it is, genetic tests may be able to predict who will get the disease. "I think that's coming pretty fast," he says.

Many experts, Singer included, also suspect that a slow virus may play a role. The theory is that the virus infects a person early in life, without causing symptoms for many years. This theory is based on studies identifying viral-like particles in osteoclasts from pagetic bone. According to Sakamuri Reddy, Ph.D., assistant professor at the University of Texas Health Science Center at San Antonio, these particles react with antibodies that detect a group of viruses which includes the measles and canine distemper viruses. Reddy and his group also have shown that osteoclasts from patients with Paget's disease contain the measles virus messenger RNA. Osteoclasts of people without Paget's disease do not contain this RNA.

This isn't to say that measles is the cause, though, says Leo Lutwak, M.D., Ph.D., an endocrinologist and medical reviewer in FDA's division of metabolism and endocrine drug products. "The agent may be related to the measles virus," he says.

How do the viral theory and genetics' role fit together? Experts in Paget's disease surmise that heredity may put people at risk for the suspected Paget's virus.

"It may be that some people inherit the tendency to have this virus affect their osteoclasts, while other people are, due to their own genetic makeup, more resistant," Siris writes in the Paget Foundation publication *A Patient's Guide to Paget's Disease of Bone*.

Accidental Diagnoses

Many patients, especially those with mild cases, first learn they have Paget's disease when a routine blood test reveals an abnormally high blood level of total alkaline phosphatase, an enzyme produced by osteoblasts, as well as cells of the intestine and liver.

When osteoblasts are more numerous or are especially active, the amount of alkaline phosphatase throughout the skeleton is increased. The increased bone alkaline phosphatase spills over into the blood, increasing the serum alkaline phosphatase.

A normal serum alkaline phosphatase ranges from 20 to 141 units per liter (U/L). Patients with severe Paget's disease may have 6 to 10 times that range. Halstead recalls that at one point his serum alkaline phosphatase rose to nearly 2,000 U/L. Jan Brown of Rockville recalls her alkaline phosphatase was more than 1,000 U/L when she was first diagnosed. "The doctor said he had never seen such a high alkaline phosphatase in as young a person," recalls Brown, who was 52 when diagnosed with Paget's disease.

Sometimes, Paget's patients first learn about their diagnosis when an X-ray taken for other reasons reveals pagetic bone.

Usually, bone pain is the first complaint of patients with symptoms. Bone deformities, arthritic pain, and hearing loss are other complaints that may lead patients to seek medical attention.

Laboratory tests, such as the serum alkaline phosphatase and urinary hydroxyproline (a measure of bone breakdown), may offer evidence of Paget's disease, but X-rays give the definitive diagnosis. Bone scans also may be taken to determine the extent and activity of Paget's disease. Bone scans involve less radiation and are more sensitive than X-rays in detecting areas of pagetic bone.

Treatments

Safe drugs for treating Paget's disease of bone became available only in the last 25 years. FDA approved the first two, calcitonin and Didronel (etidronate disodium), in the mid-1970s.

Salmon calcitonin (Calcimar and Miacalcin) and human calcitonin (Cibacalcin) are synthetic substances similar to the human hormone calcitonin. Synthetic calcitonin preparations help inhibit bone breakdown by decreasing the activity of osteoclasts. Only injectable calcitonin is approved for patients with Paget's disease, although nasal-spray calcitonin, which is approved for other uses, is under study for Paget's disease also, according to the Paget Foundation.

Didronel is taken orally in the middle of a four-hour fast. It is a bisphosphonate, a class of drugs that slows bone turnover.

Two newer bisphosphonates, Aredia (pamidronate disodium for injection) and Fosamax (alendronate sodium tablets), appear to achieve more effective results—as measured by laboratory tests— according to studies, and usually in smaller doses because they are more potent. Aredia, approved by FDA in October 1991, is given intravenously over four hours daily for three consecutive days.

Fosamax, approved by FDA in October 1995, is taken orally. Because this medicine is poorly absorbed, patients should take Fosamax with a glass of water first thing in the morning, then wait at least 30 minutes before taking other medications, eating, or drinking anything other than water. Also, to help prevent esophageal irritation and to ease delivery of the medicine to the stomach, patients should drink a glass of water and not lie down for at least 30 minutes after taking Fosamax.

In clinical studies, patients receiving Fosamax had a 20 to 25 percent greater drop in serum alkaline phosphatase levels than those receiving Didronel. The drop was up to 65 percent greater compared with placebo, which had little effect on alkaline phosphatase levels. Bone tissue studies indicated that normal bone was produced during treatment with Fosamax, even where pre-existing bone had the abnormally disorganized pattern characteristic of Paget's disease.

Fosamax and Didronel usually are taken for no longer than six months at a time. If symptoms worsen or laboratory tests indicate a worsening of the disease, the drugs may be restarted after at least a six-month break from the medications.

Additional Therapies

According to the Paget Foundation, several more bisphosphonate drugs are undergoing clinical tests. These drugs may offer greater ease of use, says Charlene Waldman, executive director of the Paget Foundation.

Because new bone formation occurs as part of the process of repair in pagetic bone, it is important that along with calcitonin and the bisphosphonates to inhibit abnormal bone breakdown, patients eat a diet that provides 1,000 to 1,500 milligrams of calcium and 400 International Units of vitamin D daily. These nutrients are needed for proper bone formation.

Calcium can be obtained by eating a well-balanced diet that includes foods that are good sources of calcium—for example, milk and milk products, dark-green leafy vegetables (such as mustard greens and kale), and canned fish with soft bones (such as sardines and salmon). Dietary supplements of calcium may be another source.

Some Paget's patients, especially those with severe bowing of legs, fractures, and degenerative arthritis, may need splints, braces, and other devices such as canes and walkers. Patients also may receive physical therapy.

Although uncommon, surgery may be required, especially in cases of fractured bones, severe arthritis, and progressive deformity of leg bones.

Exercise is important for patients with Paget's disease, just as it is for everyone. Because patients with Paget's disease are prone to bone fractures, they should consult their doctors or physical therapists before starting an exercise program.

Various laboratory tests monitor the progression of Paget's disease. The most common is the total alkaline phosphatase. FDA has cleared

two tests—Hybritech Ostase in 1994 and Metra Alkphase-B in 1995—
that measure only the alkaline phosphatase from bone, since the enzyme in the blood can come from other organs, too.

A possible future test, which is still under research, would measure osteocalcin, a byproduct of osteoblasts, to determine bone turnover rates.

Deciding When to Treat

For many years, doctors generally treated patients with Paget's
disease only if they had symptoms. In recent years, with the availability of a wider range of drugs, doctors have begun treating patients
without symptoms, as well, hoping that the drugs may prevent the
effects of Paget's disease. Factors to consider in deciding whether to
treat patients without symptoms, according to Siris, are the location
of the disease and the likelihood of its progression. Diseased bone near
joints, in the spine or skull, or in the leg bones are particularly "bad
spots," she says, and may indicate the need for drug therapy.

Patients who are told they have Paget's disease may want to seek
a medical specialist in that condition. The Paget Foundation recommends endocrinologists (doctors who specialize in hormonal and metabolic disorders) or rheumatologists (doctors who specialize in joint and
muscle disorders). Orthopedic doctors (who specialize in bone problems), neurologists (doctors who specialize in nerve disorders), and
otolaryngologists (eye, ear, nose, and throat specialists) also may be
called on to evaluate specific symptoms.

Siris and Michael McClung, M.D., an endocrinologist and director
of the Oregon Osteoporosis Center in the Oregon Health Sciences
University in Portland, say that too often doctors who aren't specialists in the disease fail to follow up on laboratory tests or X-rays that
indicate Paget's disease. "They might tell patients: 'Forget about it.
You'll just end up in a wheelchair,'" Siris says. She believes that many
doctors aren't aware of current treatments because effective drugs for
Paget's disease weren't available when they were trained.

Since Paget's disease often runs in families, medical experts recommend that people with a family history of Paget's disease have their
serum alkaline phosphatase measured after age 40, since the disease
rarely shows up in people under 40. The laboratory test can be done
as part of the routine medical exam.

With prompt medical attention and treatment, when needed,
people with Paget's disease may be able to avoid some of the disease's
serious, often painful effects.

Maryland resident Brown hopes that will be true for her. "[The disease] is foremost in my mind," she says. "I wonder: 'Am I going to suffer any deformities from this?' I don't know. But I must be treated or so many things could happen."

—by Paula Kurtzweil

Paula Kurtzweil is a member of FDA's public affairs staff.

More Information

The Paget Foundation for Paget's Disease of Bone and Related Disorders

200 Varick St., Suite 1004
New York, NY
10014-4810
(1-800) 23-PAGET
E-mail:pagetfdn@aol.com
World Wide Web: http://www.housecall.com/

Osteoporosis and Related Bone Diseases National Resource Center

1150 17th St., N.W., Suite 500
Washington, D.C.
20036-4603
(1-800) 624-BONE
TTY for hearing-impaired callers: (202) 466-4315
E-mail: orbdnrc@nof.org
World Wide Web: http://www.osteo.org/

Research Developments: Paget's Disease of Bone

The Senate Appropriations Committee, in its report accompanying the Fiscal-Year 1992 Appropriations Bill, within the section on the National Institute of Arthritis and Musculoskeletal and Skin Diseases (NIAMS), stated:

The Committee is pleased that the NIAMS has taken the lead among the NIH institutes in targeting research on Paget's disease bone disorders. The Committee requests NIAMS to provide an NIH-wide report on its plans to address this particular disease entity. Senate Report 102-104, p. 131.

In response to this request, research activities of seven NIH Institutes and Centers (ICDs) dealing with Paget's disease of bone have been reviewed. The ICDs are:

- The National Institute of Arthritis and Musculoskeletal and Skin Diseases;

- The National Institute of Diabetes and Digestive and Kidney Diseases;

- The National Cancer Institute;

- The National Institute of Dental Research;

- The National Institute on Deafness and Other Communication Disorders;

- The National Institute on Aging; and

- The National Center for Research Resources.

These NIH components were asked to describe their research in the area of Paget's disease of bone and report on their Fiscal-Year 1990 projects. The third section of this report, following the Introduction and Background sections, discusses the research and related activities, such as conferences and workshops, that are supported by these NIH components. The fourth section discusses research opportunities for the future.

This report was prepared under the auspices of the Arthritis and Musculoskeletal Diseases Interagency Coordinating Committee (AMDICC), established by Congress in the Health Research Extension Act of 1985 as part of the language authorizing establishment of the NIAMS. The Coordinating Committee consists of representatives from NIH ICDs and other Federal agencies with complementary missions.

Background

Paget's disease of bone is a chronic disease of the skeleton affecting the process that maintains healthy bone structure. It is caused by an excessively rapid rate of local bone turnover that produces weak bone structure. It is as though oak were being replaced by balsa wood. Paget's disease of bone was first described in 1876 by the English surgeon Sir James Paget. Pagetic bone has been found in the skeleton of an Egyptian mummy and also in Saxon skeletons buried around 950 A.D.

It is estimated that 1 percent to 3 percent of Americans over the age of 45 are affected with the disease. Most diagnoses are made in persons between the ages of 50 and 70. People of Western European heritage are affected most often, especially those from Great Britain, France, and Germany. The disease tends to predominate in men.

The prevalence of Paget's disease of bone is difficult to determine because most individuals affected have either no symptoms or very vague symptoms. Disabling bone deformities do develop, however, in advanced stages of the disease. Pain in the joints is the most common reason for seeking medical help. Other complaints are sensation of heat over affected areas and headache when the skull is involved. Less common complications include bowing of a limb or uneven enlargement of a leg, upper or lower curving of the spine, enlargement of the skull, hearing loss, ringing in the ears, loss of balance when the skull is involved, and muscle and sensory disturbances.

Paget's disease may occur in more than one member of a family, and the evidence suggests that, in some cases, a predisposition to acquire Paget's disease of bone is genetically transmitted. In most cases, however, the disease appears to occur spontaneously.

It is not known what causes Paget's disease of bone, but some of the mechanisms that cause the bone deformities and symptoms are now understood. In Pagetic bone, the rate of bone turnover (resorption and formation of bone, known as remodeling) speeds up from its normal course when an unidentified factor stimulates excessive bone breakdown in localized areas. This increased breakdown triggers an increase in the rate of bone formation and repair, leading to new bone being laid down in a disorderly way at these sites. With time, affected bone may become thickened and weak. The involved areas can cause pain, become deformed, and occasionally fracture spontaneously. The use of blood tests can detect malfunctions in the body's chemistry. Bone scans and x-rays are also used to detect abnormalities.

Early diagnosis and treatment help slow progress of the disease and its sometimes irreversible complications. Treatment of Paget's disease focuses on relieving pain and attempting to prevent deformity, fractures, and loss of mobility. When symptoms are mild, aspirin or other anti-inflammatory or analgesic agents are sufficient to ease pain and inflammation. Some patients may develop Paget's arthritis, a form of osteoarthritis, in joints adjacent to affected areas. Severe and disabling pain may require additional treatment. Signs other than pain that suggest more vigorous therapy include:

- progressive skeletal involvement;

- greatly increased levels of serum alkaline phosphatase in the blood or urinary hydroxyproline;

- significant involvement of weight-bearing bone or bone adjacent to joints, such as the hip or knee;

- rapidly progressing deafness; and

- nerve compression by Pagetic bone or involvement of bone where patients are at risk for such compression.

Treatments used in Paget's disease include:

Calcitonin. A hormone produced by specialized cells in the thyroid gland that slows the rate of bone breakdown and thus of bone turnover. This drug is taken by injection, but alternative routes are being examined. A nasal spray form of calcitonin is now being developed.

Bisphosphonates. A group of drugs available in pill form that block bone breakdown. One example, etidronate disodium (Didronel), is taken in six month therapeutic cycles. Bisphosphonates appear to suppress disease activity for many months after remission. A number of new bisphosphonates may soon be available for treatment.

Plicamycin (Mithramycin) and gallium nitrate. Experimental agents that have not yet been approved in the United States for treatment of Paget's disease. Plicamycin is a toxic agent, but is being used successfully in research and may have potential, especially in combination with other agents in cases of particularly resistant disease. Gallium nitrate is also currently being investigated as a possible treatment option.

Surgery. Paget's patients who have nerve involvement, joint damage, fractures, tumors, or disability, may require surgical treatment as an adjunct to drug treatment. However, the need for surgery is rare.

NIH Research and Related Activities in Paget's Disease of Bone

The National Institute of Arthritis and Musculoskeletal and Skin Diseases

Bone is a dynamic tissue that continually undergoes the processes of formation and resorption. Since the sum of these processes dictate net skeletal mass and gross bone architecture, gaining major insights into these processes is necessary to understanding diseases of bone, including Paget's disease. In Paget's disease of bone, osteoclasts, which are multinucleated cells involved in the absorption and removal of bone tissue, become greatly enlarged and increase the rate and extent of bone resorption, which, in turn, stimulates increased bone formation by osteoblasts. This quickened pace for clearing out old bone and reforming new bone creates a structure that is less compact bone and has a greater number of blood vessels, making it prone to deformity and fracture.

In December 1988, NIAMS issued a program announcement entitled "Research in Paget's Disease of Bone" to learn more about why the process goes awry. This program announcement still continues to stimulate applications. The three projects that follow were recently received in direct response to this announcement.

A team of investigators are investigating the role of a pivotal enzyme, carbonic anhydrase, in the activity of the osteoclast. This enzyme makes it possible for osteoclasts to break down bone. The absence of this enzyme leads to another serious bone disorder, osteopetrosis, in which bone breakdown is arrested. This research may provide new insights into therapeutic interventions in all bone diseases involving the function of the osteoclast.

Scientists are developing an animal model of the high bone turnover in Paget's disease, using transgenic mice expressing a gene from a virus. This study will investigate the mechanism by which viral genes can induce rapid bone turnover and will contribute to a basic understanding of the mechanism of activation of cytokine (cell growth factor) genes.

A research team is comparing the effects of two treatments for Paget's disease, calcitonin and pamidronate (a bisphosphonate). Using quantitative x-ray tomography, they will evaluate the effects of these two treatments on the bone healing process and on bone mineral redistribution. As part of this study, improved techniques for the measurement of bone density in small volumes of bone will be developed. This should have a clinical impact on the study of a variety of bone disorders.

Other research that NIAMS is currently supporting on Paget's disease of bone follows. The principal investigator on a NIAMS-supported project hopes to elucidate the functional implications of fusion in normal and pathological bone resorption and the body's defense mechanisms involved in inflammatory reactions and tumors. To accomplish this, the team is investigating the mechanisms and regulation of the cell fusion that produces osteoclasts.

Another team of NIAMS-supported researchers is also examining the activities of osteoclasts. Recent improvements in isolating and maintaining osteoclasts in culture are being used to document that these cells have the capacity to degrade bone collagen.

Other investigators are studying the factors involved in the differentiation or activation of osteoclasts. Cytokines that stimulate bone resorption and those that inhibit bone resorption are being studied. Analysis of the factors that are produced in the bone micro-environment are necessary to gain an understanding of how bone volume and normal bone remodeling are controlled.

Another project is investigating the hypothesis that Paget's disease of bone may be caused by a virus. There is some evidence to suggest that some viruses are involved in the etiology of Paget's disease. If it is confirmed that Paget's disease is caused by a viral infection, treatment regimens may be developed that utilize either systemic or local administration of antiviral agents. Vaccines might also be developed. If a virus can cause Paget's disease, such knowledge may also be important to understanding other chronic musculoskeletal diseases.

Projects funded by NIAMS that are focused on answering questions about bone cell function should contribute to better understanding the pathogenesis of Paget's disease. Areas being investigated include:

- the factors regulating cellular function;
- the origin, biology, maturation, and regulation of the osteoclast;
- molecular biology of bone growth, remodeling, and repair;
- the role of osteocalcin in resorption of bone;
- bone cell collagen production;
- mechanisms of regulation of growth factor (TGF beta) activity;
- the regulation of bone resorption; and
- the activation of cytokine genes.

A NIAMS-supported research team developed imaging and densitometry techniques precise enough to examine changes in small lesions. This methodology is being used along with biochemical measurements of metabolic activity to study Pagetic bone and its response to calcitonins and bisphosphonates, as they relate to osteoclast and osteoblast function. This study will determine whether the type of treatment affects the rate or pattern of healing and analyze the relationship between changes in bone density and certain biochemical markers of disease activity.

A study is also being funded that is examining collagen turnover in selected metabolic diseases and genetic disorders of connective tissue.

Through assays of blood and urine, rates of collagen synthesis and degradation will be measured. This study utilizes measurements of certain compounds of bone breakdown in urine to provide further information about resorption of skeletal matrix (intercellular substance of bone tissue).

A NIAMS-supported study about to begin will provide an analysis of how gallium nitrate modulates the molecular events necessary for bone formation. Gallium nitrate is a drug that inhibits osteoclastic bone resorption. It is approved by the Food and Drug Administration for the treatment of malignant hypercalcemia, but there are preliminary reports of its effectiveness in Paget's disease.

The Institute co-sponsored with the Paget's Disease Foundation the First Paget's Disease Foundation Working Group Meeting in New York City in May 1991. This meeting provided a forum for discussion of what is not currently known about Paget's disease and suggested future directions for both basic and clinical research. The meeting offered an opportunity for exchange of ideas by leaders in the field. Other cosponsors were the National Institute on Aging and the National Institute for Dental Research. The Institute has also prepared materials for health professionals and patients that are distributed through the National Arthritis and Musculoskeletal and Skin Diseases Information Clearinghouse. A brochure entitled "Understanding Paget's Disease" is available for patient use through both the Clearinghouse and the Paget's Disease Foundation. In addition, the Paget's Disease Annotated Bibliography, released by NIAMS in 1990, was added as an appendix to the recently published book, *Paget's Disease of Bone: Clinical Assessment Present and Future Therapy.*

National Institute of Diabetes and Digestive and Kidney Diseases

The National Institute of Diabetes and Digestive and Kidney Diseases (NIDDK) provides support for biomedical research on the causes, diagnosis, prevention, and treatment of bone disorders. Although no research is devoted directly to Paget's disease, NIDDK supports research in bone and mineral metabolism.

Endocrinology researchers are studying how hormones and growth factors interact with bone cells at the molecular and biochemical levels to regulate bone formation and loss. Regulation of urinary calcium excretion is also essential to maintaining appropriate calcium levels in the body and is thus a subject of study in nephrology research. In addition, regulation of calcium absorption from the diet is a crucial issue in endocrine and nutrition research.

Hormones are major factors in the regulation of bone formation and bone loss (also called bone resorption); the amount of bone present reflects the net difference between these two processes. NIDDK supports research on parathyroid hormone (PTH), the primary peptide hormone regulating blood calcium levels and the major systemic regulator of bone resorption. However, although PTH regulates bone resorption, it acts directly on bone-forming cells, and has the potential to enhance bone formation.

Recently, NIDDK grantees have identified a number of growth factors, or cytokines, that may play a role in regulating bone metabolism. These substances are produced by several types of cells, including bone cells, and there is mounting evidence that bone-active cytokines may act collectively to regulate the processes associated with bone metabolism. Ongoing research focuses on the development of model systems to study the physiological effects of cytokines at the cellular level. Ultimately, understanding the complex effects of hormones that stimulate both bone formation and resorption may lead to development of strategies to uncouple these processes and selectively stimulate bone formation in various bone diseases.

The Institute has contributed to the Paget's Disease Foundation Symposium on Disorders of Bone Resorption held in Chicago, Illinois, in November 1991.

National Cancer Institute

The National Cancer Institute (NCI) provides funding for research on cancer causes, prevention, diagnosis, treatment, and rehabilitation, and for the distribution of information. The Institute studies the means by which cancer may destroy bone. Osteogenic sarcoma, a form of bone cancer, is an extremely rare complication of Paget's disease that occurs in less than 1 percent of all patients. The following extramural research is being funded by NCI.

In a pilot study, investigators are testing whether gallium nitrate is effective in decreasing accelerated bone turnover in patients with advanced, treatment-resistant Paget's disease of bone, as this compound has been shown previously to decrease bone turnover in patients with cancer-related hypercalcemia and bone metastases. Biochemical parameters of disease activity (e.g., urinary hydroxyproline excretion and serum alkaline phosphatase activity) are being monitored to see if enzyme levels are reduced by administration of gallium nitrate. Short-term treatment with gallium nitrate appears to reduce biochemical parameters of disease activity. Long-term administration of an intermediate dose given on an intermittent schedule is currently being tested.

A project is studying the effects of gallium on bone metabolism. Researchers are testing the hypothesis that gallium blocks bone resorption and enhances bone formation by favorably altering the function of bone cells (osteoclasts and osteoblasts) as well as physicochemically altering mineral properties. Physical methods to localize traces of gallium in the bone matrix and biochemical methods to measure mineral formation and bone collagen and osteocalcin synthesis are being applied to a panel of synthetic (fabricated) and cell and organ culture *(in vitro)* systems, and *in vivo* models. Results of these efforts should provide a basis for the design of future clinical trials with gallium.

How tumor cells affect the skeleton and induce hypercalcemia, bone pain, and susceptibility to fracture is being studied. The aim is to characterize the tumor-associated factors responsible for causing hypercalcemia, determine the effects of these specific tumor-associated peptides on calcium homeostasis *in vivo* and, through *in vitro* and *in vivo* models, determine the relative importance of their specific effects on bone and renal function.

National Institute of Dental Research

The National Institute for Dental Research (NIDR) conducts and supports basic and clinical research on bones and teeth. The Institute has been a pioneer in studying the normal processes of development and turnover of the body's hard tissues and how these processes are deranged in a wide variety of disorders.

NIDR-supported scientists have been prominent in the discovery and analysis of the various collagens and non-collagenous proteins found in the extracellular matrices of bones and teeth. This research includes mapping and sequencing of associated genes, discovery of bone growth factors and other local and systemic factors important in bone growth and repair, and development of cell culture methods and animal models for bone disease. While this research may not be specifically targeted to Paget's disease, the projects focus on the cells (osteoclasts and osteoblasts), molecules, and processes involved in bone remodeling.

The Bone Research Branch of the NIDR Intramural Research Program has contributed to major advances in the genetics and molecular biology of bone. Each specific intramural research project is studying a variety of cells or molecules in both normal and abnormal conditions. Also, NIDR intramural investigators are maintaining Paget's disease cells in culture to determine if the metabolic activity of the cells is normal or has been altered by viral products. In addition, these scientists exchange a variety of reagents and antisera with Paget's disease investigators around the country in the hope of discovering biological markers indicative of Paget's disease activity.

The NIDR also contributed to the First Paget's Disease Foundation Working Group that met in New York City in May 1991.

National Institute on Deafness and Other Communication Disorders

Paget's disease can be divided into two histologic phases. The first primarily involves bone resorption and the second the formation of new bone. Since both phases frequently occur simultaneously in adjacent sections of a bone, the structure of the new bone is greatly distorted. As the disease encroaches upon the openings in bone through which nerves pass (neural foramina), neurologic symptoms such as deafness may result.

Otosclerosis is the formation of a spongy bone growth usually around the stapes (a stirrup-shaped bone in the middle ear that transmits sound waves to the inner ear). The web-like bone growth impedes the movement of the stapes, leading to gradual hearing loss.

Although the National Institute on Deafness and Other Communication Disorders (NIDCD) does not currently provide support for research directly related to Paget's disease, the following studies are indirectly related to the disease since they address otosclerosis.

Researchers are working with temporal bones acquired from human subjects who have a medical history and offer the best data of otological disease. These temporal bones are prepared for either light microscopy, electron microscopy, or histochemistry, and in some instances, more than one method is used on the same temporal bones. It is anticipated that through these studies, knowledge of the pathology and causes of otologic disease will be furthered and will lead to more effective methods of prevention and treatment.

Another project will focus on the histopathology of temporal bones. Congenital deafness, Meniere's disease, sudden deafness, and facial paralysis may result from one of many different pathological processes, and an understanding of anatomical pathology is an essential first step in determining the causes of such disorders.

A team of NIDCD investigators are directing their attention toward understanding the mechanisms controlling pathological bone remodeling in the middle ear, with the long range goal of preventing and reversing the hearing loss caused by these diseases. Specific aims include identifying the cellular and biochemical events leading to localized bone loss, and studying cochlear damage to hair cells, nerve cells, and nerve fibers in areas adjacent to localized bone loss and remodeling. In the long term, it may be determined whether factors produced in the remodeling process are toxic to the inner ear.

Another study focuses on temporal bone and central nervous system histopathologic changes in specific and general disorders due to overt or possible cochlear and/or vestibular abnormalities. This study furnishes the opportunity to correlate vestibular and auditory function with histopathologic changes of the temporal bone and membranous labyrinth. The project will lead to a better understanding of disorders of hearing and balance and possibly to more adequate clinical preventive and therapeutic measures.

National Institute on Aging

The National Institute on Aging (NIA) supports biomedical, clinical, behavioral, and social research and training on the aging process and diseases of older people. NIA is currently funding two research projects that pertain to Paget's disease.

In the first project, scientists are evaluating fundamental processes controlling physicochemical characteristics of bone mineralization and properties related to its elasticity. The study will attempt to show how physicochemical properties in human bone are affected by age and disorders like osteoporosis, renal osteodystrophy, osteomalacia, and Paget's disease.

The object of the second project is to develop and validate radioimmunoassays for measurement of "bone-specific" proteins in serum and urine. Normal values will be established in healthy individuals of both sexes from 20 to 90 years of age. These assays will be used to assess bone formation and resorption in age-related bone loss and metabolic bone disease, such as Paget's disease. In addition to these two research grants, the NIA provided funds to support the First Paget's Disease Foundation Working Group meeting in May 1991.

National Center for Research Resources

National Center for Research Resources (NCRR) programs are designed to strengthen and enhance the research environments of institutions conducting biomedical and behavioral research by developing and supporting essential resources, services, and training for the research community through a variety of extramural and intramural programs. Some Center-support research involving Paget's disease of the bone is discussed below.

The General Clinical Research Centers (GCRC) Program provides specialized facilities, equipment, and staff vital to clinical investigators and controlled clinical trials. Investigators at one of the GCRCs are studying the correlation of high blood levels of parathyroid hormone, a regulator of metabolic activity in bone, and calcium with the severity of Paget's disease. In a study of 39 patients, the seven most severely affected patients had higher levels of parathyroid hormone than the others. It is thought that the increased level of calcium with this hormone is causing even more serious malformations in the bone. At several other GCRCs, clinical trials are being performed to determine the efficacy and proper dosage for a variety of therapeutic agents including bisphosphonates and calcitonin.

The Biomedical Research Technology Program provides support to develop the latest experimental technologies for application to biomedical research problems. Researchers at the Magnetic Resonance Imaging Resource Center in Massachusetts are investigating the abnormal spatial distribution of minerals in bone as a result of Paget's disease in order to develop a non-invasive way to perform a chemical analysis and determine the distribution of calcium and phosphorous in a living organism. The present diagnostic method is an invasive biopsy that can only provide information on a small area.

The Biomedical Research Support Grant (BRSG) Program provides flexible funds to PHS-supported institutions to enhance their ongoing research endeavors and to initiate pilot projects. Three institutions are using BRSG funds to study tenascin (a glycoprotein that plays a role in the development of bone), type I collagen, and the etiology of Paget's disease.

The Shared Instrumentation Grant program supports the acquisition and updating of expensive, sophisticated instruments on a shared-use basis for NIH-supported investigators. Three of these instruments (two computers and a spectrometer) are being utilized to perform basic research on collagen peptides and the molecular basis of Paget's disease.

Research Opportunities for the Future

There were approximately 100 years between the time Paget's disease was first described and effective medical treatments became available. Much of the delay was caused by lack of knowledge about bone remodeling and the abnormality that produces this particular disorder. Through improved understanding of the pathophysiology of Paget's disease, therapies have become available and the basic and clinical research needed to provide treatment, effect a cure, or prevent the disorder is clearer. Advances in osteoclast/osteoblast biology include the development of cell culture models, the identification of receptors for hormones and growth factors, the discovery that osteoclasts are generated by a monocyte macrophage precursor, and the identification of growth factors and cytokines synthesized by bone cells. Future research needs to focus on the identification of new markers for bone formation and bone resorption and to define the details of gene regulation. There is need to delineate the origins of bone cells and determine what controls their differentiation and to identify the communication network that involves bone cells, bone matrix proteins, local factors, and hormones.

Now that there have been advances in the genetics of type I collagen, non-collagen proteins, the storage and release of growth factors by the matrix, and the description of the relationships between proteins and minerals, it is important to establish the role of specific matrix proteins, define cell matrix interactions and integrins, and understand how cells control matrix mineralization. In addition to more robust investigation of basic mechanisms, there needs to be further work in developing animal models.

Better methods are needed to determine optimal sites for predicting fracture in bone and improved technology is needed for assessing bone strength and identifying new specific markers of bone turnover. It is also important to focus research on the effect calcitonin has in reducing fracture. Clinical studies are needed to determine the optimal manner of using the new bisphosphonates and to determine whether or not the apparent long-term suppression of disease activity by this drug decreases the incidence of other complications, particularly fracture. The effectiveness of combination therapies utilizing more than one drug should be explored. There are also opportunities to examine therapeutic use of growth factors and bone morphogenetic proteins.

As research on Paget's disease of bone continues, an important companion activity is to increase public awareness of the disease and education for those who suffer from the disease and the health professionals who care for them. The publications that NIAMS has developed and made available through its clearinghouse, and its collaboration with other NIH Institutes and with the Paget's Disease Foundation enhance public awareness and encourage earlier diagnosis and treatment.

The research being carried out on bone metabolism, and the etiology, treatment and prevention of Paget's disease will contribute as well to a better understanding of many other bone diseases and disorders.

Chapter 25

Raynaud's Phenomenon

Questions and Answers about Raynaud's Phenomenon

What is Raynaud's phenomenon?

Raynaud's phenomenon is a disorder that affects the blood vessels in the fingers, toes, ears, and nose. This disorder is characterized by episodic attacks, called vasospastic attacks, that cause the blood vessels in the digits (fingers and toes) to constrict (narrow). Although estimates vary, recent surveys show that Raynaud's phenomenon may affect 5 to 10 percent of the general population in the United States. Women are more likely than men to have the disorder. Raynaud's phenomenon appears to be more common in people who live in colder climates. However, people with the disorder who live in milder climates may have more attacks during periods of colder weather.

What happens during an attack?

For most people, an attack is usually triggered by exposure to cold or emotional stress. In general, attacks affect the fingers or toes but may affect the nose, lips, or ear lobes.

Reduced Blood Supply to the Extremities: When a person is exposed to cold, the body's normal response is to slow the loss of heat

NIAMS web Document. 6/96, Office of Scientific and Health Communications. National Institute of Arthritis and Musculoskeletal and Skin Diseases. [http://www.nih.gov/niams/healthinfo/]

and preserve its core temperature. To maintain this temperature, the blood vessels that control blood flow to the skin surface move blood from arteries near the surface to veins deeper in the body. For people who have Raynaud's phenomenon, this normal body response is intensified by the sudden spasmodic contractions of the small blood vessels (arterioles) that supply blood to the fingers and toes. The arteries of the fingers and toes may also collapse. As a result, the blood supply to the extremities is greatly decreased, causing a reaction that includes skin discoloration and other changes.

Changes in Skin Color and Sensation: Once the attack begins, a person may experience three phases of skin color changes (white, blue, and red) in the fingers or toes. The order of the changes of color is not the same for all people, and not everyone has all three colors. Pallor (whiteness) may occur in response to spasm of the arterioles and the resulting collapse of the digital arteries. Cyanosis (blueness) may appear because the fingers or toes are not getting enough oxygen-rich blood. The fingers or toes may also feel cold and numb. Finally, as the arterioles dilate (relax) and blood returns to the digits, rubor (redness) may occur. As the attack ends, throbbing and tingling may occur in the fingers and toes. An attack can last from less than a minute to several hours.

How is Raynaud's phenomenon classified?

Doctors classify Raynaud's phenomenon as either the primary or the secondary form. In medical literature, "primary Raynaud's phenomenon" may also be called Raynaud's disease, idiopathic Raynaud's phenomenon, or primary Raynaud's syndrome. The terms idiopathic and primary both mean that the cause is unknown.

Primary Raynaud's Phenomenon: Most people who have Raynaud's phenomenon have the primary form (the milder version). A person who has primary Raynaud's phenomenon has no underlying disease or associated medical problems. More women than men are affected, and approximately 75 percent of all cases are diagnosed in women who are between 15 and 40 years old.

People who have only vasospastic attacks for several years, without involvement of other body systems or organs, rarely have or will develop a secondary disease (that is, a connective tissue disorder such as scleroderma) later. Several researchers who studied people who appeared to have primary Raynaud's phenomenon over long periods of time found that less than 9 percent of these people developed a secondary disease.

Secondary Raynaud's Phenomenon: Although secondary Raynaud's phenomenon is much less common than the primary form, it is often a more complex and serious disorder. Secondary means that patients have an underlying disease or condition that causes Raynaud's phenomenon. Connective tissue diseases are the most common cause of secondary Raynaud's phenomenon. Some of these diseases reduce blood flow to the digits by causing blood vessel walls to thicken and the vessels to constrict too easily. Raynaud's phenomenon is seen in approximately 85 to 95 percent of patients with scleroderma and mixed connective tissue disease, and it is present in about one-third of patients with systemic lupus erythematosus. For most people with lupus, Raynaud's phenomenon acts like the primary form of the disorder. Raynaud's phenomenon also can occur in patients who have other connective tissue diseases, including Sjögren's syndrome, dermatomyositis, and polymyositis.

Possible causes of secondary Raynaud's phenomenon, other than connective tissue diseases, are carpal tunnel syndrome and obstructive arterial disease (blood vessel disease). Some drugs, including beta-blockers (used to treat high blood pressure), ergotamine preparations (used for migraine headaches), certain agents used in cancer chemotherapy, and drugs that cause vasoconstriction such as some over-the-counter cold medications and narcotics are linked to Raynaud's phenomenon.

People in certain occupations may be more vulnerable to secondary Raynaud's phenomenon. Some workers in the plastics industry (who are exposed to vinyl chloride) develop a scleroderma-like illness, of which Raynaud's phenomenon can be a part. Workers who operate vibrating tools can develop a type of Raynaud's phenomenon called vibration-induced white finger. In addition, people whose fingers are subject to repeated stress, such as typing or playing the piano, are more vulnerable to the disorder.

People with secondary Raynaud's phenomenon often experience associated medical problems. The more serious problems are skin ulcers (sores) or gangrene (tissue death) in the fingers or toes. Painful ulcers and gangrene are fairly common and can be difficult to treat. In addition, a person may experience heartburn or difficulty in swallowing. These two problems are caused by weakness in the muscle of the esophagus (the tube that takes food and liquids from the mouth to the stomach) that can occur in people with connective tissue diseases.

How does a doctor diagnose Raynaud's phenomenon?

If a doctor suspects Raynaud's phenomenon, he or she will ask the patient for a detailed medical history. The doctor will then examine the patient to rule out other medical problems. The patient might have a vasospastic attack during the office visit, which makes it easier for the doctor to diagnose Raynaud's phenomenon. Most doctors find it fairly easy to diagnose Raynaud's phenomenon but more difficult to identify the form of the disorder. (See below for the criteria doctors use to diagnose primary or secondary Raynaud's phenomenon.)

Nailfold capillaroscopy (study of capillaries under a microscope) can help the doctor distinguish between primary and secondary Raynaud's phenomenon. During this test, the doctor puts a drop of oil on the patient's nailfolds, the skin at the base of the fingernail. The doctor then examines the nailfolds under a microscope to look for abnormalities of the tiny blood vessels called capillaries. If the capillaries are enlarged or deformed, the patient may have a connective tissue disease.

The doctor may also order two particular blood tests, an antinuclear antibody test (ANA) and an erythrocyte sedimentation rate (ESR). The ANA test determines whether the body is producing special proteins (antibodies) often found in people who have connective tissue diseases or other autoimmune disorders. The ESR test is a measure of inflammation in the body and tests how fast red blood cells settle out of unclotted blood. Inflammation in the body causes an elevated ESR.

Diagnostic Criteria for Raynaud's Phenomenon

Primary Raynaud's Phenomenon

- Periodic vasospastic attacks of pallor or cyanosis (some doctors include the additional criterion of the presence of these attacks for at least two years)

- Normal nailfold capillary pattern

- Negative antinuclear antibody test

- Normal erythrocyte sedimentation rate

- Absence of pitting scars or ulcers of the skin, or gangrene (tissue death) in the fingers or toes

Secondary Raynaud's Phenomenon

- Periodic vasospastic attacks of pallor and cyanosis
- Abnormal nailfold capillary pattern
- Positive antinuclear antibody test
- Abnormal erythrocyte sedimentation rate
- Presence of pitting scars or ulcers of the skin, or gangrene in the fingers or toes

What is the treatment for Raynaud's phenomenon?

The aims of treatment are to reduce the number and severity of attacks and to prevent tissue damage and loss in the fingers and toes. Most doctors are conservative in treating patients with primary and secondary Raynaud's phenomenon; that is, they recommend non-drug treatments and self-help measures first. Doctors may prescribe medications for some patients, usually those with secondary Raynaud's phenomenon. In addition, patients are treated for any underlying disease or condition that causes secondary Raynaud's phenomenon.

Non-drug Treatments and Self-help:

Several nondrug treatments and self-help measures can decrease the severity of Raynaud's attacks and promote overall well-being.

- **Take Action During an Attack:** An attack should not be ignored. Its length and severity can be lessened by a few simple actions. The first and most important action is to warm the hands or feet. In cold weather, people should go indoors. Running warm water over the fingers or toes or soaking them in a bowl of warm water will warm them. Taking time to relax will further help to end the attack. If a stressful situation triggers the attack, a person can help stop the attack by getting out of the stressful situation and relaxing. People who are trained in biofeedback can use this technique along with warming the hands or feet in water to help lessen the attack.

- **Keep Warm:** It is important not only to keep the extremities warm but also to avoid chilling any part of the body. In cold weather, people with Raynaud's phenomenon must pay particular attention to dressing. Several layers of loose clothing, socks, hats, and gloves or mittens are recommended. A hat is important because a great deal of body heat is lost through the scalp. Feet should be kept dry and warm. Some people find it helpful to wear mittens and socks to bed during winter. Chemical warmers, such as small heating pouches that can be placed in pockets, mittens, boots, or shoes, can give added protection during long periods outdoors. People who have secondary Raynaud's phenomenon should talk to their doctors before exercising outdoors in cold weather.

People with Raynaud's phenomenon should also be aware that air conditioning can trigger attacks. Turning down the air conditioning or wearing a sweater may help prevent attacks. Some people find it helpful to use insulated drinking glasses and to put on gloves before handling frozen or refrigerated foods.

- **Quit Smoking:** The nicotine in cigarettes causes the skin temperature to drop, which may lead to an attack.

- **Control Stress:** Because stress and emotional upsets may trigger an attack, particularly for people who have primary Raynaud's phenomenon, learning to recognize and avoid stressful situations may help control the number of attacks. Many people have found that relaxation or biofeedback training can help decrease the number and severity of attacks. Biofeedback training teaches people to bring the temperature of their fingers under voluntary control. Local hospitals and other community organizations, such as schools, often offer programs in stress management.

- **Exercise:** Many doctors encourage patients who have Raynaud's phenomenon, particularly the primary form, to exercise regularly. Most people find that exercise promotes overall well-being, increases energy level, helps control weight, and promotes restful sleep. Patients with Raynaud's phenomenon should talk to their doctors before starting an exercise program.

- **See a Doctor:** People with Raynaud's phenomenon should see their doctors if they are worried or frightened about attacks or if they have questions about caring for themselves. They should always see their doctors if attacks occur only on one side of the body (one hand or one foot) and any time an attack results in sores or ulcers on the fingers or toes.

Treatment with Medications

People with secondary Raynaud's phenomenon are more likely than those with the primary form to be treated with medications. Many doctors believe that the most effective and safest drugs are calcium-channel blockers, which relax smooth muscle and dilate the small blood vessels. These drugs decrease the frequency and severity of attacks in about two-thirds of patients who have primary and secondary Raynaud's phenomenon. These drugs also can help heal skin ulcers on the fingers or toes.

Other patients have found relief with drugs called alpha blockers that counteract the actions of norepinephrine, a hormone that constricts blood vessels. Some doctors prescribe a nonspecific vasodilator (drug that relaxes blood vessels), such as nitroglycerine paste, which is applied to the fingers, to help heal skin ulcers. Patients should keep in mind that the treatment for Raynaud's phenomenon is not always successful. Often, patients with the secondary form will not respond as well to treatment as those with the primary form of the disorder.

Patients may find that one drug works better than another. Some people may experience side effects that require stopping the medication. For other people, a drug may become less effective over time. Women of childbearing age should know that the medications used to treat Raynaud's phenomenon may affect the growing fetus. Therefore, women who are pregnant or are trying to become pregnant should avoid taking these medications if possible.

Self-Help Reminders

- Take action during an attack
- Keep warm
- Don't smoke
- Control stress
- Exercise regularly
- See a doctor if questions or concerns develop

What research is being conducted to help people who have Raynaud's phenomenon?

Researchers are studying the use of other drugs to treat Raynaud's phenomenon; for example, oral and intravenous prostaglandins, such as iloprost. Other investigators are studying the molecular mechanisms behind Raynaud's phenomenon and the anatomy of blood vessels.

Several medical centers in the United States are studying the use of biofeedback to control attacks. Researchers studying scleroderma and other connective tissue diseases are also investigating Raynaud's phenomenon in relation to these diseases.

Where can I get more information about Raynaud's phenomenon?

Arthritis Foundation
1314 Spring Street, N.W.
Atlanta, GA 30309
404/827-7100 or call your local chapter
800/283-7800

This is the main voluntary organization devoted to all forms of arthritis. The Foundation publishes a free pamphlet on Raynaud's phenomenon and also provides physician referrals.

The NIAMS gratefully acknowledges the assistance of Phillip J. Clements, M.D., of the University of California, Los Angeles, Jay D. Coffman, M.D., of the Boston University Medical Center, and Frederick M. Wigley, M.D., of The Johns Hopkins University School of Medicine in the preparation and review of this fact sheet used for this chapter.

Chapter 26

Scleroderma

What Is Scleroderma?

The word scleroderma means a "hard skin." Scleroderma is a chronic (long-lasting) disease that can affect your skin, joints, blood vessels and internal organs.

Scleroderma is a rare disease. It affects women three to five times more often than men. The disease usually starts between the ages of 30 and 50. It is sometimes seen in children and the elderly.

There are two forms of scleroderma: localized and generalized (also called systemic sclerosis).

Localized Scleroderma

Localized scleroderma mainly affects the skin. It also can affect muscles and bone, but it does not affect internal organs. This form usually is not as severe as generalized scleroderma. The two types of localized scleroderma are morphea and linear.

Morphea refers to the type of scleroderma in which hard, oval-shaped patches form on the skin. The patches usually are whitish with a purplish ring around them. They usually occur on the trunk, but can also occur on your face, arms, legs and other parts of your body. This type of scleroderma often improves by itself, over time.

Linear refers to the type of scleroderma in which a line of thickened skin forms in areas such as the arms, legs or forehead. It can occur in more than one area. The line can extend deep into the skin and affect the bones and muscles. This can affect the motion of joints and muscles as well as growth of the affected area.

Linear scleroderma usually occurs in childhood.

Generalized Scleroderma

Generalized scleroderma affects many parts of the body. It may affect your skin as well as blood vessels esophagus, stomach, bowel, heart, lungs, kidneys, muscles and joints. In rare cases, scleroderma may affect only some internal organs, leaving the skin and joints untouched.

There are two types of generalized scleroderma: limited (also called the CREST syndrome) and diffuse.

CREST stands for a combination of symptoms: calcinosis, Raynaud's phenomenon, esophageal dysfunction, sclerodactyly (sklare-oh-DACK-till-ee) and telangiectasia (tah-lan-jec-TAY-shah). (Each is defined later.) This type of scleroderma usually has a slow onset, with the first symptoms appearing 10 to 20 years before the full syndrome occurs. It usually affects the skin on the face, fingers and hands. Later it may affect internal organs, such as the esophagus, the lungs and bowels.

Diffuse scleroderma occurs throughout the body. It usually affects the skin on the arms, thighs, chest and abdomen in addition to the face, hands and thighs. Other body parts, such as your lungs, kidneys, heart, bowels, blood vessels and joints, also can be affected. This type also can cause problems such as high blood pressure, muscle weakness, trouble swallowing or shortness of breath.

Diffuse scleroderma may progress slowly in some people and more rapidly in others. However, it usually can be controlled.

What Causes Scleroderma?

The cause is unknown. It is known that in scleroderma the body produces too much of a protein called collagen. Excess collagen is deposited in the skin and in body organs. This causes thickening and hardening of the skin and affects the function of internal organs. Scientists think the body's immune system plays a part in causing these excess collagen deposits.

In addition, small blood vessels are damaged by scleroderma. There may be a connection between the build-up of excess collagen and blood vessel changes.

What Happens in Scleroderma?

Scleroderma affects everyone differently. It can be mild or severe. Following are examples of how it may affect the body.

Skin Changes

Skin changes can include hardening and thickening of your skin, especially on your hands, arms and face, ulcers on your fingers, loss of hair, and a change in skin color.

Swelling

Swelling, puffiness, or tightening of the skin of the hands and feet often happens in the morning. Skin may become shiny in appearance.

Sclerodactyly

Sclerodactyly means "hardness of the digits" (fingers and toes) and contractures of finger joints into bent positions.

Raynaud's Phenomenon

If you are affected by Raynaud's phenomenon you may notice that your fingers, toes and sometimes the tips of your ears, nose or tongue being very sensitive to cold.

Note If you smoke, stop! Smoking can trigger attacks of Raynaud's phenomenon.

Telangiectasia

Telangiectasia happens when tiny blood vessels near the surface of the skin become dilated and show through the skin. It involves small reddish spots appearing on your fingers, palms, face, lips and/or tongue.

The spots are not harmful and can be hidden with cosmetics.

Calcinosis

Calcinosis happens when small white calcium lumps form under the skin. This is due to scleroderma and is NOT caused by too much calcium in your diet. Calcinosis involves the formation of hard white lumps under the skin on your fingers or other areas of your body.

The lumps may break through the skin and leak a chalky white liquid. They can become infected when injured or drained.

Arthritis and Muscle Weakness

Arthritis and muscle weakness also may be symptoms of scleroderma. Arthritis occurs when joints become painful and swollen and when contractures occur.

Sjogren's Syndrome

Sjogren's (SHO-grens) syndrome is a condition leading to a decrease in secretions from the tear ducts, salivary glands and other areas of your body, such as the vagina. This happens if scleroderma affects the glands that produce these fluids.

Digestive Problems

Scleroderma can weaken your esophagus and bowels. It can also cause a build-up of scar tissue in your esophagus, which narrows the tube leading to difficulty swallowing, heartburn, nausea, weight loss, diarrhea or constipation.

Heart and Lung Problems

Scleroderma may cause the heart to slow down and, in some cases, can lead to heart failure or other problems. When the lungs are affected, they cannot function as well as in a healthy person.

Kidney Problems

Scleroderma can cause high blood pressure and kidney failure. If not treated, this can be a serious problem. You should be aware of the signs of kidney problems listed here. You may happen to notice sudden onset of:

- Severe headache;
- Shortness of breath;
- Visual disturbances;
- Chest pain;
- Mental confusion.

How Is Scleroderma Treated?

See Parts VI and VII for more detailed explanations of treatments and coping strategies.

Medication

Although there's not yet a cure for scleroderma, there are many drugs that help control it. They include aspirin in large doses, nonsteroidal anti-inflammatory drugs (NSAIDS), steroids, antacids, blood pressure medication, and drugs that increase blood flow to your fingers and toes.

Exercise

Regular exercise helps improve overall health and fitness. For people who have scleroderma, it also helps keep the skin and joints flexible, maintain better blood flow and prevent contractures.

Joint Protection

Joint protection means protecting swollen and painful joints from stresses and strains that can make them hurt more. Joint protection includes learning to perform daily activities in ways that will help your joints rather than strain them. Joint protection also may include resting individual joints in removable, lightweight splints to help control inflammation.

Skin Protection

The goal of skin protection is to keep a good supply of blood flowing to your skin and to protect your skin from injury. Dressing warmly will help do this. Keeping your body warm helps open the blood vessels in your arms, hands, legs and feet. Other ways to protect your skin include:

- Use a cold-water room humidifier to keep your skin moist.
- Avoid using strong detergents or other substances that irritate your skin.
- Try soap, creams and bath oils that are designed to prevent dry skin.
- Do not attempt to remove calcium deposits
- Enlist help from family and friends.

Chapter 27

Avascular Necrosis

What is avascular necrosis?

Avascular necrosis is a disease resulting from the temporary or permanent loss of the blood supply to the bones. Without blood, the bone tissue dies and causes the bone to collapse. If the process involves the bones near a joint, it often leads to collapse of the joint surface. This disease also is known as osteonecrosis, aseptic necrosis, and ischemic bone necrosis.

Although it can happen in any bone, avascular necrosis most commonly affects the ends (epiphysis) of long bones such as the femur, the bone extending from the knee joint to the hip joint. The disease may affect just one bone, more than one bone at the same time, or more than one bone at different times. Avascular necrosis usually affects people between 30 and 50 years of age; about 10,000 to 20,000 people develop avascular necrosis each year.

The amount of disability that results from avascular necrosis depends on what part of the bone is affected, how large an area is involved, and how effectively the bone rebuilds itself. The process of bone rebuilding takes place after an injury as well as during normal growth. Normally, bone continuously breaks down and rebuilds old bone is torn away and reabsorbed, and replaced with new bone. The process keeps the skeleton strong and helps it to maintain a balance of minerals.

National Institute of Arthritis and Musculoskeletal and Skin Diseases web document. [http:\ \www.nih.gov/niams/healthinfo/avnecqa.htm].

In the course of avascular necrosis, however, the healing process is usually ineffective and the bone tissues break down faster than the body can repair them. If left untreated, the disease progresses, the bone collapses, and the joint surface breaks down, leading to pain and arthritis.

What causes avascular necrosis?

Avascular necrosis has several causes. Loss of blood supply to the bone can be caused by an injury (trauma-related avascular necrosis) or by certain risk factors (non-traumatic avascular necrosis), such as some medications (steroids) or excessive alcohol use. Increased pressure within the bone also is associated with avascular necrosis. The pressure within the bone causes the blood vessels to narrow, making it hard for the vessels to deliver enough blood to the bone cells.

Injury

When a joint is injured, as in a fracture or dislocation, the blood vessels may be damaged. This can interfere with the blood circulation to the bone and lead to trauma-related avascular necrosis. Studies suggest that this type of avascular necrosis may develop in more than 20 percent of people who dislocate their hip joint.

Steroid Medications

Corticosteroids such as prednisone are commonly used to treat diseases in which there is inflammation, such as systemic lupus erythematosus, rheumatoid arthritis, and vasculitis. Studies suggest that long-term, systemic (oral or intravenous) corticosteroid use is associated with 35 percent of all cases of non-traumatic avascular necrosis. However, there is no known risk of avascular necrosis associated with the limited use of steroids. Patients should discuss concerns about steroid use with their doctor.

Doctors aren't sure exactly why the use of corticosteroids sometimes lead to avascular necrosis. They may interfere with the body's ability to break down fatty substances. These substances then build up in and clog the blood vessels, causing them to narrow. This reduces the amount of blood that gets to the bone. Some studies suggest that corticosteroid-related avascular necrosis is more severe and more likely to affect both hips (when occurring in the hip) than avascular necrosis resulting from other causes.

Alcohol Use

Excessive alcohol use and corticosteroid use are two of the most common causes of non- traumatic avascular necrosis. In people who drink an excessive amount of alcohol, fatty substances may block blood vessels causing a decreased blood supply to the bones that results in avascular necrosis.

Other Risk Factors

Other risk factors or conditions associated with non-traumatic avascular necrosis include Gaucher's disease, pancreatitis, radiation treatments and chemotherapy, decompression disease, and blood disorders such as sickle cell disease.

Who is likely to develop avascular necrosis?

Avascular necrosis strikes both men and women and affects people of all ages. It is most common among people in their thirties and forties. Depending on a person's risk factors and whether the underlying cause is trauma, it also can affect younger or older people.

What are the symptoms?

In the early stages of avascular necrosis, patients may not have any symptoms. As the disease progresses, however, most patients experience joint pain at first, only when putting weight on the affected joint, and then even when resting. Pain usually develops gradually and may be mild or severe. If avascular necrosis progresses and the bone and surrounding joint surface collapses, pain may develop or increase dramatically. Pain may be severe enough to limit the patient's range of motion in the affected joint. The period of time between the first symptoms and loss of joint function is different for each patient, ranging from several months to more than a year.

How is avascular necrosis diagnosed?

After performing a complete physical examination and asking about the patient's medical history (for example, what health problems the patient has had and for how long), the doctor may use one or more imaging techniques to diagnose avascular necrosis. As with many other diseases, early diagnosis increases the chances of treatment success.

It is likely that the doctor first will recommend a radiograph, commonly called an x-rays. X-rays can help identify many causes of joint pain, such as a fracture or arthritis. If the x-ray is normal, the patient may need to have more tests. Research studies have shown that magnetic resonance imaging, or MRI, is the most sensitive method for diagnosing avascular necrosis in the early stages. The tests described below may be used to determine the amount of bone affected and how far the disease has progressed.

X-rays

An x-ray is a common tool that the doctor may use to help diagnose the cause of joint pain. It is a simple way to produce pictures of bones. The x-rays of a person with early avascular necrosis is likely to be normal because x-rays are not sensitive enough to detect the bone changes in the early stages of the disease. X-rays can show bone damage in the later stages, and once the diagnosis is made, they are often used to monitor the course of the condition.

Magnetic Resonance Imaging (MRI)

MRI is quickly becoming a common method for diagnosing avascular necrosis. Unlike x-rays, bone scans, and CT (computed/computerized tomography) scans, MRI detects chemical changes in the bone marrow and can show avascular necrosis in its earliest stages. MRI provides the doctor with a picture of the area affected and the bone rebuilding process. In addition, MRI may show diseased areas that are not yet causing any symptoms.

Bone Scan

Also known as bone scintigraphy, bone scans are used most commonly in patients who have normal x-rays. A harmless radioactive dye is injected into the affected bone and a picture of the bone is taken with a special camera. The picture shows how the dye travels through the bone and where normal bone formation is occurring. A single bone scan finds all areas in the body that are affected, thus reducing the need to expose the patient to more radiation. Bone scans do not detect avascular necrosis at the earliest stages.

Computed / Computerized Tomography

A CT scan is an imaging technique that provides the doctor with a three-dimensional picture of the bone. It also shows slices of the bone, making the picture much clearer than x-rays and bone scans. Some doctors disagree about the usefulness of this test to diagnose avascular necrosis. Although a diagnosis usually can be made without a CT scan, the technique may be useful in determining the extent of bone damage.

Biopsy

A biopsy is a surgical procedure in which tissue from the affected bone is removed and studied. Although a biopsy is a conclusive way to diagnose avascular necrosis, it is rarely used because it requires surgery.

Functional Evaluation of Bone

Tests to measure the pressure inside a bone may be used when the doctor strongly suspects that a patient has avascular necrosis, despite normal results of x-rays, bone scans, and MRIs. These tests are very sensitive for detecting increased pressure within the bone, but they require surgery.

What treatments are available?

Appropriate treatment for avascular necrosis is necessary to keep joints from breaking down. If untreated, most patients will suffer severe pain and limitation in movement within two years.

Several treatments are available that can help prevent further bone and joint damage and reduce pain. To determine the most appropriate treatment, the doctor considers the following aspects of a patient's disease:

- The age of the patient.
- The stage of the disease—early or late.
- The location and amount of bone affected—a small or large area.
- The underlying cause of avascular necrosis—with an ongoing cause such as corticosteroid or alcohol use, treatment may not work unless use of the substance is stopped.

The goal in treating avascular necrosis is to improve the patient's use of the affected joint, stop further damage to the bone, and ensure bone and joint survival. To reach these goals, the doctor may use one or more of the following treatments:

- **Reduced Weight Bearing.** If avascular necrosis is diagnosed early, the doctor may begin treatment by having the patient remove weight from the affected joint. The doctor may recommend limiting activities or using crutches. In some cases, reduced weight bearing can slow the damage caused by avascular necrosis and permit natural healing. When combined with medication to reduce pain, reduced weight bearing can be an effective way to avoid or delay surgery for some patients. Most patients eventually will need surgery, however, to repair the joint permanently.

- **Core Decompression.** This surgical procedure removes the inner layer of bone, which reduces pressure within the bone, increases blood flow to the bone, and allows more blood vessels to form. Core decompression works best in people who are in the earliest stages of avascular necrosis, often before the collapse of the joint. This procedure sometimes can reduce pain and slow the progression of bone and joint destruction in these patients.

- **Osteotomy.** This surgical procedure reshapes the bone to reduce stress on the affected area. There is a lengthy recovery period, and the patient's activities are very limited for 3 to 12 months after an osteotomy. This procedure is most effective for patients with advanced avascular necrosis and those with a large area of affected bone.

- **Bone Graft.** A bone graft may be used to support a joint after core decompression. Bone grafting is surgery that transplants healthy bone from one part of the patient, such as the leg, to the diseased area. There is a lengthy recovery period after a bone graft, usually from 6 to 12 months. This procedure is complex and its effectiveness is not yet proven. Clinical studies are under way to determine its effectiveness.

- **Arthroplasty/Total Joint Replacement.** Total joint replacement is the treatment of choice in late-stage avascular necrosis and when the joint is destroyed. In this surgery, the diseased joint is replaced with artificial parts. It may be recommended for people who are not good candidates for other treatments, such as patients who do not do well with repeated attempts to preserve the joint. Various types of replacements are available, and people should discuss specific needs with their doctor.

In addition to the above treatments, doctors are exploring the use of medications, electrical stimulation, and combination therapies to increase the growth of new bone and blood vessels. These treatments have been used experimentally alone and in combination with other treatments, such as osteotomy and core decompression.

For most people with avascular necrosis, treatment is an ongoing process. Doctors may first recommend the least complex and invasive procedure, such as protecting the joint by limiting movement, and watch the effect on the patient's condition. Other treatments then may be used to prevent further bone destruction and reduce pain. It is important that patients carefully follow instructions about activity limitations and work closely with their doctors to ensure that appropriate treatments are used.

What research is being done to help people with avascular necrosis?

With proper treatment, most people with avascular necrosis can lead normal lives. But there is still a lot to learn about prevention, diagnosis, and treatment. For example, researchers are studying:

- New ways to diagnose avascular necrosis in its earliest stages, when non-surgical treatment is most likely to help.

- The various causes of avascular necrosis so that, someday, it may be possible to prevent the disease.

- Treatments and improvement of the treatments that are available. In the future, medication may be an effective treatment for avascular necrosis.

- Improvements to the various types of hip replacements, to prevent younger patients from needing more than one hip replacement during their life.

Where can people find more information about avascular necrosis?

Arthritis Foundation
1330 West Peachtree Street
Atlanta, GA 30309
404/872-7100
800/283-7800 or call your local chapter (listed in the telephone directory)
World Wide Web address: http://www.arthritis.org

The Hip Society
c/o Richard B. Welch, M.D.
One Shrader Street, Suite 650
San Francisco, CA 94117
415/221-0665
Fax: 415/221-4023

The Society maintains a list of physicians who are specialists in problems of the hip and provides physician referrals by geographic area.

Acknowledgments

The NIAMS gratefully acknowledges the assistance of Thomas D. Brown, Ph.D., of the University of Iowa; James Panagis, M.D., M.P.H., of the National Institutes of Health; and Harry E. Rubash, M.D., of the University of Pittsburgh Medical Center, in the preparation and review of the fact sheet that makes up this chapter.

Part Four

Arthritis-like Pains
in Specific Joints

Chapter 28

Back Pain

Back pain is one of the most common health problems in the United States, yet its cause is generally unidentified. It is estimated that 50 to 80 percent of adults have had back pain at some time and that 10 percent of all Americans have back pain in a given year. Back pain can occur at any age in both men and women. However, it may occur slightly more often in women beginning at middle age, probably due to osteoporosis.

Back pain is one of the leading causes of disability and time lost from work. Studies indicate that direct medical costs for lower back pain approach $24 billion each year, with indirect costs (work loss, compensation) reaching approximately $35 billion for a combined total of nearly $60 billion.

Back pain can be a symptom of arthritis or many other conditions. This chapter is for anyone who has back pain, regardless of the cause. For more detailed information see the Omnigraphics' volumes *Head Trauma Sourcebook*, *Back and Neck Disorders Sourcebook*, and *Pain Sourcebook*.

Is There Only One Kind of Back Pain?

Everyone's back pain is different. For some people, back pain involves mild pain (pain that is bothersome, aching, sore). For other people, back pain involves severe pain (pain that hurts all the time, even when resting).

Most doctors refer to back pain as acute (generally severe, but short-lived), subacute or chronic (long-lasting or occurring often). Acute back pain usually lasts from one to seven days. Pain may be mild or severe and occasionally may be caused by an accident or injury. About 80 percent of all back pain is acute. Subacute back pain usually lasts from seven days to seven weeks and usually is mild; occasionally it's severe. This pain generally is unrelated to other illnesses you may have. About 10 to 20 percent of all back pain is subacute. Chronic back pain usually lasts more than three months and may be mild or severe. It may be related to other illnesses you may have or may have no identifiable cause. About 5 to 10 percent of all back pain is chronic.

What Is the Structure of the Back?

Your back is held upright by muscles attached to the backbone. Doctors often refer to the backbone as the spine, spinal column or vertebral column. The backbone isn't one long bone, but actually 24 separate bones called vertebrae. These vertebrae are stacked one on top of another to form the backbone.

The points where two vertebrae or bones fit together are called joints. They enable the spine to move and turn in different directions.

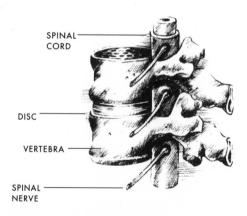

SPINAL CORD

DISC

VERTEBRA

SPINAL NERVE

Figure 28.1. Portion of the spinal cord

What keeps joints and bones from rubbing against each other and wearing out? Look at the diagram of the backbone (Figure 28.1) and find the discs located between each vertebra. These discs are made of cartilage, which is a soft, elastic material. Discs act as cushions, or shock absorbers. Their main job is to protect the joints from wearing out. Most joints contain a slippery substance called synovial fluid that keeps them moving smoothly.

The spinal cord is very important because it transmits electrical signals between the brain and the nerves in your legs, arms, back and other parts of your body. The spinal cord runs through a hole in each vertebra of the upper and middle parts of your backbone, much like a piece of string through a beaded necklace (see Figure 28.1). The space it runs through is called the spinal canal. At times, a message might signal pain or discomfort. The pain signal is an important one, because pain tells you that some part of your body needs attention.

What Causes Back Pain?

Anything that puts pressure on your back muscles or nerves can cause pain. Any illness or damage to your spine also can cause pain. The cause of most acute back pain is unknown, but probably is due to minor strains, sprains and overuse. Emotional stress may add to the pain, especially since it slows the rate of recovery. Other possible causes of back pain are included in the following sections.

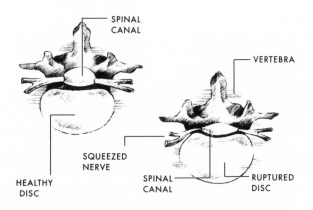

Figure 28.2. Healthy disc versus ruptured disc

Ruptured Intervertebral Disc. This may be the most painful, yet easiest condition to identify. A ruptured or herniated disc is one that bulges into the spinal canal, pressing on the nerve roots (see Figure 28.2). This causes the nerve roots to become irritated. A disc can rupture after you have done excessive bending over and lifting, or it may occur for no apparent reason.

A ruptured disc may cause back pain and muscle spasms, but a more common symptom is sciatic (SY-at-ick) pain. This is severe pain spreading down one leg and often into the foot. Sometimes it is the only symptom of a ruptured disc.

Spinal Stenosis. In spinal stenosis, the spinal canal becomes narrowed. This squeezes the back nerves and puts pressure on them. It is this pressure that causes the back pain. Numbness, pain and weakness in the legs also can occur. The most common symptom of spinal stenosis is pain that worsens when walking and subsides when sitting down.

Osteoarthritis. Osteoarthritis is just one form of arthritis that can cause back pain. It breaks down the cartilage that cushions the spinal joints and other joints in the body. Lower back pain can become more intense when osteoarthritis affects the hips or the knees. Osteoarthritis also can directly affect the spine, causing muscles, tendons or ligaments to become strained, which can lead to back and/or neck pain.

Ankylosing Spondylitis. This form of arthritis causes the joints in the spine to become stiff and swollen. In time, stiff joints can fuse (grow together). The most common symptoms are pain and stiffness in the buttocks and lower back (particularly in the morning) that continue for more than three months.

Injury or Accident. Have you ever moved a piece of furniture that didn't seem too heavy, only to feel pain in your back the next day? Have you ever stretched for something that was just a little out of your reach and felt a twinge in your back? Many back injuries are caused by an unexpected twist or sudden motion. This usually results in muscle strain.

With either an injury or accident, severe muscle spasms usually last 48 to 72 hours, followed by days or weeks of less severe pain. It usually takes two to four weeks to heal completely from a mild back injury. It could take from 6 to 12 weeks if there are strained ligaments or if the strain is more severe. Severe back injury from a fall or accident may require hospitalization and a longer recovery period.

Other Rheumatic Problems. Osteoarthritis and ankylosing spondylitis are only two of the more than 100 kinds of rheumatic diseases. Other rheumatic diseases, such as those in the following list, also can cause back pain.

Osteoporosis. This bone disorder causes bones to become thin and weak due to calcium loss. Fragile bones, especially those bones in the spinal column, can break more easily, and there is an increased tendency for this to happen in older women. Osteoporosis also contributes to compression fractures, or spinal fractures in which the vertebrae become flattened. Falls, lifting heavy objects or moving the wrong way can result in a compression fracture.

Rheumatoid Arthritis. This form of arthritis causes any joint to become stiff, painful and swollen. It can affect the neck but almost never the joints in the lower back.

Polymyalgia Rheumatica (PMR). This rheumatic disorder causes muscle pain, aching and stiffness in the neck and shoulders, lower back, thighs and hips. It can last a few months or many years. Most people with PMR experience severe stiffness in the morning.

Fibromyalgia. People with fibromyalgia feel pain and stiffness in muscles and tendons, especially in the neck and upper back. The pain can last for weeks, months or years. The symptoms may disappear by themselves. This condition often is related to sleep problems, poor conditioning or an old injury.

Paget's Disease. This is a disorder in which the calcium in the bone spreads unevenly. The bones most commonly affected are in the lower back, pelvis, tailbone, skull and long bones of the legs.

Back pain may be a symptom, but most often there are no obvious symptoms. Paget's disease usually is discovered on an X-ray or bone scan done for reasons other than pain.

Other Conditions

Sometimes pain felt in the back actually originates elsewhere in the body. Such problems may include:

- prostate trouble in men;
- problems with reproductive organs in women;
- kidney diseases, such as an infection or kidney stone;
- diseases of the intestines or pancreas, such as cancer or a blockage;
- cancer that has spread to the spine;
- multiple myeloma, a form of cancer of the bone and bone marrow;
- curvature of the spine; or
- rarely, a tumor on the spinal cord.

Factors That Can Make Back Pain Worse

Stress, poor posture, lack of exercise and being overweight all can contribute to back pain. In terms of stress, people react to it in different ways. Some may feel tired, sleep poorly, overeat or feel irritable. Some clench their jaw. Others tighten their neck and shoulders. Still others get a headache or an upset stomach when they are tense.

Many people tighten their back muscles when they are worried or tense. This can make existing back problems worse. Take a minute now to think about what happens in your own body when you worry or get tense. Do you think stress is affecting your back? If so, look in the stress management section of Omnigraphics' *Pain Sourcebook* for some helpful tips.

Think about the extra pounds people carry every day due to their being overweight. This puts added pressure and strain on the back and stomach muscles, causing them to stretch and weaken. Weak back and stomach muscles cannot support the back properly. Poor posture can shift your body out of balance. This forces only a few muscles and joints to do all the work. Without proper exercise, muscles become weak and tire easily. Exercise is necessary to keep the back strong and limber.

A good conditioning exercise program led by a trained instructor can be particularly helpful. An effective program includes a warmup period; about 30 minutes of aerobic activity (exercise that results in a sustained heart rate of 100 or more beats per minute); isolated muscle group work (including abdominal muscle toning); and a cooldown period. Over a period of time, the rewards of regular aerobic workouts can include a slimmer waistline and healthier back.

How Is a Diagnosis Made?

It often is difficult for doctors to find the exact cause of back pain, especially since there are so many possible causes. If the cause is unclear, your family doctor may suggest that you see a rheumatologist (doctor specializing in arthritis), orthopedist, neurosurgeon, neurologist, physiatrist or other medical specialist for diagnosis. If your back pain is accompanied by any of the following, see a doctor today:

- weakness or numbness in one or both legs,
- pain going down one leg below the knee;
- back pain from a fall or injury;
- back pain accompanied by fever without flu-like aches;
- pain that continues to interrupt sleep after three nights; or
- back pain that remains after six weeks of home treatment.

Medical History

Your doctor first will ask you a number of questions, the most common of which are:

- What are your symptoms—that is, what aches or pains do you have?
- Exactly where is the pain?
- Where is the pain the most severe?
- When did the pain begin?
- How long have you had it?
- Did something specific cause your back pain, such as an accident or injury?
- What home treatments have you used?
- Were you under any additional stress when the pain began?
- Do you have any other health problems,
- What kind of work do you do? In what types of recreational activities do you participate?

Physical Exam

Your doctor will perform a physical examination of muscles and joints, and attempt to identify the location of specific pains and in what body positions they occur.

Special Tests

If the doctor needs more specific information, he or she may ask you to undergo one or more of the following tests:

- **X-ray.** X-rays can confirm injuries to back bones, tumors, deformity in the spine, or ankolysing spondylitis.

- **CT Scan (computer axial tomography).** A computer interprets an x-ray scan into a three-dimensional view of the back to reveal conditions not apparent on regular x-rays like spinal stenosis, tumors, and infections of the spinal cord.

- **MRI (magnetic resonance imaging).** MRI is another way to make very clear pictures of parts of the spine. The MRI does not use X-rays or radioactive dyes. It can provide clearer pictures of soft tissues such as muscles, cartilage, ligaments, tendons and blood vessels, in addition to bone structure.

- **Myelogram.** During a myelogram, a special liquid dye called contrast medium is injected into the spinal canal. X-rays are then taken of the area. The contrast medium can make problem areas show up more clearly on the X-ray.

  A doctor may order a myelogram to detect problems such as spinal stenosis or spinal cord tumors. If surgery is being considered, particularly for a person who has had a serious back injury, many neurosurgeons will require a myelogram beforehand.

- **Bone Scan.** During a bone scan, a very small amount of radioactive liquid is injected into a vein and concentrates in the bones for a short time. A special radioactive detecting machine then will scan the area of concern to produce a picture.

  Occasionally bone scans are done to look for damage or tumors in the bones themselves. However, back pain is rarely due to diseases of the bones.

- **Electrodiagnostic Studies.** Electrodiagnostic studies are used to help confirm the presence of nerve compression in the spine. An electrodiagnostic study consists of two tests. One is an electrical test, which is designed to study nerve conduction. In this test the nerve is given an electrical stimulation, and the speed of the impulse is measured. The other test is a needle test called an electromyogram, or EMG. The purpose of this test is to study the muscles for primary disease or for the effect of nerve compression on the muscle. The compression is especially seen in herniated discs or spinal stenosis.

- **Blood Tests.** If your doctor orders blood tests for you, a laboratory technician will carefully draw a small amount of blood from a vein in your arm, which then will be tested in the laboratory. Any one of the following blood tests may be ordered:

—erythrocyte sedimentation rate (sed rate);
—hematocrit and hemoglobin;
—white blood cell count;
—HLA B-27 test; or
—chemical profile (SMAC).

Your doctor may order other blood tests. Ask for an explanation of the tests before you have them.

Treatment for Back Pain

More than 85 percent of people with lower back pain improve with minimal treatment in a matter of days. However, if back problems persist, doctors generally prescribe one or more of the following treatments: proper exercise, rest, heat and cold, posture training, weight loss, stress management and relaxation exercises, medication, spinal manipulation and/or surgery. For some back conditions, the doctor may refer you to another specialist such as an orthopedist, rheumatologist, physiatrist, physical or occupational therapist, psychologist, psychiatrist or surgeon.

For more detailed information, see the Omnigraphics' Health Reference Series Sourcebooks, *Back and Neck Disorders Sourcebook*, and *Pain Sourcebook*.

Chapter 29

Knee Problems

This chapter contains general information about knee problems. It includes descriptions of the different parts of the knee, including bones, cartilage, muscles, ligaments, and tendons. Individual sections of the chapter describe the symptoms, diagnosis, and treatment of specific types of knee injuries and conditions. Information is also provided on the prevention of knee problems.

How common are knee problems? What causes them?

According to the American Academy of Orthopaedic Surgeons, more than 4.1 million people seek medical care each year for a knee problem.

Some knee problems result from wear of parts of the knee, such as occurs in osteoarthritis. Other problems result from injury, such as a blow to the knee or sudden movements that strain the knee beyond its normal range of movement.

How can people prevent knee problems?

Some knee problems, such as those resulting from an accident, cannot be foreseen or prevented. However, a person can prevent many knee problems by following these suggestions:

NIH Web Publication 09/97. National Institute of Arthritis and Musculoskeletal and Skin Diseases, Office of Scientific and Health Communications. [http://www.nih.gov/niams/healthinfo/kneeprobs/kneeqa.htm]

- First warm up by walking or riding a stationary bicycle, then do stretches before exercising or participating in sports. Stretching the muscles in the front of the thigh (quadriceps) and back of the thigh (hamstrings) reduces tension on the tendons and relieves pressure on the knee during activity.

- Strengthen the leg muscles by doing specific exercises (for example, by walking up stairs or hills, or by riding a stationary bicycle). A supervised workout with weights is another pathway to strengthening leg muscles that benefit the knee.

- Avoid sudden changes in the intensity of exercise. Increase the force or duration of activity gradually.

- Wear shoes that both fit properly and are in good condition to help maintain balance and leg alignment when walking or running. Knee problems may be caused by flat feet or overpronated feet (feet that roll inward). People can often reduce some these problems by wearing special shoe inserts (orthotics). Maintain appropriate weight to reduce stress on the knee. Obesity increases the risk of degenerative (wearing) conditions such as osteoarthritis of the knee.

What kinds of doctors treat knee problems?

Extensive injuries and diseases of the knees are usually treated by an orthopaedic surgeon, a doctor who has been trained in the nonsurgical and surgical treatment of bones, joints, and soft tissues (for example, ligaments, tendons, and muscles). Patients seeking nonsurgical treatment of arthritis of the knee may also consult a rheumatologist (a doctor specializing in the diagnosis and treatment of arthritis and related disorders).

What are the major structures of the knee? What do they do?

The knee joint works like a hinge to bend and straighten the lower leg. It permits a person to sit, stand, and pivot. The knee is composed of the following parts:

Structures of the Knee

Bones and Cartilage

The knee joint is the junction of three bones—the femur (thigh bone or upper leg bone), the tibia (shin bone or larger bone of the lower leg), and the patella (kneecap). The patella is about 2 to 3 inches wide and 3 to 4 inches long. It sits over the other bones at the front of the knee joint and slides when the leg moves. It protects the knee and gives leverage to muscles.

The ends of the three bones in the knee joint are covered with articular cartilage, a tough, elastic material that helps absorb shock and allows the knee joint to move smoothly. Separating the bones of the knee are pads of connective tissue called menisci, which are divided into two crescent-shaped discs positioned between the tibia and femur on the outer and inner sides of each knee. The two menisci in each knee act as shock absorbers, cushioning the lower part of the leg from the weight of the rest of the body, as well as enhancing stability.

Muscles

There are two groups of muscles at the knee. The quadriceps muscle comprises four muscles on the front of the thigh that work to straighten the leg from a bent position. The hamstring muscles, which bend the leg at the knee, run along the back of the thigh from the hip to just below the knee.

Ligaments

Ligaments are strong, elastic bands of tissue that connect bone to bone. They provide strength and stability to the joint. Four ligaments connect the femur and tibia:

- The medial collateral ligament (MCL) provides stability to the inner (medial) aspect of the knee.

- The lateral collateral ligament (LCL) provides stability to the outer (lateral) aspect of the knee.

- The anterior cruciate ligament (ACL), in the center of the knee, limits rotation and the forward movement of the tibia.

- The posterior cruciate ligament (PCL), also in the center of the knee, limits backward movement of the tibia.

Other ligaments are part of the knee capsule, which is a protective, fiber-like structure that wraps around the knee joint. Inside the capsule, the joint is lined with a thin, soft tissue, called synovium.

Tendons

Tendons are tough cords of tissue that connect muscle to bone. In the knee, the quadriceps tendon connects the quadriceps muscle to the patella and provides power to extend the leg. The patellar tendon connects the patella to the tibia. Technically, it is a ligament, but it is commonly called a tendon.

How are knee problems diagnosed?

Doctors use several methods to diagnose knee problems:

- **Medical history**—the patient tells the doctor details about symptoms and about any injury, condition, or general health problem that might be causing the pain.

- **Physical examination**—the doctor bends, straightens, rotates (turns), or presses on the knee to feel for injury and discover the limits of movement and location of pain.

- **Diagnostic tests**—the doctor uses one or more tests to determine the nature of a knee problem.

- **X-ray (radiography)**—an x-ray beam is passed through the knee to produce a two-dimensional picture of the bones.

- **Computerized axial tomography (CAT) scan**—x-rays lasting a fraction of a second are passed through the knee at different angles, detected by a scanner, and analyzed by a computer. This produces a series of clear cross-sectional images ("slices") of the knee tissues on a computer screen. CAT scan images show soft tissues more clearly than normal x-rays. Individual images can be combined by computer to give a three-dimensional view of the knee.

- **Bone scan (radionuclide scanning)**—a very small amount of radioactive material is injected into the patient's bloodstream and detected by a scanner. This test detects blood flow to the bone and cell activity within the bone, and can show abnormalities in these processes that may aid diagnosis.

- **Magnetic resonance imaging (MRI)**—energy from a powerful magnet (rather than x-rays) stimulates tissues of the knee to produce signals that are detected by a scanner and analyzed by computer. This creates a series of cross-sectional images of a specific part of the knee. An MRI is particularly sensitive for detecting damage or disease of soft tissues, such as ligaments and muscles. As with a CAT scan, a computer can be used to produce three-dimensional views of the knee during MRI.

- **Arthroscopy**—the doctor manipulates a small, lighted optic tube (arthroscope) that has been inserted into the joint through a small incision in the knee. Images of the inside of the knee joint are projected onto a television screen.

Knee Injuries and Problems

Cartilage Injuries and Disorders

Chondromalacia

What is chondromalacia?

Chondromalacia (pronounced KON-DRO-MAH-LAY-SHE-AH), also called chondromalacia patellae, refers to softening of the articular cartilage of the kneecap. The disorder occurs most often in young adults and may be caused by trauma, overuse, parts out of alignment, or muscle weakness. Instead of gliding smoothly across the lower end of the thigh bone, the kneecap rubs against it, thereby roughening the cartilage underneath the kneecap. The damage may range from a slight abnormality of the surface of the cartilage to a surface that has been worn away completely to the bone. Traumatic chondromalacia occurs when a blow to the knee cap tears off either a small piece of articular cartilage or a large fragment containing a piece of bone (osteochondral fracture).

What are the symptoms of chondromalacia? How is it diagnosed?

The most frequent symptom of chondromalacia is a dull pain around or under the kneecap that worsens when walking down stairs or hills. A person may also feel pain when climbing stairs or during other activities when the knee bears weight as it is straightened. The disorder is common in runners and is also seen in skiers, cyclists, and soccer players. A patient's description of symptoms and a follow-up x-ray usually help the doctor make a diagnosis. Although arthroscopy can confirm the diagnosis of chondromalacia, it is not performed unless the condition requires extensive treatment.

How is chondromalacia treated?

Many doctors recommend that patients with chondromalacia perform low-impact exercises that strengthen muscles, particularly the inner part of the quadriceps, without injuring joints. Swimming, riding a stationary bicycle, and using a cross-country ski machine are acceptable as long as the knee is not bent more than 90 degrees. Electrical stimulation may also be used to strengthen the muscles. If these treatments fail to improve the condition, the physician may perform arthroscopic surgery to smooth the surface of the articular cartilage and "wash out" cartilage fragments that cause the joint to catch during bending and straightening. In more severe cases of chondromalacia, surgery may be necessary to correct the angle of the kneecap and relieve friction involving the cartilage or to reposition parts that are out of alignment.

Injuries to the Meniscus

What is the cause of injuries to the meniscus?

The two menisci are easily injured by the force of rotating the knee while bearing weight. A partial or total tear of a meniscus may occur when a person quickly twists or rotates the upper leg while the foot stays still (for example, when dribbling a basketball around an opponent or turning to hit a tennis ball). If the tear is tiny, the meniscus stays connected to the front and back of the knee; if the tear is large, the meniscus may be left hanging by a thread of cartilage. The seriousness of a tear depends on its location and extent.

What are the symptoms of injury?

Generally, when people injure a meniscus, they feel some pain, particularly when the knee is straightened. The pain may be mild, and the person may continue activity. Severe pain may occur if a fragment of the meniscus catches between the femur and tibia. Swelling may occur soon after injury if blood vessels are disrupted, or swelling may occur several hours later if the joint fills with fluid produced by the joint lining (synovium) as a result of inflammation. If the synovium is injured, it may become inflamed and produce fluid to protect itself. This causes swelling of the knee. Sometimes, an injury that occurred in the past but was not treated becomes painful months or years later, particularly if the knee is injured a second time. After any injury the knee may click, lock, or feel weak. Symptoms of meniscal injury may disappear on their own but frequently, symptoms persist or return and require treatment.

How is meniscal injury diagnosed?

In addition to listening to the patient's description of the onset of pain and swelling, the physician may perform a physical examination and take x-rays of the knee. The examination may include a test in which the doctor flexes (bends) the leg then rotates the leg outward and inward while extending it. Pain or an audible click suggests a meniscal tear. An MRI test may be recommended to confirm the diagnosis. Occasionally, the doctor may use arthroscopy to help diagnose and treat a meniscal tear.

How is an injured meniscus treated?

If the tear is minor and the pain and other symptoms go away, the doctor may recommend a muscle-strengthening program. Exercises for meniscal problems are best performed with initial guidance from a doctor and physical therapist or exercise therapist. The therapist will make sure that the patient does the exercises properly and without risk of new or repeat injury. The following exercises after injury to the meniscus are designed to build up the quadriceps and hamstring muscles and increase flexibility and strength:

- Warming up the joint by riding a stationary bicycle, then straightening and raising the leg (but avoiding straightening the leg too much).

- Extending the leg while sitting (a weight may be worn on the ankle for this exercise).

- Raising the leg while lying on the stomach.

- Exercising in a pool, including walking as fast as possible in chest-deep water, performing small flutter kicks while holding onto the side of the pool, and raising each leg to 90 degrees in chest-deep water while pressing the back against the side of the pool.

If the tear to a meniscus is more extensive, the doctor may perform either arthroscopic surgery or open surgery to see the extent of injury and to repair the tear. The doctor can suture (sew) the meniscus back in place if the patient is relatively young, the injury is in an area with a good blood supply, and the ligaments are intact. Most young athletes are able to return to vigorous sports with meniscus-preserving repair.

If the patient is elderly or the tear is in an area with a poor blood supply, the doctor may cut off a small portion of the meniscus to even the surface. In some cases, the doctor removes the entire meniscus. However, degenerative changes, such as osteoarthritis, are more likely to develop in the knee if the meniscus is removed. Medical researchers are currently investigating a procedure called an allograft, in which the surgeon replaces the meniscus with one from a cadaver. A grafted meniscus is fragile and may shrink and tear easily. Researchers have also attempted to replace a meniscus with an artificial one, but the procedure is even less successful than an allograft.

Recovery after surgery to repair a meniscus takes several weeks longer and post-operative activity is slightly more restricted than when the meniscus is removed. Nevertheless, putting weight on the joint actually fosters recovery. Regardless of the form of surgery, rehabilitation usually includes walking, bending the legs, and doing exercises that stretch and build up the leg muscles. The best results of treatment for meniscal injury are obtained in people who do not show articular cartilage changes and who have an intact anterior cruciate ligament.

Arthritis of the Knee

What is arthritis of the knee?

Arthritis of the knee is most often osteoarthritis, a degenerative disease where cartilage in the joint gradually wears away. In rheumatoid arthritis, which can also affect the knees, the joint becomes inflamed and cartilage may be destroyed. Arthritis not only affects joints, it may also affect supporting structures such as muscles, tendons, and ligaments.

Osteoarthritis may be caused by excess stress on the joint, such as from repeated injury, deformity, or if a person is overweight. It most often affects middle-aged and older people. A young person who develops osteoarthritis may have an inherited form of the disease or may have experienced continuous irritation from an unrepaired torn meniscus or other injury. Rheumatoid arthritis usually affects people at an earlier age than osteoarthritis.

What are the signs of knee arthritis and how is it diagnosed?

A person who has arthritis of the knee may experience pain, swelling, and a decrease in knee motion. A common symptom is morning stiffness that lessens after moving around. Sometimes the knee joint locks or clicks when the knee is bent and straightened, but these signs may also occur in other knee disorders. The doctor may confirm the diagnosis by performing a physical examination and taking x-rays, which typically show a loss of joint space. Blood tests may be helpful for diagnosing rheumatoid arthritis, but other tests may be needed as well. Analysis of fluid from the knee joint may be helpful in diagnosing some kinds of arthritis. The doctor may use arthroscopy to directly visualize damage to cartilage, tendons, and ligaments and to confirm a diagnosis, but arthroscopy is usually done only if a repair procedure is to be performed.

How is arthritis of the knee treated?

Most often osteoarthritis of the knee is treated with analgesics (pain-reducing medicines), such as aspirin or acetaminophen (Tylenol):* nonsteroidal anti-inflammatory drugs (NSAIDs), such as ibuprofen (Motrin, Nuprin, Advil); and exercises to restore joint movement and strengthen the knee. Losing excess weight can also help people with osteoarthritis. Rheumatoid arthritis of the knee may require a treatment plan that includes physical therapy and use of more powerful medications. In people with arthritis of the knee, a seriously damaged joint may need to be surgically replaced with an artificial one. (Note: A new procedure designed to stimulate the growth of cartilage using a patient's own cartilage cells is being used experimentally to repair cartilage injuries at the end of the femur at the knee. It is not a treatment for arthritis.)

Ligament Injuries

Anterior and Posterior Cruciate Ligament Injury

What are the causes of injury to the cruciate ligaments?

Injury to the cruciate ligaments of the knee is sometimes referred to as a "sprain." The anterior cruciate ligament is most often stretched, torn, or both by a sudden twisting motion (for example, when the feet are planted one way and the knees are turned another way). The posterior cruciate ligament is most often injured by a direct impact, such as in an automobile accident or football tackle.

What are the symptoms of cruciate ligament injury? How is injury diagnosed?

Injury to a cruciate ligament may not cause pain. Rather, the person may hear a popping sound, and the leg may buckle when he or she tries to stand on it. To diagnose an injury, the doctor may perform several tests to see if the parts of the knee stay in proper position when pressure is applied in different directions. A thorough examination is essential to the diagnosis. An MRI is very accurate in detecting a complete tear, but arthroscopy may be the only reliable means of detecting a partial tear.

How are cruciate ligament tears treated?

For an incomplete tear, the doctor may recommend that the patient begin an exercise program to strengthen surrounding muscles. The doctor may also prescribe a protective knee brace for the patient to wear during activity. For a completely torn anterior cruciate ligament in an active athlete and motivated patient, the doctor is likely to recommend surgery. The surgeon may reattach the torn ends of the ligament or reconstruct the torn ligament by using a piece (graft) of healthy ligament from the patient (autograft) or from a cadaver (allograft). Although repair using synthetic ligaments has been tried experimentally, the procedure has not yielded as good results as use of human tissue. One of the most important elements in a patient's successful recovery after cruciate ligament surgery is following an exercise and rehabilitation program for four to six months that may involve the use of special exercise equipment at a rehabilitation or sports center. Successful surgery and rehabilitation will allow the patient to return to a normal full lifestyle.

Medial and Lateral Collateral Ligament Injury

What is the most common cause of injury to the medial collateral ligament?

The medial collateral ligament is more easily injured than the lateral collateral ligament. It is most often caused by a blow to the outer side of the knee, which often happens in contact sports like football or hockey, that stretches and tears the ligament on the inner side of the knee.

What are the symptoms of collateral ligament injury? How is injury diagnosed?

When injury to the medial collateral ligament occurs, a person may feel a pop and the knee may buckle sideways. Pain and swelling are common. A thorough examination is essential to determine the nature and extent of injury. To diagnose a collateral ligament injury, the doctor exerts pressure on the side of the knee to determine the degree of pain and looseness of the joint. An MRI is helpful in diagnosing injuries to these ligaments.

How are collateral ligament injuries treated?

Most sprains of the collateral ligaments will heal if the patient follows a prescribed exercise program. In addition to exercise, the doctor may recommend that the patient apply ice packs to reduce pain and swelling and wear a small sleeve-type brace to protect and stabilize the knee. A sprain may take 2 to 4 weeks to heal. A severely sprained or torn collateral ligament may be accompanied by a torn anterior cruciate ligament, which usually requires surgical repair.

Tendon Injuries and Disorders

Tendinitis and Ruptured Tendons

What are the causes of tendinitis and ruptured tendons?

Knee tendon injuries range from tendinitis (inflammation of a tendon) to a ruptured (torn) tendon. If a person overuses a tendon during certain activities such as dancing, cycling, or running, the tendon stretches like a worn-out rubber band and becomes inflamed. Movements such as trying to break a fall may cause excessive contraction of the quadriceps muscles and tear the quadriceps tendon above the patella or the patellar tendon below the patella. This type of injury is most likely to happen in older people whose tendons tend to be weaker. Tendinitis of the patellar tendon is sometimes called jumper's knee. This is because in sports requiring jumping, such as basketball, the muscle contraction and force of hitting the ground after a jump strain the tendon. The tendon may become inflamed or tear after repeated stress.

What are the symptoms of tendon injuries? How are injuries diagnosed?

People with tendinitis often have tenderness at the point where the patellar tendon meets the bone. They also may feel pain during faster movements, such as running, hurried walking, or jumping. A complete rupture of the quadriceps or patellar tendon is not only painful but also makes it difficult for a person to bend, extend, or lift the leg against gravity. If there is not much swelling, the doctor will be able to feel a defect in the tendon near the tear during a physical examination. An x-ray will show that the patella is lower in position than normal in a quadriceps tendon tear and higher than normal in a patellar tendon tear. The doctor may use an MRI to confirm a partial or total tear.

How are knee tendon injuries treated?

Initially, the doctor may ask a patient with tendinitis to rest, elevate, and apply ice to the knee and to take medicines such as aspirin or ibuprofen to relieve pain and decrease inflammation and swelling. If the quadriceps or patellar tendon is completely ruptured, a surgeon will reattach the ends. After surgery, the patient will wear a cast for three to six weeks and use crutches. If the tear is only partial, the doctor might apply a cast without performing surgery.

A partial or complete tear of a tendon requires an exercise program as part of rehabilitation that is similar to but less vigorous than that prescribed for ligament injuries. The goals of exercise are to restore the ability to bend and straighten the knee and to strengthen the leg to prevent a repeat knee injury. A rehabilitation program may last six months, although the patient can return to many activities before then.

Osgood-Schlatter Disease

What are the causes of Osgood-Schlatter Disease?

Osgood-Schlatter disease is caused by repetitive stress or tension on a part of the growth area of the upper tibia (the apophysis). It is characterized by inflammation of the patellar tendon and surrounding soft tissues at the point where the tendon attaches to the tibia. The disease may also be associated with an avulsion injury, in which the tendon is stretched so much that it tears away from the tibia and takes a fragment of bone with it. The disease most commonly affects active young people, particularly boys between the ages of 10 and 15, who play games or sports that include frequent running and jumping.

What are the symptoms of Osgood-Schlatter disease? How is it diagnosed?

People with this disease experience pain just below the knee joint that usually worsens with activity and is relieved by rest. A bony bump that is particularly painful when pressed may appear on the upper edge of the tibia (below the knee cap). Usually, motion of the knee is not affected. Pain may last a few months and may recur until a child's growth is completed.

Osgood Schlatter disease is most often diagnosed by the symptoms. An x-ray may be normal, or show an avulsion injury, or, more typically, show that the apophysis is in fragments.

How is Osgood-Schlatter disease treated?

Usually, the disease disappears without treatment. Applying ice to the knee when pain first begins helps relieve inflammation and is sometimes used along with stretching and strengthening exercises. The doctor may advise the patient to limit participation in vigorous sports. Children who wish to continue participating in moderate or less stressful sports may need to wear knee pads for protection and apply ice to the knee after activity. If a great deal of pain is felt during sports activities, participation may be limited until any remaining discomfort is tolerable.

Iliotibial band syndrome

What causes iliotibial band syndrome?

This is an overuse inflammatory condition due to friction (rubbing) of a band of a tendon over the outer bone (lateral condyle) of the knee. Although iliotibial band syndrome may be caused by direct injury to the knee, it is most often caused by the stress of long-term overuse, such as sometimes occurs in sports training.

What are the symptoms of iliotibial band syndrome and how is it diagnosed?

A person with this syndrome feels an ache or burning sensation at the side of the knee during activity. Pain may be localized at the side of the knee or radiate up the side of the thigh. A person may also feel a snap when the knee is bent and then straightened. Swelling is usually absent and knee motion is normal. The diagnosis of this disorder is usually based on the patient's symptoms, such as pain at the lateral condyle, and exclusion of other conditions with similar symptoms.

How is iliotibial band syndrome treated?

Usually, iliotibial band syndrome disappears if the person reduces activity and performs stretching exercises followed by muscle-strengthening exercises. In rare cases when the syndrome doesn't disappear, surgery may be necessary to split the tendon so it is not stretched too tightly over the bone.

Other Knee Injuries

Osteochondritis Dissecans

What is Osteochondritis Dissecans?

Osteochondritis Dissecans results from a loss of the blood supply to an area of bone underneath a joint surface and usually involves the knee. The affected bone and its covering of cartilage gradually loosen and cause pain. A person with this disruption of the joint may eventually develop osteoarthritis. This disorder usually arises spontaneously in an active adolescent or a young adult. It may be due to a slight blockage of a small artery or to an unrecognized injury or tiny fracture that damages the overlying cartilage.

The bone undergoes avascular necrosis (degeneration from lack of a blood supply). The involvement of several joints or the appearance of Osteochondritis Dissecans in several family members may indicate that the disorder is inherited.

What are the symptoms of Osteochondritis Dissecans? How is it diagnosed?

If spontaneous healing doesn't occur, cartilage eventually separates from the diseased bone and a fragment breaks loose into the knee joint, causing locking of the joint, weakness, and sharp pain. An x-ray, MRI, or arthroscopy can determine the condition of the cartilage and be used to diagnose Osteochondritis Dissecans.

How is Osteochondritis Dissecans treated?

If cartilage fragments have not broken loose, a surgeon may fix them in place with pins or screws that are sunk into the cartilage to stimulate a new blood supply. If fragments are loose, the surgeon may scrape down the cavity to reach fresh bone and add a bone graft and fix the fragments in position. Fragments that cannot be mended are removed, and the cavity is drilled or scraped to stimulate new growth of cartilage. Research is currently being done to assess the use of cartilage cell transplants and other tissues to treat this disorder.

Plica Syndrome

Plica (pronounced PLI-KAH) syndrome occurs when plicae (bands of remnant synovial tissue) are irritated by overuse or injury. Synovial plicae are remnants of tissue pouches found in the early stages of fetal development. As the fetus develops, these pouches normally combine to form one large synovial cavity. If this process is incomplete, plicae remain as four folds or bands of synovial tissue within the knee. Injury, chronic overuse, or inflammatory conditions are associated with development of this syndrome.

What are the symptoms of plica syndrome? How is it diagnosed?

People with this syndrome are likely to experience pain and swelling, a clicking sensation, and locking and weakness of the knee. Because the symptoms are similar to symptoms of some other knee problems, plica syndrome is often misdiagnosed. Diagnosis usually depends on the exclusion of other conditions that cause similar symptoms.

How is plica syndrome treated?

The goal of treatment is to reduce inflammation of the synovium and thickening of the plicae. The doctor usually prescribes medicine such as ibuprofen to reduce inflammation. The patient is also advised to reduce activity, apply ice and compression wraps (elastic bandage) to the knee, and do strengthening exercises. If this treatment program fails to relieve symptoms within three months, the doctor may recommend arthroscopic or open surgery to remove the plicae. A cortisone injection into the region of the plica folds helps about half of the patients treated. The doctor can also use arthroscopy to confirm the diagnosis and treat the problem.

Other Sources of Information on Knee Problems

American Academy of Orthopaedic Surgeons
6300 N. River Road
Rosemont, IL 60018-4262
847/823-7186
800/346-2267
World Wide Web address: http://www.aaos.org

The academy publishes several brochures on the knee, including "Knee Arthroscopy" and "Total Knee Replacement," which doctors can obtain and give to their patients. Single copies of two other pamphlets, "Arthroscopy" and "Total Joint Replacement," are available free to the public if a self-addressed, stamped envelope is provided.

American Physical Therapy Association
1111 N. Fairfax Street
Alexandria, VA 22314
800/999-APTA (2782)
World Wide Web address: http://www.apta.org

The association has published a free brochure titled "Taking Care of the Knees."

Arthritis Foundation
1330 Peach Tree Street
Atlanta, GA 30309
404/872-7100
800/283-7800 or call your local chapter (listed in the local telephone directory)
World Wide Web address: http://www.arthritis.org

The Foundation has several free brochures about coping with arthritis, taking nonsteroid and steroid medicines, and exercise. A free brochure on protecting your joints is titled "Using Your Joints Wisely." The foundation also provides doctor referrals.

American College of Rheumatology/Association of Rheumatology Health Professionals
60 Executive Park South, Suite 150
Atlanta, GA 30329
phone: 404/633-3777
Fax: 404/633-1870
World Wide Web address: http://www.rheumatology.org

This national professional organization can provide referrals to rheumatologists and allied health professionals, such as physical therapists. One-page fact sheets are available on various forms of arthritis. Lists of specialists by geographic area and fact sheets are also available on ACR's web site.

National Arthritis and Musculoskeletal and Skin Diseases Information Clearinghouse (NAMSIC)
National Institutes of Health
1 AMS Circle
Bethesda, MD 20892-3675
Phone: 301/495-4484
TTY: 301/ 565-2966
Automated faxback system: 301/881-2731
World Wide Web address: http://www.nih.gov/niams

The Clearinghouse has additional information about some of the knee problems described in this chapter, including osteoarthritis and avascular necrosis, as well as information about total knee replacement and arthritis and exercise. Single copies of fact sheets and information packages on these topics are available free upon request.

Brand names included in this chapter are provided as examples only, and their inclusion does not mean that these products are endorsed by the National Institutes of Health or any other Government agency or Omnigraphics. Also, if a particular brand name is not mentioned, this does not mean or imply that the product is unsatisfactory.

Acknowledgments

The NIAMS gratefully acknowledges the assistance of Frank A Pettrone, M.D., of Arlington/Vienna,Virginia; W. Norman Scott, M.D., of Beth Israel Medical Center in New York, New York; and James Panagis, M.D., M.P.H., and John H. Klippel, M.D., of the National Institutes of Health, in the preparation and review of the fact sheet that makes up this chapter.

The National Arthritis and Musculoskeletal and Skin Diseases Information Clearinghouse (NAMSIC) is a public service sponsored by the NIAMS that provides health information and information sources. The NIAMS, a part of the National Institutes of Health (NIH), leads the Federal medical research effort in arthritis and musculoskeletal and skin diseases. The NIAMS sponsors research and research training throughout the United States as well as on the NIH campus in Bethesda, MD, and disseminates health and research information.

Chapter 30

Shoulder Problems

This chapter first answers general questions about the shoulder and shoulder problems. It then answers questions about specific shoulder problems (dislocation, separation, tendinitis, bursitis, impingement syndrome, torn rotator cuff, frozen shoulder, and fracture) as well as diseases that can cause shoulder pain (arthritis, myofascial pain, reflex sympathetic dystrophy, and thoracic outlet syndrome).

How common are shoulder problems?

According to the American Academy of Orthopaedic Surgeons, about four million people in the U.S. seek medical care each year for shoulder sprain, strain, dislocation, or other problems. Each year, shoulder problems account for about 1.5 million visits to orthopaedic surgeons—doctors who treat disorders of the bones, muscles, and related structures.

What are the structures of the shoulder and how does the shoulder function?

The shoulder joint is composed of three bones: the clavicle (collarbone), the scapula (shoulder blade), and the humerus (upper arm bone). Two joints facilitate shoulder movement. The acromioclavicular (AC)

National Institute of Arthritis and Musculoskeletal and Skin Diseases, 8/97, Office of Scientific and Health Communications, Web document. [http://www.nih.gov/niams/healthinfo/shoulderprobs/shoulderqa.htm].

285

joint is located between the acromion (part of the scapula that forms the highest point of the shoulder) and the clavicle. The glenohumeral joint, commonly called the shoulder joint, is a ball-and-socket type joint that helps move the shoulder forward and backward and allows the arm to rotate in a circular fashion or hinge out and up away from the body. (The ball is the top, rounded portion of the upper arm bone or humerus; the "socket," or glenoid, is a dish-shaped part of the outer edge of the scapula into which the ball fits.) The capsule is a soft tissue envelope that encircles the glenohumeral joint. It is lined by a thin, smooth synovial membrane.

The bones of the shoulder are held in place by muscles, tendons, and ligaments. Tendons are tough cords of tissue that attach the shoulder muscles to bone and assist the muscles in moving the shoulder. Ligaments attach shoulder bones to each other, providing stability. For example, the front of the joint capsule is anchored by three glenohumeral ligaments.

Structures of the Shoulder

The rotator cuff is a structure composed of tendons that, with associated muscles, holds the ball at the top of the humerus in the glenoid socket and provides mobility and strength to the shoulder joint. Two filmy sac-like structures called bursae permit smooth gliding between bone, muscle, and tendon. They cushion and protect the rotator cuff from the bony arch of the acromion.

What are the origin and causes of shoulder problems?

The shoulder is the most movable joint in the body. However, it is an unstable joint because of the range of motion allowed. It is easily subject to injury because the ball of the upper arm is larger than the shoulder socket that holds it. To remain stable, the shoulder must be anchored by its muscles, tendons, and ligaments. Some shoulder problems arise from the disruption of these soft tissues as a result of injury or from overuse or underuse of the shoulder. Other problems arise from a degenerative process in which tissues break down and no longer function well.

Shoulder pain may be localized or may be referred to areas around the shoulder or down the arm. Disease within the body (such as gallbladder, liver, or heart disease, or disease of the cervical spine of the neck) also may generate pain that travels along nerves to the shoulder.

How are shoulder problems diagnosed?

Following are some of the ways doctors diagnose shoulder problems:

- Medical history (the patient tells the doctor about an injury or other condition that might be causing the pain).

- Physical examination to feel for injury and discover the limits of movement, location of pain, and extent of joint instability.

Tests to confirm the diagnosis of certain conditions. Some of these tests include:

- **x-ray**

- **arthrogram**—Diagnostic record that can be seen on an x-ray after injection of a contrast fluid into the shoulder joint to outline structures such as the rotator cuff. In disease or injury, this contrast fluid may either leak into an area where it does not belong, indicating a tear or opening, or be blocked from entering an area where there normally is an opening.

- **MRI (magnetic resonance imaging)**—A non-invasive procedure in which a machine produces a series of cross-sectional images of the shoulder.

Other diagnostic tests, such as injection of an anesthetic into and around the shoulder joint, are discussed in specific sections of this chapter.

What is a shoulder dislocation?

The shoulder joint is the most frequently dislocated major joint of the body. In a typical case of a dislocated shoulder, a strong force that pulls the shoulder outward (abduction) or extreme rotation of the joint pops the ball of the humerus out of the shoulder socket. Dislocation commonly occurs when there is a backward pull on the arm that either catches the muscles unprepared to resist or overwhelms the muscles. When a shoulder dislocates frequently, the condition is referred to as shoulder instability. A partial dislocation where the upper arm bone is partially in and partially out of the socket is called a subluxation.

What are the signs of a dislocation and how is it diagnosed?

The shoulder can dislocate either forward, backward, or downward. Not only does the arm appear out of position when the shoulder dislocates, the dislocation also produces pain. Muscle spasms may increase the intensity of pain. Swelling, numbness, weakness, and bruising are likely to develop. Problems seen with a dislocated shoulder are tearing of the ligaments or tendons reinforcing the joint capsule and, less commonly, nerve damage. Doctors usually diagnose a dislocation by a physical examination, and x-rays may be taken to confirm the diagnosis and to rule out a related fracture.

How is a dislocated shoulder treated?

Doctors treat a dislocation by putting the ball of the humerus back into the joint socket—a procedure called a reduction. The arm is then immobilized in a sling or a device called a shoulder immobilizer for several weeks. Usually the doctor recommends resting the shoulder and applying ice three or four times a day. After pain and swelling have been controlled, the patient enters a rehabilitation program that includes exercises to restore the range of motion of the shoulder and strengthen the muscles to prevent future dislocations. These exercises may progress from simple motion to the use of weights.

After treatment and recovery, a previously dislocated shoulder may remain more susceptible to re-injury, especially in young, active individuals. Ligaments may have been stretched or torn, and the shoulder may tend to dislocate again. A shoulder that dislocates severely or often, injuring surrounding tissues or nerves, usually requires surgical repair to tighten stretched ligaments or reattach torn ones.

Sometimes the doctor performs surgery through a tiny incision into which a small scope (arthroscope) is inserted to observe the inside of the joint. After this procedure, called arthroscopic surgery, the shoulder is generally immobilized for about six weeks and full recovery takes several months. Arthroscopic techniques involving the shoulder are relatively new and many surgeons prefer to repair a recurrent dislocating shoulder by the time-tested open surgery under direct vision. There are usually fewer repeat dislocations and improved movement following open surgery, but it may take a little longer to regain motion.

Separation

What is a shoulder separation?

A shoulder separation occurs where the collarbone (clavicle) meets the shoulder blade (scapula). When ligaments that hold the joint together are partially or completely torn, the outer end of the clavicle may slip out of place, preventing it from properly meeting the scapula. Most often the injury is caused by a blow to the shoulder or by falling on an outstretched hand.

What are the signs of a shoulder separation and how is it diagnosed?

Both shoulder pain or tenderness and, occasionally, a bump in the middle of the top of the shoulder (over the AC joint), are signs that a separation may have occurred. Sometimes the severity of a separation can be detected by taking x-rays while the patient holds a light weight that pulls on the muscles, making a separation more pronounced.

How is a shoulder separation treated?

A shoulder separation is usually treated conservatively by rest and wearing a sling. Soon after injury, an ice bag may be applied to relieve pain and swelling. After a period of rest, a therapist helps the patient perform exercises that put the shoulder through its range of motion. Most shoulder separations heal within two or three months without further intervention. However, if ligaments are severely torn, surgical repair may be required to hold the clavicle in place. A doctor may wait to see if conservative treatment works before deciding whether surgery is required.

Tendinitis, Bursitis, and Impingement Syndrome

What are tendinitis, bursitis, and impingement syndrome of the shoulder?

These conditions are closely related and may occur alone or in combination. If the rotator cuff and bursa are irritated, inflamed, and swollen, they may become squeezed between the head of the humerus and the acromion. Repeated motion involving the arms, or the aging process involving shoulder motion over many years, may also irritate and wear down the tendons, muscles, and surrounding structures.

Tendinitis is inflammation (redness, soreness, and swelling) of a tendon. In tendinitis of the shoulder, the rotator cuff and/or biceps tendon become inflamed, usually as a result of being pinched by surrounding structures. The injury may vary from mild inflammation to involvement of most of the rotator cuff. When the rotator cuff tendon becomes inflamed and thickened, it may get trapped under the acromion. Squeezing of the rotator cuff is called impingement syndrome.

Tendinitis and impingement syndrome are often accompanied by inflammation of the bursa sacs that protect the shoulder. An inflamed bursa is called bursitis. Inflammation caused by a disease such as rheumatoid arthritis may cause rotator cuff tendinitis and bursitis. Sports involving overuse of the shoulder and occupations requiring frequent overhead reaching are other potential causes of irritation to the rotator cuff or bursa and may lead to inflammation and impingement.

What are the signs of tendinitis and bursitis?

Signs of these conditions include the slow onset of discomfort and pain in the upper shoulder or upper third of the arm and/or difficulty sleeping on the shoulder. Tendinitis and bursitis also cause pain when the arm is lifted away from the body or overhead. If tendinitis involves the biceps tendon (the tendon located in front of the shoulder that helps bend the elbow and turn the forearm), pain will occur in the front or side of the shoulder and may travel down to the elbow and forearm. Pain may also occur when the arm is forcefully pushed upward overhead.

How are these conditions diagnosed?

Diagnosis of tendinitis and bursitis begins with a medical history and physical examination. X-rays do not show tendons or the bursae but may be helpful in ruling out bony abnormalities or arthritis. The doctor may remove and test fluid from the inflamed area to rule out infection. Impingement syndrome may be confirmed when injection of a small amount of anesthetic (lidocaine hydrochloride) into the space under the acromion relieves pain.

How are tendinitis, bursitis, and impingement syndrome treated?

The first step in treating these conditions is to reduce pain and inflammation with rest, ice, and anti-inflammatory medicines such as aspirin, naproxen (Naprosyn*), or ibuprofen (for example, Advil, Motrin, or Nuprin). In some cases the doctor or therapist will use ultrasound (gentle sound-wave vibrations) to warm deep tissues and improve blood flow. Gentle stretching and strengthening exercises are added gradually. These may be preceded or followed by use of an ice pack. If there is no improvement, the doctor may inject a corticosteroid medicine into the space under the acromion. While steroid injections are a common treatment, they must be used with caution because they may lead to tendon rupture. If there is still no improvement after 6 to 12 months, the doctor may perform either arthroscopic or open surgery to repair damage and relieve pressure on the tendons and bursae.

Torn Rotator Cuff

What is a torn rotator cuff?

One or more rotator cuff tendons may become inflamed from overuse, aging, a fall on an outstretched hand, or a collision. Sports requiring repeated overhead arm motion or occupations requiring heavy lifting also place a strain on rotator cuff tendons and muscles. Normally tendons are strong, but a longstanding wearing down process may lead to a tear.

What are the signs of a torn rotator cuff?

Typically, a person with a rotator cuff injury feels pain over the deltoid muscle at the top and outer side of the shoulder, especially when the arm is raised or extended out from the side of the body. Motions like those involved in getting dressed can be painful. The shoulder may feel weak, especially when trying to lift the arm into a horizontal position. A person may also feel or hear a click or pop when the shoulder is moved.

How is a torn rotator cuff diagnosed?

Pain or weakness on outward or inward rotation of the arm may indicate a tear in a rotator cuff tendon. The patient also feels pain when lowering the arm to the side after the shoulder is moved backward and the arm is raised. A doctor may detect weakness but may not be able to determine from a physical examination where the tear is located. X-rays, if taken, may appear normal. An MRI can help detect a full tendon tear, but does not detect partial tears. If the pain disappears after the doctor injects a small amount of anesthetic into the area, impingement is likely to be present. If there is no response to treatment, the doctor may use an arthrogram, rather than an MRI, to inspect the injured area and confirm the diagnosis.

How is a torn rotator cuff treated?

Doctors usually recommend that patients with a rotator cuff injury rest the shoulder, apply heat or cold to the sore area, and take medicine to relieve pain and inflammation. Other treatments might be added, such as electrical stimulation of muscles and nerves, ultrasound, or a cortisone injection near the inflamed area of the rotator cuff. The patient may need to wear a sling for a few days. If surgery is not an immediate consideration, exercises are added to the treatment program to build flexibility and strength and restore the shoulder's function. If there is no improvement with these conservative treatments and functional impairment persists, the doctor may perform arthroscopic or open surgical repair of the torn rotator cuff.

Frozen Shoulder (Adhesive Capsulitis)

What is a frozen shoulder?

As the name implies, movement of the shoulder is severely restricted in people with a frozen shoulder. This condition, which doctors call adhesive capsulitis, is frequently caused by injury that leads to lack of use due to pain. Intermittent periods of use may cause inflammation. Adhesions (abnormal bands of tissue) grow between the joint surfaces, restricting motion. There is also a lack of synovial fluid, which normally lubricates the gap between the arm bone and socket to help the shoulder joint move. It is this restricted space between the capsule and ball of the humerus that distinguishes adhesive capsulitis from a less complicated painful, stiff shoulder. There are a number of risk factors for frozen shoulder, including diabetes, stroke, accidents, lung disease, and heart disease. The condition rarely appears in people under 40 years old.

What are the signs of a frozen shoulder and how is it diagnosed?

With a frozen shoulder, the joint becomes so tight and stiff that it is nearly impossible to carry out simple movements, such as raising the arm. People complain that the stiffness and discomfort worsens at night. A doctor may suspect the patient has a frozen shoulder if a physical examination reveals limited shoulder movement. An arthrogram may confirm the diagnosis.

How is a frozen shoulder treated?

Treatment of this disorder focuses on restoring joint movement and reducing shoulder pain. Usually, treatment begins with nonsteroidal anti-inflammatory drugs and the application of heat, followed by gentle stretching exercises. These stretching exercises, which may be performed in the home with the help of a therapist, are the treatment of choice. In some cases, transcutaneous electrical nerve stimulation (TENS) with a small battery-operated unit may be used to reduce pain by blocking nerve impulses. If these measures are unsuccessful, the doctor may recommend manipulation of the shoulder under general anesthesia. Surgery to probe into the joint and cut the adhesions is only necessary in some cases.

Fracture

What happens when the shoulder is fractured?

A fracture involves a partial or total crack through a bone. The break in a bone usually occurs as a result of an impact injury, such as a fall or blow to the shoulder. A fracture usually involves the clavicle or the neck (area below the ball) of the humerus.

What are the signs of a shoulder fracture and how is it diagnosed?

A shoulder fracture that occurs after a major injury is usually accompanied by severe pain. Within a short time, there may be redness and bruising around the area. Sometimes a fracture is obvious because the bones appear out of position. Both diagnosis and severity can be confirmed by x-rays.

How is a shoulder fracture treated?

When a fracture occurs, the doctor tries to bring the affected parts into a position that will promote healing and restore arm movement. If the clavicle is fractured, the patient must at first wear a strap and sling to keep the clavicle in place. After removing the strap and sling, the doctor will prescribe exercises to strengthen the shoulder and restore movement. Surgery is occasionally needed for certain clavicle fractures.

Fracture of the neck of the humerus is usually treated with a sling or shoulder immobilizer. If the bones are out of position, surgery may be necessary to reset them. Exercises are also part of restoring shoulder strength and motion.

Arthritis of the Shoulder

What is arthritis of the shoulder?

Arthritis is a degenerative disease caused by either wear and tear (osteoarthritis) or an inflammation (rheumatoid arthritis) of one or more joints. Arthritis not only affects joints; it may secondarily affect supporting structures such as muscles, tendons, and ligaments.

What are the signs of shoulder arthritis and how is it diagnosed?

The usual signs of arthritis of the shoulder are pain, particularly over the AC joint, and a decrease in shoulder motion. A doctor may suspect the patient has arthritis when there is both pain and swelling in the joint. The diagnosis may be confirmed by a physical examination and x-rays. Blood tests may be helpful for diagnosing rheumatoid arthritis, but other tests may be needed as well. Analysis of synovial fluid from the shoulder joint may be helpful in diagnosing some kinds of arthritis. Although arthroscopy permits direct visualization of damage to cartilage, tendons, and ligaments, and may confirm a diagnosis, it is usually only done if a repair procedure is to be performed.

How is arthritis of the shoulder treated?

Most often osteoarthritis of the shoulder is treated with nonsteroidal anti-inflammatory drugs such as aspirin or ibuprofen. (Rheumatoid arthritis of the shoulder may require physical therapy and additional medicine, such as corticosteroids.) When conservative treatment of osteoarthritis of the shoulder fails to relieve pain or improve function, or when there is severe deterioration of the joint causing parts to loosen and move out of place, shoulder joint replacement (arthroplasty) may provide better results. In this operation, a surgeon replaces the shoulder joint with an artificial ball for the humerus and a cap (glenoid) for the scapula. Passive shoulder exercises (where someone else moves the arm to rotate the shoulder joint) are started soon after surgery. Patients begin exercising on their own about three to six weeks after surgery. Eventually, stretching and strengthening exercises become a major part of the rehabilitation program. The success of the operation often depends on the condition of rotator cuff muscles prior to surgery and the degree to which the patient follows the exercise program.

Where can people get additional information about shoulder problems?

American Academy of Orthopaedic Surgeons
P.O. Box 2058
Des Plaines, IL 60017
847/823-7186
800/346-2267
Fax: 847/823-8026
E-mail: julitz@mac.aaos.org
World Wide Web address: http://www.aaos.org

The American Academy of Orthopaedic Surgeons (AAOS) is a not-for-profit organization that provides education programs for orthopaedic surgeons, allied health professionals, and the public and is an advocate for improved patient care. The AAOS has the following educational brochures on the shoulder: Shoulder Pain, Arthroscopy, and Joint Replacement. Single copies are free upon submission of a business-size, stamped, self-addressed envelope.

American Physical Therapy Association
1111 North Fairfax Street
Alexandria, VA 22314-1488
703/684-2782
800/999-2782 x3395
World Wide Web address: http://www.apta.org

The American Physical Therapy Association (APTA) is a national professional organization representing physical therapists, allied personnel, and students. Its objectives are to improve research, public understanding, and education in the physical therapies. APTA provides a free brochure titled "Taking Care of Your Shoulder: A Physical Therapist's Perspective" upon submission of a business-size, stamped, self-addressed envelope.

Arthritis Foundation
1330 West Peachtree Street
Atlanta, GA 30309
404/872-7100
800/283-7800 or call your local chapter (listed in the telephone directory)
World Wide Web address: http://www.arthritis.org

This is the major voluntary organization devoted to arthritis. The Foundation publishes pamphlets on arthritis, such as "Arthritis Answers," that may be obtained by calling the toll-free telephone number. The Foundation also can provide physician and clinic referrals. Local chapters also provide information and organize exercise programs for people who have arthritis.

American College of Rheumatology/Association of Rheumatology Health Professionals
60 Executive Park South, Suite 150
Atlanta, GA 30329
404/633-3777
Fax: 404/633-1870
World Wide Web address: http://www.rheumatology.org

This national professional organization can provide referrals to rheumatologists and allied health specialists, such as physical therapists. One-page fact sheets are also available on various forms of arthritis. Lists of specialists by geographic area and fact sheets are also available on ACR's web site.

Brand names included in this chapter are provided as examples only, and their inclusion does not mean that these products are endorsed by the National Institutes of Health or any other Government agency or Omnigraphics. Also, if a particular brand name is not mentioned, this does not mean or imply that the product is unsatisfactory.

Acknowledgments

The NIAMS gratefully acknowledges the assistance of Frank A. Pettrone, M.D., of Arlington, Virginia; Thomas J. Neviaser, M.D., of Fairfax, Virginia; and James Panagis, M.D., M.P.H., of the National Institutes of Health, in the preparation and review of the fact sheet that makes up this chapter's text.

The National Arthritis and Musculoskeletal and Skin Diseases Information Clearinghouse (NAMSIC) is a public service sponsored by the NIAMS that provides health information and information sources. The NIAMS, a part of the National Institutes of Health (NIH), leads the Federal medical research effort in arthritis and musculoskeletal and skin diseases. The NIAMS sponsors research and research training throughout the United States as well as on the NIH campus in Bethesda, MD, and disseminates health and research information.

Chapter 31

Carpal Tunnel Syndrome

What is carpal tunnel syndrome?

Carpal tunnel syndrome occurs when tendons in the wrist become inflamed after being aggravated. A tunnel of bones and ligaments in the wrist narrows, pinching nerves that reach the fingers and the muscle at the base of the thumb. The first symptoms usually appear at night. Symptoms range from a burning, tingling numbness in the fingers, especially the thumb and the index and middle fingers, to difficulty gripping or making a fist.

Is there any treatment?

Carpal tunnel syndrome is treated by immobilizing the wrist in a splint to minimize or prevent pressure on the nerves. If that fails, patients are sometimes given anti-inflammatory drugs or injections of cortisone in the wrist to reduce the swelling. There is also a surgical procedure in which doctors can open the wrist and cut the ligament at the bottom of the wrist to relieve the pressure. However, only a small percentage of patients require surgery.

What is the prognosis?

Approximately 1 percent of individuals with carpal tunnel syndrome develop permanent injury. The majority recover completely and

NIH Web Publication, National Institutes of Health, Bethesda, Maryland 20892 Written April 1996, (Last Updated April 7, 1998).

can avoid re-injury by changing the way they do repetitive movements, the frequency with which they do the movements, and the amount of time they rest between periods when they perform the movements.

What research is being done?

Much of the on-going research on carpal tunnel syndrome is aimed at prevention and rehabilitation. The National Institute of Arthritis and Musculoskeletal and Skin Diseases (NIAMS) funds research on carpal tunnel syndrome.

These articles, available from a medical library, may provide more in-depth information on carpal tunnel syndrome:

Kasdan, ML, Lane, C, Merritt, WH, and Nathan, PA. "Carpal tunnel syndrome: management techniques." *Patient Care*, 111-138 (April 1993).

Medalie, JH. "Joint injections: some very good recommendations." *Modern Medicine*, 56; 3 (June 1988).

"Testing for carpal tunnel syndrome." *The Lancet*. 338:8762; 479-480 (August 1991).

Wilke, WS, and Tuggle, CJ. "Optimal techniques for intra-articular and periarticular joint injections." *Modern Medicine*, 56; 58-72 (June 1988).

Information may also be available from the following organizations (last updated April 7, 1998):

Association for Repetitive Motion Syndromes (ARMS)
P.O. Box 514
Santa Rosa, CA 95402
(707) 571-0397

American Chronic Pain Association
P.O. Box 850
Rocklin, CA 95677
(916) 632-0922

National Chronic Pain Outreach Association Inc.
P.O. Box 274
Millboro, VA 24460
(540) 997-5004

National Institute of Arthritis and Musculoskeletal and Skin Diseases
Building 31, Room 4C05
Bethesda, MD 20892-2350
(301) 496-8188

National Institute of Neurological Disorders and Stroke
National Institutes of Health
Bethesda, MD 20892

Chapter 32

Getting a Grip on Hand Problems

A trip to the supermarket or signing a paycheck didn't used to rank high on the list of 31-year-old Wanda Wood's concerns. But now, everyday chores like pumping gas and carrying groceries to the car are ordeals for her.

Wood can't hold a pen long enough to finish signing her check. She has trouble grasping a nozzle to fill her gasoline tank. And she can't grip her groceries to keep them from falling out of her hands.

"It's when a jar of tomato sauce cracks all over the pavement that I get real embarrassed," said Wood, a Richmond, Va., former postal worker. "It's pretty tough to handle when you're standing in a parking lot covered with red goo."

Like Wood, an increasing number of American workers are experiencing the sudden onset of one of several cumulative trauma disorders affecting the hands, according to James McGlothlin, Ph.D., a research hygienist at the National Institute for Occupational Safety and Health in Cincinnati. Doctors often call them repetitive strain injuries (RSIs).

RSI is a catch-all term used to refer to many painful conditions, such as trigger finger, nerve spasms, and carpal tunnel syndrome. They can cause stiffness, swelling, tingling, weakness, numbness, and, in some cases, irreversible nerve damage.

Carpal tunnel syndrome is the most frequently reported RSI, with 192 cases per 100,000 workers in 1989, according to the U.S. Public

FDA Consumer, July-August 1993.

Health Service. It occurs when tissues on the palm side of the hand swell, compressing or entrapping the important median nerve, which runs through this area. Numbness and tingling usually start in the wrist, and can radiate down to the thumb and fingers, or up to the elbow. Many patients feel pins and needles when their wrist is tapped. Weakness occurs on effort. For example, patients may suddenly drop objects they are holding. A nerve conduction test, a recording of the electrical activity of the hand and arm muscles, is helpful in diagnosing this disorder.

Other RSIs include nerve spasm and "trigger finger." When nerve entrapment and the pressure caused by it occurs over a long period, the nerve can become irritated and go into spasms, stimulating muscle activity that eventually causes pain similar to severe muscle cramps.

When finger tendons, fibrous bands of tissue that connect muscle to bone, get irritated, they can grow nodules, which, at the points of attachment, get caught in the lubricating sheath that surrounds them. When this happens, the finger can become stuck; this condition is called trigger finger.

RSIs are self-limiting conditions that result from excessive use of the muscles and tendons of the hands, wrists and forearms. Meat cutters, auto workers, cashiers, journalists, keyboard operators, and others who spend long hours at repetitive chores are particularly vulnerable.

Wood used to spend long shifts operating a letter sorter, typing hours at a time at a computer keyboard to route the mail to its destination.

"My pain eventually became so severe that it worked its way from my fingers to my wrist to my elbow until it felt like a constant crook in my neck," she said.

Hopes for Help

Because the consequences of these disorders are so high, the goal of safety and health professionals across the country is to collect information on which to base decisions about the best ways to prevent and treat these illnesses.

But this is not an easy task. For example, some proposed treatments have not been substantiated by controlled clinical trials.

According to John Vanderveen, Ph.D., director of the Food and Drug Administration's division of nutrition, "We have from time to time dealt with claims for the use of nutrients to prevent or treat carpal tunnel syndrome, but could only find anecdotal reports."

He said, "It's difficult to do such studies because animal models are more tenuous to tease out pain and performance data from than humans. So right now we don't know if basic clinical research is likely to support such claims."

In addition to RSIs, various forms of arthritis can cause hand problems. Rheumatoid arthritis, for example, is a chronic, autoimmune disease affecting the entire musculo-skeletal system. Osteoarthritis, a degenerative, "wear and tear" condition can also affect the hands.

Vanderveen said researchers are investigating the innovative use of omega-3 fatty acids, found in fish oils, to help suppress the disease by curtailing production of prostaglandins, a series of hormone-like substances associated with inflammation that occurs in arthritis. Vanderveen cautions that it's still premature at this time to think that these fatty acids will be therapeutic for many arthritis patients.

Today the best bet for RSI patients is to cope with the condition in ways similar to patients with arthritis. Such coping skills include protecting and caring for their joints and using OTC drugs such as aspirin or ibuprofen (Advil, Nuprin, Motrin IB) for mild to moderate symptoms or prescription NSAIDs (nonsteroidal anti-inflammatory drugs) for stronger anti-inflammatory relief.

A general practitioner can treat these disorders, in most patients with either exercise, rest, aspirin, or NSAIDs, such as Motrin or Naprosyn. But if relief does not occur within a few weeks, the physician may refer the patient to a specialist.

Occupational therapists can also help patients with these disorders to practice "joint protection," according to Jan Chmela, director of Sheltering Arms Day Rehabilitation Program in Richmond, Va.

Chmela, herself an occupational therapist, said that patients can learn to use their hands in "non-deforming positions." For example, instead of grabbing a key with a thumb and twisting, patients can learn to turn a key with adaptive equipment. They can learn to use their largest joints for a job, rather than their smaller, more vulnerable ones, for opening a jar, for example. She advocates teaching patients to use their hands closest to their anatomical position, outstretched as much as possible instead of twisting and turning them, because bending the hands stresses the joints.

As with most other disorders, however, prevention, where possible, is the best cure.

The National Institute for Occupational Safety and Health is focusing research on ways to redesign the workplace to make RSIs less likely.

The agency's McGlothlin said, "We don't want to try and fit the worker to the job, but the job to the worker, and that can best be done through engineering controls so that both the worker and the company benefit."

For instance, he suggests adjustable height tables to accommodate workers of different heights and builds. McGlothlin also stressed that employers must be sensitive to the extreme demands on many of their workers and allow for recovery time.

"There are more and more demands on people these days. Many work two jobs or through the night. Women in the workplace may also be raising families. Employees need time off to rest. In order for ideas that we've developed to succeed, there has to be a partnership between workers and their companies to make it a more productive and helpful workplace," he said.

Employers can also cut down on RSIs by providing their workers with chairs that give them better postural support and adjustable work stations that allow them to adjust their screen, keyboard and wrists.

Diagnosis Important

Forty-three-year-old Barbara McGhee, a public affairs specialist at a Virginia Department of Health and Human Services Social Security Administration office, was diagnosed with rheumatoid arthritis at age 19.

Over the years, her hand joints have become rigid and misshapen by chronic inflammation. Her hand dexterity is poor— just shuffling through the pages of a book is difficult.

When McGhee first heard the diagnosis, she said she refused to despair. "I went to the library and learned all I could about it." Because unrealistic expectations only make it that much harder on patients, McGhee said she "needed information so I could make some important decisions. I needed to learn what I would and would not be able to do."

"I realized my attribute was my high energy level and if I cultivated it, I could put it to good use." Twenty-four years later, she is unable to waterski or horseback ride or participate in other sports she used to adore, but she has nevertheless found her niche. McGhee not only holds down a full-time job, but also volunteers for her local chapter of the Arthritis Foundation and the Richmond Mayor's Commission for Disabilities.

McGhee said she only wishes that she hadn't waited five years from the onset of her problems to seek the help of a physician. She said she wonders if she had paid attention to her condition earlier whether she could have avoided having one wrist and one ankle replaced, and the other ankle fused.

Because aches and pains are commonplace, people with early morning stiffness, difficulty in movement, or tenderness in one or more joints sometimes do not realize that they may need to see a doctor.

But it's important that people whose symptoms last longer than several weeks see their physicians immediately. For example, in some cases of moderate to severe carpal tunnel syndrome, early treatment can prevent significant permanent damage to nerves.

Hayes Willis, assistant professor of medicine, division of rheumatology, allergy and immunology at the Medical College of Virginia, explained that "damaged nerves just don't heal well."

He added that for both arthritis and RSIs, the earlier a diagnosis is made, the greater the likelihood of minimizing disability.

—by Cheryl Platzman Weinstock

Cheryl Platzman Weinstock is a writer in Long Island, N.Y., who specializes in health and science issues.

Part Five

Osteoporosis:
Not Another Form of Arthritis

Chapter 33

Arthritis and Osteoporosis: A Common, and Deadly, Confusion

Women Delay Osteoporosis Diagnosis, Treatment Because They Confuse Bone-thinning Disease with Arthritis

Research Findings Prompt NOF to Issue Public Health Advisory

Washington, D.C. (July 2, 1997)—New research suggests that confusion surrounding osteoporosis and arthritis is so extensive that many women may be waiting for the swollen joints, stiffness and pain typically associated with arthritis to occur before they become concerned about osteoporosis, according to an urgently issued Public Health Advisory from the National Osteoporosis Foundation (NOF). Since osteoporosis is a symptomless, painless disease until a fracture occurs, the advisory warns women against waiting for symptoms to develop before seeking a diagnosis or discussing their risk for osteoporosis with their doctors.

"As health professionals, we need to do everything we can to make clear distinctions between osteoporosis and arthritis," says Robert Lindsay, M.D., Ph.D., president of NOF and chief of internal medicine at Helen Hayes Hospital in New York. "We've made significant progress in preventing, diagnosing and treating osteoporosis, yet many women still fail to take adequate steps to protect themselves

---

from the disease and its debilitating effects. We're concerned that confusion surrounding these two diseases leads many women to ignore their risk for osteoporosis, thereby jeopardizing their long-term health, mobility and independence."

The newly issued Public Health Advisory suggests that in addition to educating themselves about osteoporosis and assessing personal risk with their doctors, women also should ask their physicians about the need for a bone density measurement test, the only currently available means to assess the state of the bones and potential risk for future fractures. Although highly accurate in predicting fracture risk, bone density measurements are under-utilized perhaps because, as this new research points out, women may be waiting for symptoms before taking the risk of osteoporosis seriously. In general, six in ten women think that osteoporosis has warning signs or symptoms when in fact, the disease progresses without signs or symptoms until a fracture occurs. Of those surveyed, 71 percent cited pain, half mentioned stiffness, and a third referred to swollen joints, as symptoms of osteoporosis, but those are actually symptoms of arthritis. In addition, half of the women surveyed indicated they believe there are similar treatment approaches for arthritis and osteoporosis, although the treatments are vastly different. The research findings were compiled through a telephone survey of 505 American women and have a margin of error of + 5 percentage points.

Osteoporosis is characterized by the exaggerated loss of bone mass and by poor bone quality. Over time, bones become fragile and susceptible to fractures. Arthritis, on the other hand, affects the joints and surrounding tissue. Osteoarthritis and rheumatoid arthritis are the most common forms of arthritis and are entirely separate conditions from osteoporosis. Yet, this new research shows that more than 40 percent of women think that osteoporosis and osteoarthritis are related diseases, possibly misled by the similar names.

"Since more than 28 million Americans either have or are at high risk for osteoporosis, it is crucial for everyone—women and men, young and old—to understand that osteoporosis is a disease that is an entirely separate condition from osteoarthritis," says Dr. Lindsay. "NOF urges the American public to take action against this debilitating disease by following the recommended steps outlined in the Public Health Advisory issued today."

Many individuals can prevent osteoporosis and treatments are available to slow bone loss and prevent fractures caused by osteoporosis. If you are diagnosed as having osteoporosis, your doctor will prescribe a treatment program that is right for you.

"It is important for people who think they are at risk or who already have osteoporosis to see a doctor and be properly diagnosed and treated, since osteoporosis and arthritis have different causes and different treatments," added Sandra C. Raymond, executive director of NOF. "In fact, in some cases the treatment for one of these diseases may cause or worsen the other. For example, a common drug used for treating one form of arthritis is corticosteroid medication, which can lead to osteoporosis when used in high doses for long periods of time."

At the same time, a program of regular, weight-bearing exercises, which are highly beneficial for preventing osteoporosis and maintaining strong bones, may worsen the condition of joints affected by osteoarthritis.

Osteoporosis: The "Silent" Disease

Osteoporosis-related fractures typically develop in the hip, spine and wrist, but any bone can be affected. While the majority of sufferers of this disease are women, 20 percent of those affected by osteoporosis are men.

Osteoporosis has been considered a "silent" disease because of the way it progresses without symptoms or pain until a fracture occurs. Currently, this silent disease causes a total of 1.5 million fractures every year in the United States. Osteoporosis leads annually to more than half a million vertebral fractures, 300,000 hip fractures, 200,000 broken wrists and 300,000 fractures of other bones. An estimated 37,500 people die each year following fracture-related complications. The disease also takes an enormous personal and economic toll—with estimated costs of nearly $14 billion annually for direct medical treatment for osteoporotic fractures.

To provide additional information on the differences between osteoporosis and arthritis, the National Osteoporosis Foundation has published a new brochure, "What People With Arthritis Need to Know About Osteoporosis." Single copies are available at no charge by contacting NOF, PO Box 96616, Dept. ART, Washington, D.C., 20077-7456.

The National Osteoporosis Foundation is the nation's only scientific and medically based nonprofit, voluntary health agency exclusively dedicated to reducing the widespread prevalence of osteoporosis through programs of research, education and advocacy. The National Osteoporosis Foundation has information to help people better understand, prevent, and treat the disease. To stay informed about osteoporosis, contact the National Osteoporosis Foundation at the above address.

Public Health Advisory on Osteoporosis Arthritis

American women confuse osteoporosis and arthritis and may be jeopardizing their long-term bone health by failing to take action as a result of inaccurate and incomplete information.

The National Osteoporosis Foundation is issuing this urgent advisory to the public regarding confusion surrounding osteoporosis and arthritis. Recent research and clinical observation has confirmed that many potential osteoporosis patients associate the symptoms and treatments for arthritis with osteoporosis. Consequently, many women may not take the necessary steps to protect themselves against the debilitating effects of osteoporosis.

It is critically important that the public recognize that osteoporosis and arthritis are separate diseases with distinct treatments. Adding to the seriousness of this situation is the fact that many people are unaware that some of the treatment approaches for arthritis actually can accelerate the osteoporosis process. NOF is issuing this advisory to eliminate this dangerous confusion and to offer the public some specific recommendations to minimize their risk of developing osteoporosis or complicating its treatment.

Need for an Advisory:

Although osteoporosis has gained significant media attention and public visibility in the last ten years, many patients still are undiagnosed and millions of American women have failed to act on the advice of experts to prevent osteoporosis, or diagnose and treat it early.

Because osteoporosis is a symptomless, painless disease until a fracture occurs, many women may be waiting for the swollen joints, stiffness and pain typically associated with arthritis to occur before they become concerned about osteoporosis. An osteoporotic fracture of a vertebrae in the spine can cause considerable pain, even when the fracture itself goes undetected, and this often is the first time individuals experience pain from osteoporosis.

Although multiple factors may influence this situation, new research and clinical experience suggest that basic confusion surrounding osteoporosis and arthritis may be one of the reasons people fail to take effective action to prevent and treat osteoporosis.

Symptoms Adult Women Incorrectly Associate with Osteoporosis

This new research found, for example, that:

312

- Many people incorrectly assume that osteoporosis has symptoms similar to arthritis. In general, six in ten people think osteoporosis has warning signs or symptoms; in fact however, osteoporosis has no signs or symptoms until a bone fractures.

- One in two women incorrectly believe that there are similar treatment approaches for osteoporosis and arthritis.

- A plurality of women (42 percent) mistakenly believe that osteoporosis and osteoarthritis are related.

Simply put, individuals who believe that arthritis and osteoporosis are related or are similar in nature may be waiting for pain or other symptoms to develop before they ask their physicians whether they are at risk for osteoporosis. However, osteoporosis is a symptomless disease that progresses without warning until a fracture occurs. It is important to understand that bone loss occurs without pain. Once pain occurs, individuals already have suffered one or more osteoporosis related fractures. Individuals who wait for symptoms to appear typically don't take steps to prevent osteoporosis. Ultimately, they are delaying diagnosis and compromising the potential effectiveness of any future treatment, since osteoporosis is best treated when detected early.

It's also important to note that certain medications used to treat rheumatoid arthritis increase the risk of developing osteoporosis.

Call to Action:

In light of this situation, NOF recommends to women that they:

- **Get the Facts**. Understand the differences between osteoporosis and arthritis, especially if you are at risk for or have either of these diseases. Keep in mind that unlike arthritis, osteoporosis does not cause pain (prior to fractures), swollen joints, stiffness or any other symptoms.

- **Understand your risk of osteoporosis**. Assess your personal risk for developing osteoporosis by considering your risk factors. The following risk factors have been identified:

  — Being female
  — Thin and/or small frame
  — Advanced age
  — A family history of osteoporosis

— Early menopause
— Abnormal absence of menstrual periods (amenorrhea)
— Anorexia nervosa or bulimia
— A diet low in calcium
— Use certain medications, such as corticosteroids and anti-convulsants
— Low testosterone levels in men
— An inactive lifestyle
— Cigarette smoking or excessive alcohol use
— Caucasian or Asian, although African Americans and Hispanic Americans are at significant risk as well

- **Ask your doctor about getting a bone density measurement**. Currently, a bone density measurement is the only way to assess the state of your bones and the potential for future fractures. Since osteoporosis is a symptomless disease, this non-invasive, painless test can tell you if you need to be concerned about osteoporosis.

- **Know the side effects for medications.** This is especially important if you are taking medication to treat arthritis, since some of these medications actually can increase the risk of developing osteoporosis.

- **If you are at all confused or unsure about your risk of osteoporosis, seek help.** Ask your doctor or NOF to answer your questions if you are unsure about your risk for osteoporosis. Don't wait for symptoms to occur. NOF has a toll-free number available to provide further information—call 1-800/223-9994.

- **Review your approach to managing the disease if you've already been diagnosed.** Think about how you're coping with osteoporosis. Make sure you're not self-medicating with drugs that may complicate your condition. Discuss your current medications (both for osteoporosis and other conditions) and lifestyle with your doctor to ensure that you are on the right track in managing osteoporosis.

To provide additional information on the differences between osteoporosis and arthritis, the National Osteoporosis Foundation has published a new brochure, "What People With Arthritis Need to Know About Osteoporosis." Single copies are available at no charge by contacting NOF, PO Box 96616, Dept. ART, Washington, D.C., 20077-7456.

Chapter 34

Osteoporosis

Introduction

Osteoporosis is a major underlying cause of bone fractures in post-menopausal women and older persons in general. It is a condition in which bone mass decreases, causing bones to be more susceptible to fracture. A fall, blow, or lifting action that would not bruise or strain the average person can easily cause one or more bones to break in a person with severe osteoporosis.

Medical practitioners and patients alike are concerned with the optimum approach to the treatment and prevention of osteoporosis. The appropriate timing and proper use of agents, such as calcium, vitamin D, estrogens, and fluorides, as well as the role of exercise are issues that have generated major research efforts and considerable controversy.

In an effort to resolve some of the questions surrounding these issues, the National Institutes of Health convened a Consensus Development Conference on Osteoporosis on April 24, 1984. After a day and a half of presentations by experts in the field, a consensus panel including representatives of orthopaedics, endocrinology, gynecology, rheumatology, epidemiology, nutrition, biochemistry, family medicine, and the general public considered the evidence and agreed on answers to the following key questions:

NIH Publication, Consensus Development Conference Statement, April, 1984.

315

- What is osteoporosis?
- What are the clinical features of osteoporosis, and how is it detected?
- Who is at risk for developing osteoporosis?
- What are the possible causes of osteoporosis?
- How can osteoporosis be prevented and treated?
- What are the directions for future research?
- Panel's Conclusions

Osteoporosis is a major public health problem. Although all bones are affected, fractures of the spine, wrist, and hip are typical and most common. The risk of developing osteoporosis increases with age and is higher in women than in men and in whites than in blacks. Its cause appears to reside in the mechanisms underlying an accentuation of the normal loss of bone, which follows the menopause in women and occurs in all individuals with advancing age. There are no laboratory tests for defining individuals at risk or those with mild osteoporosis. The diagnosis of primary osteoporosis is established by documentation of reduced bone density or mass in a patient with a typical fracture syndrome after exclusion of known causes of excessive bone loss. Prevention of fracture in susceptible patients is the primary goal of intervention. Strategies include assuring estrogen replacement in postmenopausal women, adequate nutrition including an elemental calcium intake of 1,000-1,500 mg a day, and a program of modest weight-bearing exercise. There is great need for additional research on understanding the biology of human bone, defining individuals at special risk, and developing safe, effective, low-cost strategies for fracture prevention.

What is osteoporosis?

Primary osteoporosis is an age-related disorder characterized by decreased bone mass and by increased susceptibility to fractures in the absence of other recognizable causes of bone loss.

Osteoporosis is a common condition affecting as many as 15-20 million individuals in the United States. About 1.3 million fractures attributable to osteoporosis occur annually in people age 45 and older. Among those who live to be age 90, 32 percent of women and 17 percent of men will suffer a hip fracture, most due to osteoporosis. The cost of osteoporosis in the United States has been estimated at $3.8 billion annually.

Bone is composed of a collagen-rich organic matrix impregnated with mineral—largely calcium and phosphate. Two major forms of bone exist. Compact cortical bone forms the external envelopes of the skeleton; trabecular or medullary bone forms plates that traverse the internal cavities of the skeleton. The proportions of cortical and trabecular bone vary at different sites. Vertebral bodies contain predominantly trabecular bone, while the proximal femur contains predominantly cortical bone. The responses of the two forms of bone to metabolic influences and their susceptibility to fracture differ.

Bone undergoes continuous remodeling (turnover) throughout life. Osteoclasts resorb bone in microscopic cavities; osteoblasts then reform the bone surfaces, filling the cavities. Normally, bone resorption and formation are linked closely in space, time, and degree. Mechanical and electrical forces, hormones, and local regulatory factors influence remodeling.

Peak bone mass is achieved at about 35 years of age for cortical bone and earlier for trabecular bone. Sex, race, nutrition, exercise, and overall health influence peak mass. Bone mass is approximately 30 percent higher in men than in women and approximately 10 percent higher in blacks than in whites. In each group, bone mass varies among individuals.

After reaching its peak, bone mass declines throughout life due to an imbalance in remodeling. Bones lose both mineral and organic matrix but retain their basic organization. In women, bone mass decreases rapidly for three to seven years after menopause. Bone loss also is enhanced in a variety of diseases.

Women have more fractures than men, and whites have more fractures than blacks. Three factors determine the likelihood of fractures:

1. The magnitude, direction, and duration of the applied force;
2. The dissipation of that force by muscle contraction and soft tissue absorption;
3. Bone strength.

Injuries are more frequent and energy dissipation diminishes with advancing age. Reduction in bone mass is the most important reason for the increased frequency of bone fractures in postmenopausal women and in the elderly.

Classifying primary osteoporosis into clinical, histological, or biochemical subsets may be useful from the standpoints of etiology, prevention, and treatment. There is clinical and histological evidence for different subsets. Vertebral fractures occur most frequently in women aged 55 to 75 with accelerated loss of trabecular bone. Hip fractures occur most frequently in older men and women who slowly have lost

317

both cortical and trabecular mass. Bone biopsies from some individuals with primary osteoporosis show high turnover rates; biopsies from others show low or intermediate rates of turnover.

What are the clinical features of osteoporosis, and how is it detected?

The clinical manifestations of osteoporosis include fractures and their vertebral bodies, the neck and intertrochanteric regions of the femur, and the distal radius. Osteoporotic individuals may fracture any bone more easily than their non-osteoporotic counterparts.

Vertebral compression fractures occur more frequently in women than in men, and typically affect T8-L3. These fractures may develop during routine activities, such as bending, lifting, or rising from a chair or bed. Immediate, severe, local back pain often results. Pain usually subsides within several months. Some individuals experience persistent pain due to altered spinal mechanics. In contrast, some vertebral fractures do not cause pain. Gradual asymptomatic vertebral compression may be detected only upon radiographic examination. Loss of body height and/or the development of kyphosis may be the only signs of multiple vertebral fractures. Discomfort, debility, and, rarely, pulmonary dysfunction may accompany thoracic shortening. Abdominal symptoms may include early satiety, bloating, and constipation.

Hip fractures are another important manifestation of osteoporosis. The affected population tends to be older and the sex distribution more even than is the case in vertebral fracture. Acute complications—hospitalization, depression, and mechanical failure of the surgical procedure—are common. Most patients fail to recover normal activity, and mortality within one year approaches 20 percent. Distal radial fractures limit use of the extremity for four to eight weeks, although long-term disability is uncommon. These fractures promote fear of loss of independent living, fear of additional falls and fractures, and depression.

Detection of low skeletal mass and/or a fracture after minor trauma should alert the physician to the presence of metabolic bone disease. The physician should evaluate further to exclude osteomalacia, hyperparathyroidism, hyperthyroidism, multiple myeloma, metastatic disease, syndromes of glucocorticoid excess, and other causes of secondary osteoporosis. No blood or urine test establishes specifically the diagnosis of primary osteoporosis, but such tests may exclude secondary causes.

Several non-invasive methods are available to evaluate bone density. These vary widely in cost, availability, and radiation dose. Standard radiographs of the spine are most widely available. Roentgenograms are, however, insensitive indicators of bone loss, since bone density must be decreased by at least 20 to 30 percent before the reduction can he appreciated. Characteristic abnormalities on standard roentgenograms are sufficient for establishing the diagnosis of osteoporosis if secondary causes are excluded clinically or radiographically. If the spine film is not diagnostic but clinical suspicion is high, a variety of other procedures may be indicated. These include radiogrammetry for measurement of cortical thickness, photodensitometry, the Singh Index of femoral trabecular pattern, single and dual photon absorptiometry, neutron activation, Compton scattering, and single and dual energy computed tomography. Use of these techniques will depend on their availability, cost, and further studies of their discriminatory capabilities and sensitivity.

With histomorphometry, usually performed on a bone biopsy from the iliac crest, bone mass can be evaluated and osteomalacia and certain forms of secondary osteoporosis excluded. Bone biopsy is safe but requires specialized equipment and expert analysis that are not widely available.

Who is at risk for developing osteoporosis?

The correlation of osteoporosis with the following factors is well documented. Bone mass declines with age in all people and is related to sex, race, menopause, and body weight-for-height.

Women are at higher risk than men in that they have less bone mass and, for several years following natural or induced menopause, the rate of bone mass decline is accelerated. Early menopause is one of the strongest predictors for the development of osteoporosis. White women are at much higher risk than black women, and white men are at higher risk than black men. Women who are underweight also have osteoporosis more often than overweight women. Cigarette smoking may be an additional predictor of risk. Calcium deficiency has been implicated in the pathogenesis of this disease.

Immobilization and prolonged bed rest produce rapid bone loss, while exercise involving weight bearing has been shown both to reduce bone loss and to increase bone mass. The optimal type and amount of physical activity that will prevent osteoporosis have not been established. Exercise sufficient to induce amenorrhea in young women may lead to decreased bone mass.

The relationship of osteoporosis to hereditary and dietary factors, such as alcohol, vitamins A and C, magnesium, and protein, is less firmly established. Some of these factors may act indirectly through their effect on calcium metabolism or body weight.

What are the possible causes of osteoporosis?

Because primary osteoporosis is characterized by decreased bone mass, the causes of the disorder must be sought among the factors that determine the quantity and quality of bone, including the magnitude of maximum bone mass at maturity and the rate of bone loss with aging.

Complex cellular, physiologic, and metabolic factors may underlie the pathogenesis of osteoporosis. Discrete cell types, anatomically and functionally connected, are continually renewed and maintain the complex skeletal tissue. Several systemic hormones and an increasingly recognized number of local (paracrine) factors regulate bone cell activity. Diet, as well as intestinal and renal function, influences mineral ion homeostasis needed to maintain the skeleton. The formation and resorption of bone and their coupling also are modified by external physical forces such as those generated by body weight and exercise.

Osteoporosis is histologically, biochemically, and kinetically heterogeneous; rapid bone turnover or reduced rates of bone formation have been documented in patients with primary osteoporosis. Multiple etiologies would not be surprising, considering the complex factors regulating normal bone metabolism. Among the many possible etiologies of primary osteoporosis, current data point to two probable causes: deficiency of estrogen and deficiency of calcium. Rapid bone loss often accompanies menopause, and premature osteoporosis follows bilateral oophorectomy. Estrogen replacement prevents bone loss in both conditions. The following observations support a causal relationship between calcium deficiency and osteoporosis: Calcium deficiency in experimental animals causes osteoporosis; a low calcium intake is common among the elderly in the United States; and calcium supplementation reduces bone loss.

How can osteoporosis be prevented and treated?

Physicians must emphasize measures that retard or halt the progress of osteoporosis before irreversible structural defects occur. The mainstays of prevention and management of osteoporosis are estrogen and calcium: exercise and nutrition may be important adjuncts.

Estrogen replacement therapy is highly effective for preventing osteoporosis in women. Estrogen reduces bone resorption and retards or halts postmenopausal bone loss. Case-controlled studies have shown a substantial reduction in hip and wrist fractures in women whose estrogen replacement was begun within a few years of menopause. Studies also suggest that estrogen reduces the rate of vertebral fractures. Even when started as late as six years after menopause, estrogen prevents further loss of bone mass but does not restore it to premenopausal levels. Oral estrogen protects at low doses, such as 0.625 mg of conjugated equine estrogen, (25 micrograms of mestranol and 2 mg of estradiol valcrate daily exemplify other protective regimens reviewed by the panel).

All of the above data on efficacy are based almost exclusively on studies in white women. Therefore, the following recommendations on therapy for osteoporosis pertain to that group. Cyclic estrogen therapy should be given to women whose ovaries are removed before age 50 in whom there are no specific contraindications. Women who have had a natural menopause also should be considered for cyclic estrogen replacement if they have no contraindications and if they understand the risks and agree to regular medical evaluations. The duration of estrogen therapy need not be limited. There is no convincing evidence that initiating estrogen therapy in elderly women will prevent osteoporosis. The decision to treat women of other racial backgrounds should be determined on a case-by-case basis.

Estrogen-associated endometrial cancer is usually manifested at an early stage and is rarely fatal when managed appropriately. The bulk of evidence indicates that estrogen use is not associated with an increased risk of breast cancer. Adding a progestogen probably reduces the risk of endometrial cancer, but there is little information about the safety of long-term combined estrogen and progestogen treatment in postmenopausal women. Younger patients receiving progestogens in oral contraceptives experienced an increased risk of hypertension and cardiovascular disease. Some progestogens may blunt or eliminate the favorable effects of estrogen on lipoproteins.

Until more data on risks and benefits are available, physicians and patients may prefer to reserve estrogen (with or without progestogen) therapy for conditions that confer a high risk of osteoporosis, such as the occurrence of premature menopause.

The usual daily intake of elemental calcium in the United States, 450 mg to 550 mg, falls well below the National Research Council's (NRC) recommended dietary allowance (RDA) of 800 mg; the RDA is designed to meet the needs of approximately 95 percent or more of the population. Calcium metabolic balance studies indicate a daily requirement of about 1,000 mg of calcium for premenopausal and estrogen-treated women. Postmenopausal women who are not treated with estrogen require about 1,500 mg daily for calcium balance. Therefore, the RDA for calcium is evidently too low, particularly for postmenopausal women and may well be too low in elderly men. In some studies, high dietary calcium suppresses age-related bone loss and reduces the fracture rate in patients with osteoporosis. It seems likely that an increase in calcium intake to 1,000 to 1,500 mg a day beginning well before the menopause will reduce the incidence of osteoporosis in postmenopausal women. Increased calcium intake may prevent age-related bone loss in men as well.

The major sources of calcium in the U.S. diet are milk and dairy products. Each 8 ounce glass (240 ml) of milk contains 275-300 mg calcium. Skim or low fat milk is preferred to minimize fat intake. For those unable to take 1,000 to 1,500 mg calcium by diet, supplementation with calcium tablets is recommended with special attention to their *elemental* calcium content.

Levels of calcium intake greater than those recommended herein could cause urinary tract stones in susceptible people. Anyone with a history of kidney stones should only undertake calcium supplementation with the guidance of a physician.

Normal levels of vitamin D are required for optimal calcium absorption. The requirement for vitamin D increases with age. Persons who do not receive adequate daily sunlight exposure, such as those confined to home or to a nursing facility, are at special risk for vitamin D deficiency. Vitamin D has dangerous effects at high doses. Although the toxic dose varies among individuals, toxicity has occurred at levels as low as 2,000- 5,000 international units [I.U.] daily. No one should consume more than 15 to 20 micrograms (600 to 800 units, twice the daily RDA) without a doctor's recommendation.

Inactivity leads to bone loss. Some recent studies suggest that weight-bearing exercise may reduce bone loss. Modest weight-bearing exercise, such as walking, is recommended.

Several agents and modalities of treatment are currently under investigation, but their efficacy and/or safety have not been established. These include sodium fluoride, calcitriol, calcitonin, weakly androgenic anabolic steroids, thiazides, bisphosphonates, the 1-34 fragment of parathyroid, and "ADFR," a complex system of several drugs. Sodium fluoride, in association with a high calcium intake, may have a role to play in patients afflicted with severe osteoporosis, but its efficacy and safety are unproven; prospective studies are now under way.

Strategies to prevent falls are important in elderly patients who may fall frequently for a variety of reasons, such as from effects of drugs. Specific environmental interventions can minimize home hazards that increase the chances of falling.

Physicians treating fractures in osteoporotic patients should recognize the benefits of rapid return to function and avoidance of prolonged immobilization.

What are the directions for future research?

Future research in osteoporosis should approach the currently unanswered basic research questions concerning the development and maintenance of bone as a tissue. At the same time, there is great need for clinical and epidemiological research to further explore and extend the current potential for practical prevention and treatment of the disease. A deeper knowledge of factors controlling bone cell activity and regulation of bone mineral and matrix formation and remodeling should contribute ultimately to our understanding of the etiology of osteoporosis. This understanding will permit a more rational choice and evaluation of therapies even as current treatments are evaluated clinically.

The panel recommends:

1. Observational and epidemiological studies to determine the impact of multiple demographic and behavioral factors on bone mass and fracture frequency. Such studies could be conducted by appropriate additions to existing population-based studies.

2. Clinical studies to determine whether the observed age, sex, and skeletal distribution differences in osteoporosis reflect different mechanisms and predict different responses to intervention.

3. Studies to develop accurate, safe, inexpensive methods for determining the level of risk for osteoporosis in an individual, to establish early diagnosis, and to assess the clinical course of the disease.

4. Studies to develop safe, effective, low-cost strategies which might be applicable to populations at large for maximizing peak bone mass, minimizing bone loss, and preventing fractures.

5. Studies to determine the optimal regimen of gonadal hormones for prevention of bone loss and fracture.

6. Studies to elucidate further the mechanisms of bone growth and remodeling, their local and systemic regulation, and their alteration in osteoporosis.

7. Studies to understand alterations in the structure and biomechanical properties of bone in osteoporosis and the relationship of these alterations to the mechanisms and management of fractures.

Chapter 35

Corticosteroid-Induced Osteoporosis

Corticosteroid Induced Osteoporosis Is a Serious and Common Complication of Arthritis Treatment

NOF Comments on New Data Presented at the American College of Rheumatology Meeting

Washington, D.C. (November 9, 1997)—New data presented today at the American College of Rheumatology's National Scientific Meeting offers hope for arthritis sufferers who may develop osteoporosis as a result of taking corticosteroids for their primary disease—arthritis. The use of corticosteroids increases the risk of developing osteoporosis—a major public health problem affecting one in two women and one in eight men over the age of fifty in America today

"Exciting new research shows that bisphosphonate medications, which are already available, may prevent the bone loss caused by corticosteroid medications such as prednisone and cortisone, commonly used to treat rheumatoid arthritis and other diseases. Osteoporosis is a serious and common complication of corticosteroid therapy at any age," said Robert Lindsay, MD, PhD, president of the National Osteoporosis Foundation. "Anyone about to go on corticosteroids, or anyone who has been on them, should have a bone density test. These studies offer new hope to people who must use these medications and we look forward to FDA consideration of bisphosphonates for this indication."

Osteoporosis is a preventable and treatable disease that causes bones to thin and weaken, leaving people susceptible to fractures. Anyone at risk for osteoporosis, including people who must take corticosteroids, should ask their doctor about a bone density test, a painless test to detect bone loss and diagnose osteoporosis. Some other osteoporosis risk factors include being female, being menopausal or postmenopausal, having a family history of osteoporosis, a personal history of fractures, a thin or small build, and being Caucasian or Asian.

Many people confuse osteoporosis and osteoarthritis. For a free booklet "What People with Arthritis Need to Know About Osteoporosis" write to The National Osteoporosis Foundation, Department ART, P.O. Box 96616, Washington, D.C. 20077-7456.

The National Osteoporosis Foundation is the only scientific and medically-based nonprofit, voluntary health organization devoted to the prevention, diagnosis and treatment of osteoporosis. With more than 200,000 members and donors nationwide, NOF's mission is to eradicate the disease through research, education, and advocacy.

Chapter 36

Fractures

Treatment Methods Are Tailored to the Break

It happened so fast. You took a wrong step, slipped and fell. Before you knew it, you had a broken wrist.

Although it's little comfort, your situation is not unique. An estimated 5.6 million fractures occur in the United States each year. Fortunately, with a little help your body can usually repair a fracture. Natural processes ordinarily ensure a sound union within a few months.

But if the break is severe or doesn't heal properly, some type of intervention may be necessary. This often involves surgery, but may include devices intended to stimulate natural healing. In addition, researchers are studying promising new repair methods, such as using glue-like substances. But so far, these techniques remain experimental.

A Natural Healer

Bone is composed of two types of tissue—an inner layer of spongy (cancellous) bone and an outer layer of hard (cortical) bone. Bone maintains its shape and strength by continually absorbing and rebuilding its cells. This process also provides for healing following a fracture.

When you break a bone, it immediately begins to repair itself. A temporary blood clot seals off damaged blood vessels. A fibrous protein (collagen) develops within the fracture.

As the collagen matures, bone-forming cells (osteoblasts) build a mesh of spongy bone on the tissue, linking the ends of the fractured bone. Gradually, denser, harder bone replaces the mesh, resulting in a healed fracture.

Straightening out the Problem

Immobilizing the limb in a cast is often the only treatment required if the ends of your fractured bone are aligned properly.

Most casts today are made from strips of fiberglass or plastic and are stronger and lighter than traditional plaster of Paris casts.

But because plastic casting tape has sharper edges and can be more abrasive, it may be hard on clothing and skin. Also, the tape doesn't mold to your body quite as easily as plaster. For a break that requires a particularly snug mold, your doctor may still prefer a plaster cast.

If the ends of your broken bone are not aligned, the bone must first be returned to its proper position. Your doctor may be able to work the bone back into place, or surgery may be necessary. Fractures adjacent to or extending into a joint sometimes require metal pins, rods, plates or screws to hold the bone in position. Two methods are used:

- *Internal fixation* — This involves surgically placing the pins or plates inside or along your fractured bone. Your doctor is most likely to recommend this technique.

- *External fixation* — In some instances, such as certain wrist fractures, your doctor may recommend this method. In external fixation, metal pins are inserted through slits in your skin and into the fractured bone away from the break.

The pins are attached to an external metal or plastic frame that holds the bone in place.

Because the procedure is less invasive, there's little additional injury to nearby muscle and skin, and the risk of infection deep in the bone is reduced. Your doctor can also adjust the pins during the healing process if the fracture is not mending properly. External fixators are worn an average of 6 to 12 weeks for a wrist fracture.

External fixators may eliminate the need for a cast, and can be quite comfortable because they hold the bone very still in its normal position while it heals.

But there are trade-offs. Occasionally, the pins can cause minor bone and skin infections.

Stimulating Natural Healing

For reasons doctors don't fully understand, broken bones sometimes fail to heal. Called a fracture nonunion, the condition is more common among adults with severe fractures and appears to occur more often among smokers.

At one time, a bone graft (bone tissue grafted onto the fracture) was the only way to treat these fractures. But devices that encourage healing through stimulation of your bones may provide another option. They can sometimes be tried in place of surgery or when a graft fails.

When you break a bone, your body naturally produces small electrical signals that stimulate growth hormones in the bone. In turn, these hormones trigger the natural healing process. In fractures that don't heal, that process fails. Your doctor may try to encourage that process by using:

- **Electromagnetic stimulation**—One common type of stimulator is a battery-operated unit you wear on your body. The unit produces an undetectable electromagnetic current that travels along a wire to a coil. The coil emits a pulsating current over the fracture site for several hours a day. You still usually wear a cast to keep the fracture stable.

  Nationwide, electromagnetic stimulation is used annually on approximately 35,000 arm and leg fractures that won't heal. However, the role of these devices and their effectiveness remain controversial, even among orthopedic surgeons.

  Mayo Clinic doctors have found the devices to be helpful in some fractures, but less so in others. And it may take three or more months for a fracture to heal.

- **Ultrasound**—The Food and Drug Administration (FDA) approved the first ultrasound device for treating fractures last year.

  A transducer emitting low-intensity pulses of sound is applied to your skin over the fracture for about 20 minutes daily. The sound waves jiggle the bone, which is thought to hasten healing. Unlike electromagnetic treatment, ultrasound is intended to speed healing of fresh fractures.

Due to the cost involved and the fact most breaks eventually heal on their own, ultrasound and electromagnetic stimulation are usually reserved for fractures where doctors anticipate healing problems.

Gluing the Pieces Together

If current research is successful, doctors may someday be able to treat broken bones simply by injecting materials into the fracture area.

Clinical studies are under way on two types of injectable compounds:

- **Bone paste**—This cement-like material with a chemistry similar to bone could one day reduce the need for casts. When injected into a fracture, the paste forms carbonated apatite, the main ingredient of bone.

  Preliminary studies show it takes just 10 minutes for the paste to solidify. It's as hard as normal bone within 12 hours. Your body seems to treat the material as if it were bone, so side effects may be few. The paste eventually dissolves and is replaced with natural bone.

  Bone paste is being tested on wrist fractures. Future studies will evaluate its effectiveness on knee and hip fractures. The paste is already approved in the Netherlands.

- **Growth factors**—Created from collagen and ceramic materials, these compounds are intended to stimulate natural bone growth and provide a framework on which new bone can develop.

  Researchers are now evaluating six to eight different types. Scientists hope that growth factors will repair fractures that won't heal, reducing the need for bone grafts. But so far, there's no clear evidence they're effective.

Health Tips

Eating Healthier

What should you eat to stay healthy? Your fruits and vegetables, among other things.

New guidelines from the U.S. Departments of Agriculture and Health and Human Services recommend that you:

- **Eat a variety of foods**—No single food can supply all the nutrients you need.

- **Balance diet with *physical activity*; maintain or improve your weight**—Get 30 minutes of moderate exercise daily, and don't gain weight as you age.

- **Eat grain, vegetables and fruits**—These foods, low in fat and high in nutrients, can reduce disease risk. Eat six to 11 servings of grain products, 3 to 5 servings of vegetables and 2 to 4 servings of fruit daily.

- **Follow a low-fat, low-cholesterol diet**—Limit fat to no more than 30 percent of daily calories.

- **Eat sugars in moderation**—High-sugar foods supply calories but few nutrients.

- **Limit salt and sodium**—Reducing sodium intake can lower blood pressure. Consume less than 2,400 milligrams of sodium daily.

- **Drink alcoholic beverages in moderation**—If you drink, moderate consumption (one drink daily for women, two for men) may reduce your risk of coronary artery disease. However, larger quantities can increase your risk for many illnesses.

Part Six

Arthritis Treatments

Chapter 37

Therapies for People with Arthritis

Therapy for arthritis depends on the type of disease being treated, its severity, and patient response. Here are some common forms of treatments being used to treat the major types of arthritis.

Arthritis Medicines

According to research conducted by the Food and Drug Administration, the medicines taken most by people over 45 are those used to relieve the discomfort of arthritis. This is hardly news to older Americans, who know only too well the pain and discomfort caused by this condition.

Of the more than 100 forms of arthritis, osteoarthritis, rheumatoid arthritis, and gout are the most common. According to the Arthritis Foundation, more than nine million Americans over 65 have some symptoms of osteoarthritis. This condition strikes the joints of the hands, feet, knees, hips, neck, and back. Pain may come and go and can vary from mild to severe. Although rheumatoid arthritis often begins during middle age, it can develop at any age. This type of arthritis, which tends to occur more often in women than men, most commonly affects the joints of the wrists, hands, and feet, but can affect any movable joint. Gout causes sudden swelling and extreme pain, usually in only one joint, often the big toe.

NIH Pub No. 1990:241-292/00003, prepared by the National Institute on Aging, Food and Drug Administration as part of its series *Age Page. FDA Consumer Reprint DHHS Pub. No 89-1080.*

335

Table 37.1. Salicylates

Generic Name	Sample Brand Names
Aspirin	Bayer, Bufferin, Easprin, Ecotrin, and others
Choline magnesium trisalicylate	Trilisate
Choline salicylate	Arthropan
Diflunisal	Dolobid
Magnesium salicylate	Magan
Salicylsalicylic acid	Disalcid, Mono-Gesic

Table 37.2. Nonsalicylates

Generic Name	Sample Brand Names
Diclofenac	Voltaren
Fenoprofen	Nalfon
Flurbiprofen	Ansaid
Ibuprofen	Motrin, Rufen, and over-the-counter brands such as Advil and Nuprin
Indomethacin	Indocin
Ketoprofen	Orudis
Meclofenamate	Meclomen
Mefenamic acid	Ponstel
Naproxen	Naprosyn
Naproxen sodium	Anaprox
Piroxicam	Feldene
Sulindac	Clinoril
Tolmetin	Tolectin

Most forms of arthritis cannot be prevented or cured, so the goals of treatment are to relieve pain and maintain or restore the function of the arthritic joint. A treatment program may include rest, weight control, heat therapy, exercise, and drug therapy. Appropriate treatment depends on the type of arthritis, the stage of the disease, and the general health of the patient.

Nonsteroidal Anti-Inflammatory Drugs

Nonsteroidal anti-inflammatory drugs (NSAIDs) are commonly used to relieve arthritis pain. These drugs block the production of prostaglandins, chemicals in the body that cause pain and inflammation, which is the stiffness, swelling, and warmth felt by people with arthritis. Although some NSAIDs are available without a prescription, most are prescription drugs. It often takes a few days to a week before NSAIDs start to work and two to three weeks before the full benefits of treatment are felt.

Some of the most frequently used NSAIDs are listed below. These drugs are divided into two groups: salicylates and nonsalicylates. Although both groups of drugs have similar pain-relieving effects, they may have somewhat different side effects.

Side Effects of NSAIDs

Along with much-needed pain relief, NSAIDs may cause unwanted side effects in some people. However, side effects do not occur in everyone. They are listed here so that you will know they are possible and so that you can recognize them early and report them to your doctor. In some cases, it may be necessary to adjust treatment to keep side effects to a minimum.

NSAIDs can cause stomach ulcers. Because ulcers sometimes don't cause symptoms, it's important for people taking NSAIDs to see their doctor for regular checkups. Other stomach problems caused by these drugs include heartburn, nausea, stomach pain, vomiting, diarrhea, and occasionally gastro-intestinal (GI) bleeding. GI bleeding, which can be especially serious for older people, is signaled by black or very dark stools or blood in the stool. NSAIDs also can cause headaches, dizziness, and blurred vision.

Coated aspirin tablets and long-acting aspirin products may lessen stomach irritation. NSAIDs should be taken with a full glass of water (or milk), food, or antacids to reduce stomach upset. In addition, an antiulcer drug—misoprostol (brand name Cytotec)—is approved for preventing stomach ulcers which can be brought on by NSAIDs in people at high risk of ulcer complications (for example, older people or those who have had ulcers in the past). Ulcers and other serious stomach problems are more common in smokers and people who drink alcohol while taking these drugs. People who have stomach problems should see their doctor as soon as possible.

Corticosteroids

Corticosteroids also may reduce arthritis inflammation. These drugs closely resemble cortisone, a natural hormone produced by the body. They can be taken by mouth or by injection directly into a stiff, swollen joint.

Although corticosteroids rapidly relieve the pain, swelling, and redness caused by arthritis, these powerful drugs have serious side effects. Lowered resistance to infection, indigestion, weight gain, loss of muscle mass and strength, mood changes, blurred vision, cataracts, diabetes, thinning of bones (osteoporosis), and increased blood pressure can be caused by this treatment. Other side effects may develop and should be discussed with your doctor. Also, serious stomach problems may occur in people who take corticosteroids along with NSAIDs.

Table 37.3. Commonly Prescribed Corticosteroids

Generic Name	Sample Brand Names
Betamethasone	Celestone
Cortisone	Cortone
Dexamethasone	Decadron
Hydrocortisone	Hydrocortone
Methylprednisolone	Medrol
Prednisolone	Hydeltrasol
Prednisone	Deltasone
Triamcinolone	Aristocort

Disease-Modifying Drugs

Researchers believe that disease-modifying, antirheumatic agents slow the progress of rheumatoid arthritis, but these drugs are not used for osteoarthritis. These prescription drugs include gold compounds, D-penicillamine, and antimalarial medications.

Gold compounds. Gold compounds can help people with mild to moderate rheumatoid arthritis. Auranofin (Ridaura) is taken by mouth. Aurothioglucose (Solganol) and gold sodium thiomalate (Myochrysine) are available in injection form. It may be two to six months before relief is felt. Possible side effects are blood in the urine, easy bruising, sores in the mouth, skin rash, and numbness in the hands and feet. Diarrhea often occurs in those who take gold by mouth, and many people receiving injectable gold notice a metallic taste.

Penicillamine. Penicillamine (Depen and Cuprimine) is also used to treat rheumatoid arthritis. This drug may take two to six months to work. Side effects include blood in the urine, fever, joint pain, skin rash, sores in the mouth, easy bruising, weight gain, and, in rare cases, muscle weakness. People taking gold compounds or penicillamine should be checked regularly by their doctor.

Hydroxychloroquine. Hydroxychloroquine (Plaquenil) and other drugs originally developed to treat malaria can be used to relieve swelling, stiffness, and joint pain caused by rheumatoid arthritis. People taking these drugs should have regular eye exams because these medicines can permanently damage the retina (the light-sensitive tissue at the back of the eye). Diarrhea, headaches, loss of appetite, skin rash, and stomach pain are other possible side effects. Liver problems may develop in people who drink alcohol while taking antimalarial drugs.

Immunosuppressants

The immune system normally protects the body against foreign invaders such as viruses. Some researchers believe that rheumatoid arthritis is an autoimmune disease, a disease in which the immune system reacts against the body's own tissues. Immunosuppressants, drugs that suppress the immune system, can ease the symptoms of rheumatoid arthritis. Azathioprine (Imuran) and methotrexate are immunosuppressants used to treat this form of arthritis. Side effects, which include mouth sores, infection, fever, chills, sore throat, nausea, diarrhea, and unusual tiredness, should be reported to your doctor.

Gout Medications

Uric acid is a normal waste product found in the body. When uric acid levels become extremely high, crystals form in and around joints causing gout. The pain and swelling caused by this form of arthritis are treated with two types of drugs: one to reduce inflammation and the other to lower uric acid levels. For example, colchicine blocks inflammation. Allopurinol (Zyloprim and Lopurin) reduces uric acid production. Sulfinpyrazone (Anturane) and probenecid (Benemid) increase uric acid elimination. Allopurinol, sulfinpyrazone, and probenecid can help prevent gout attacks, but they must be taken for several months to work effectively. (In fact, allopurinol can actually make gout worse if this drug is started during an attack.) Common side effects may include diarrhea, nausea, vomiting, stomach pain, and a rash.

Over-the-Counter Drugs

Over-the-counter (OTC) products such as aspirin and low-dose forms of acetaminophen (e.g., Tylenol) and ibuprofen (e.g., Advil and Nuprin) temporarily relieve minor arthritis pain. "Extra strength" and "arthritis formula" aspirin products contain more aspirin in each tablet than regular aspirin. As with prescription drugs, these drugs can cause side effects, particularly when directions are not followed carefully. For example, long-term, high-dose use of acetaminophen, ibuprofen, or aspirin may cause liver or kidney damage. Do not take OTC products for long periods without consulting a doctor. Combinations of OTC products, or OTC products and prescription drugs, should not be taken without checking with your doctor first.

In addition, some OTC ointments offer short-term relief of minor arthritis pain. However, these ointments, which are rubbed over painful joints, do not reduce swelling and should not be used for long periods of time.

Taking Arthritis Drugs Safely

Because arthritis drugs may interact with other types of medicine, it is important to let your doctor know if you are taking any other prescription or over-the-counter medications. Be sure to follow your doctor's instructions exactly when taking your medicine—take only the amount specified, ask what to do if you miss a dose, and do not suddenly stop taking your medicine without consulting your doctor. It is also important to keep all appointments with your doctor so that your progress can be checked regularly.

Beware of Unproven Remedies

Americans spend over a billion dollars each year on useless pills, gadgets, and diets hoping to find a cure for arthritis. Because arthritis pain can come and go, many people believe that these phony "cures" really work. Beware of any pill or device that promises miracles. Don't be misled by products that are supposed to cure many different diseases. If you have questions about the safety and usefulness of a treatment, ask your doctor. *See the following chapter: "Hocus Pocus As Applied to Arthritis."*

Treatment Without Drugs

Medication at times is not the best or only choice of treatment for arthritis. Physical therapy or surgery may be indicated, or prescribed in combination with drugs. A decision should be made by the patient, physician, and any other members of the treatment team.

- **Physical therapy** can be performed at home or with professional supervision.

- **Rest** is important in treatment of painful, inflamed and fatigued joints, but it can lead to temporary stiffening of diseased joints.

- **Moist heat or cold** often reduces pain and increases the range of motion. A shower, a bath, heat packs, hydrotherapy, and paraffin treatments are examples. Occasionally, for acutely inflamed joints, ice packs are an initial treatment.

- **Exercise** helps maintain range of motion in affected joints. Special daily exercises also can strengthen the muscles that surround an arthritic joint.

- **Devices** like splints, braces and crutches may give relief by resting or supporting painful joints. Aids for daily activity can help by supporting a joint that is painful, weak or impaired.

341

Surgery

Sometimes orthopedic surgery is indicated. Surgeons can correct some deformities, remove inflamed tissue, repair ligament damage associated with arthritis, or replace a diseased joint.

For More Information

Learning about arthritis and arthritis medicines will help you make informed decisions about your health care. The Arthritis Foundation has free booklets on many forms of arthritis and most arthritis medications. This material is available from local chapters, which are listed in the telephone directory, or from the national headquarters at P.O. Box 19000, Atlanta, Georgia 30326; telephone (404) 872-7100.

Free information about arthritis is also available from the National Institute of Arthritis and Musculoskeletal and Skin Diseases, Building 31, Room 4C05, 9000 Rockville Pike, Bethesda, Maryland 20892; telephone (301) 496-8188.

To learn more about drugs and their side effects, contact the Food and Drug Administration, HFD-365, 5600 Fishers Lane, Rockville, Maryland 20857; telephone (301) 295-8012.

The National Institute on Aging (NIA) distributes a number of free Age Pages, including:

* *Arthritis Advice,*
* *Safe Use of Medicines by Older People,*
* *Finding Good Medical Care for Older Americans,*
* *Who's Who in Health Care,* and
* *Health Quackery.*

To receive these publications and other material on health and aging, contact the NIA Information Center, P.O. Box 8057, Gaithersburg, Maryland 20898-8057.

Chapter 38

Modern Treatment for That Old Pain in the Joints

The human skeleton and muscles help to make possible the grace-ful gyrations of the dancer and the prowess of the athlete, as well as the many more mundane movements of our everyday lives. We tend to take for granted the normally smooth sliding motion of our joints until it is hampered. One of the most common ills arthritis affects this vital function. Arthritis is a disorder of the joints, the junctions be-tween bones.

About 50 million people in the United States have arthritis. Al-though many suffer only intermittently, according to the National Institute of Arthritis and Musculoskeletal and Skin Diseases, the con-dition interferes with day-to-day activities for 4.4 million people, and causes partial disability in 1.5 million and complete disability in an-other 1.5 million individuals. The Arthritis Foundation estimates that 70 million person-days of missed work can be chalked up to arthritis in the United States each year, as can 500 million days of restricted activity.

Symptoms of the more than 100 types of arthritis range from mi-nor stiffness to grave disability and deformity. Although arthritis can-not be cured, its course can be slowed and symptoms relieved. And, with increasing understanding of the disease process underlying at least some forms of the illness, the outlook for new, more effective drugs is promising.

FDA Consumer, July August 1991.

The Synovial Joint

Arthritis affects the synovial joint, a liquid-filled capsule built of fibrous bands of connective tissue the ligaments that attach adjoining movable bones. The capsule is lined on the inside with a membrane that secretes the cushioning synovial fluid, which is stored in membrane-lined packets called bursae. In healthy joints between movable bones, only a thin film of synovial fluid covers the surfaces. A decrease in synovial fluid is associated with the joint stiffness that we normally feel as we age. In arthritis, the amount of synovial fluid increases, swelling the joint.

Opposing bones facing a joint are capped by cartilage, a flexible, bloodless tissue. In a healthy synovial joint, the slipperiness of the cartilage tips and the fluid in the joint allow the bones to move nearly friction-free.

Joint deterioration can be hereditary or can result from injury, infection, autoimmune disease (attack by the individual's own immune system), or even a drug reaction. Although the physical changes behind some forms of arthritis are well understood, we know relatively little about how those changes begin.

Of the more than 100 types of arthritis, by far the most prevalent are osteoarthritis (with nearly 16 million sufferers) and rheumatoid arthritis (with nearly 3 million sufferers). It is not surprising that the rarer forms of arthritis may initially be misdiagnosed as one of these more prevalent two.

This was the case with 10-year-old Christopher Green, of Scotia, N.Y., who had a fever for two weeks and then rapidly developed near-crippling arthritis in his legs and hips. Chris's condition was first diagnosed as juvenile rheumatoid arthritis, but the appearance of other symptoms soon led his physicians to suspect Kawasaki disease, a condition first identified in Japan in 1974, where several epidemics have occurred. Kawasaki disease includes arthritis 15 percent of the time. Chris fully recovered the use of his joints after three weeks, and his doctors do not expect the arthritis to recur although the condition is so recently identified that they cannot be certain.

Another rare form of arthritis is on the rise. It begins with infection by Streptococcus pyogenes, also known as strep A. The incidence is 4 to 5 cases per 100,000 people, and the death rate is a whopping 20 to 25 percent. From the initial symptoms of a sore throat and pneumonia, the illness can progress to meningitis (inflammation of the membrane covering the brain). If the patient survives, arthritis may develop.

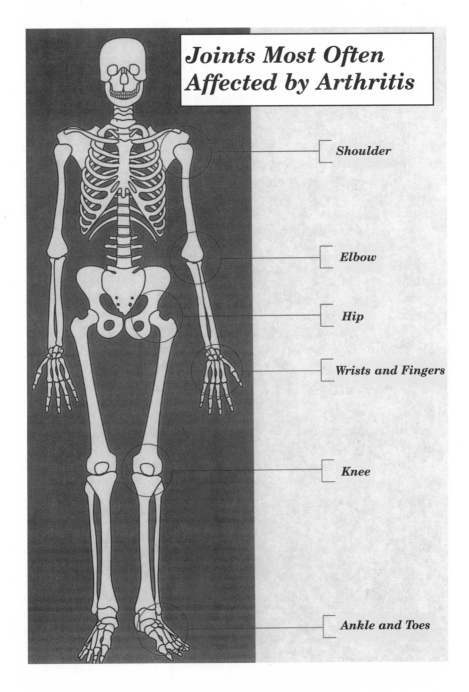

Figure 38.1. Joints Most Often Affected by Arthritis

Setting Therapy Goals

Arthritis therapy aims to protect the affected joints, maintain as much mobility as possible, and strengthen neighboring muscles to minimize loss of function. These goals can be approached by lifestyle changes, use of support devices and drugs, and, finally, by surgery.

Eating fish (such as salmon and other deep sea fish) rich in the oils eicosapentaenoic acid and ocosahexanoic acid improves symptoms of rheumatoid arthritis, says Charles Dinarello, M.D., at the Tufts University School of Medicine. "Our work on the mechanism of fish oil action suggests that its anti-inflammatory properties are at least partly due to lowering tumor necrosis factor," Dinarello says, referring to one of the immune system biochemicals that collects in rheumatoid arthritis joints.

Over the past decade, more and more rheumatologists have suggested that their patients exercise. Regular activity that does not place weight on affected joints, but strengthens surrounding bones, muscles and ligaments, can be valuable for many types of arthritis. With the help of a physical therapist, isometric and isotonic exercises and massaging can be tailored to the specific affected joints. For example, exercise that rotates the neck can relieve stiffness and pain and improve mobility in a person with an arthritic spine.

Devices and Drugs

An "activities of daily living" evaluation can help an arthritic patient identify painful movements, which will assist in the development of devices that can be used at home or in the workplace. A person with arthritic hands might use extensions long handles on utensils and pens. Shelves can be rearranged so that the most frequently used items are within easy reach of someone with arthritic shoulders. Crutches and canes can help those with arthritic knees or hips. Special thumb, hand or wrist splints and gloves can temporarily restore hand function. Wearing loose-fitting clothes that avoid putting pressure on sensitive joints and avoiding obesity make life for the arthritic patient a little easier.

In the 1940s, it was discovered that crude extracts from adrenal glands of animals could rapidly relieve the inflammation of arthritis. In the 1950s, drug companies developed the anti-inflammatory agents cortisone and hydrocortisone. These potent drugs resemble the human adrenal hormone cortisol. But their use is limited today.

"Cortisone has adverse effects that were originally discovered in the early 1950s. It is an immune suppressant, weakening the body's defense against infections," says Dottie Pease, consumer safety officer at FDA's pilot drug evaluation department. Cortisone taken by mouth can lead to osteoporosis, and direct injection into joints can damage the cartilage. Further, it can cause cataracts, skin thinning, diabetes, fluid retention, poor wound healing, and increased susceptibility to infection. Still, cortisone can offer great, albeit temporary, relief.

Today, the first pharmaceutical line of defense against arthritis is the NSAIDs (nonsteroidal anti-inflammatory drugs), which include the salicylates, such as aspirin, prescribed at higher than usual doses. Coated and timed-release preparations can lessen the risk of gastrointestinal bleeding, the major side effect of these drugs.

The NSAIDs block release of prostaglandins, which trigger inflammation. Some more commonly used NSAIDs include ibuprofen, flurbiprofen, indomethacin, and naproxen. Currently, 15 NSAIDs are available.

Drugs called disease modifiers are used in rheumatoid arthritis patients who have had symptoms for at least six months and for whom NSAIDs no longer control swelling of joints. One such treatment is gold injected into a joint, which helps about 50 percent of patients, but unfortunately remains effective in only 5 to 15 percent of them after five years of use.

"No one knows how it works, but it is not an anti-inflammatory," says Pease. The physical presence of gold in the joint may reduce swelling, or the metal may chemically react with a biochemical in some as yet unknown way.

Another disease modifier is methotrexate, an anti-cancer drug that tempers the runaway cell division in the synovial joint. If these disease modifiers do not work, agents that suppress the immune response, such as cyclophosphamide, may be tried.

Biologics Block Cytokines

Unraveling the immune imbalances that underlie some forms of arthritis, and investigating how drugs alter immune function to quell inflammation are opening up an entirely new avenue to treating arthritis the use of "Biologics," or body chemicals. A prime target for new arthritis drugs is blocking cytokine production, a different approach to halting prostaglandin synthesis, which is the mechanism of most existing arthritis drugs.

Innovative approaches under way include work at Nova Pharmaceuticals in Baltimore with unusual amino acids that, in test animals, block the release of inflammation-provoking cytokines from activated

T cells (a specialized type of white blood cell). Laboratory research at Immunex Corporation in Seattle, Synergen Corporation in Boulder, Colo., and Hoffmann-La Roche in Nutley, N.J., focuses on using interleukin-1 to prevent inflammation. Interleukin-1 is an immune system chemical that must bind to the lining inside joints to start the inflammatory process.

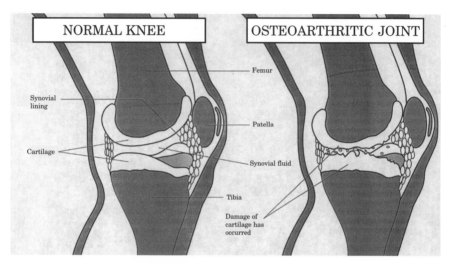

Figure 38.2. *Normal Knee Osteoarthritic Knee*

Joint Replacement

For advanced arthritis, joints can be replaced with synthetic materials, usually metals like cobalt-chrome and titanium alloys in the larger joints and polymers (long-chained molecules) such as silicone in the smaller joints, such as in the fingers. The devices must be durable and must not stimulate attack by the already overactive immune system, interfere with healing, or push surrounding structures out of their normal position.

Before the advent of implants, surgeons would remove joint surfaces, hoping that the scar tissue filling in the area would allow more mobility than the arthritic joint. This type of surgery often failed. Implants proved far more successful. They were pioneered by an army surgeon from Grand Rapids, Mich., Alfred Swanson, M.D. He fashioned the first such devices in the late 1950s out of silicone elastomers, polymers made from the element silicone, which is found in quartz.

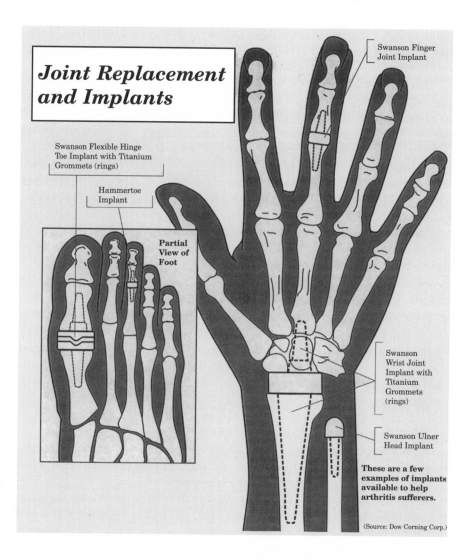

Figure 38.3. Joint Replacement and Implants

Research to fine-tune the implants continued in the 1960s, and in 1969, the first silicone-based joint implants came on the market. These implants provided a flexible hinge for the joints of the fingers, wrists and toes. Since then, more than two dozen models have been developed, several by Swanson, who is now a professor of surgery at Michigan State University. More than a million people have received joint replacements mostly in the hip and they are still based on silicone.

During implant surgery, technically called "implant resection arthroplasty," the surgeon first removes the surface of the joint bones as well as excess cartilage. The centers of the tips of abutting bones are hollowed out, and the stems of the implant are inserted here. Between the bones lies the hinge part of the implant, which both aligns the bones and allows them to bend at the joint. The implant is "fixed," or held in place, with bone cement and, finally, the tendons, muscles and ligaments are repaired. As the site heals, the patient must exercise, but it can take a year of physical therapy to achieve maximum rehabilitation.

A new type of hand surgery replaces joints and realigns fingers at the same time. "All rheumatoid arthritis patients who have a severe deviation of their fingers away from the thumb are candidates for this procedure," says Robert Pearl, M.D., associate professor of plastic surgery at Stanford University Medical Center.

He recently introduced an operation that repositions the tendon at the base of the little finger. He finds that holding the pinky in place forces the other fingers to align properly. Pearl's patients start moving the hand the night after the operation, and wear a splint-like support device for the next three weeks. "By six weeks after the operation, patients are able to do most of their usual activities especially the simple tasks that most of us take for granted, but were virtually impossible for these individuals," he says.

Newer joint replacements use materials that resemble body components. "Recent hip implants have been coated with calcium phosphate materials, like hydroxylapatite, which interact with bone. The aim is to enhance the attachment of the implant to the bone with a biologically active material," says Tom Callahan, Ph.D., of FDA's Center for Devices and Radiological Health. Rather than filling in the spaces with cement, investigators are testing a variety of porous coatings that allow "biological fixation," in which bone can grow into the implant area.

Hope, but No Miracles

Arthritis treatment seems to attract charlatans peddling "miracle cures," folk remedies, and superstition. Over the years, people with arthritis have been advised to cover themselves with horse manure, wear copper bracelets, sit in abandoned radium mines, and swallow any number of magic elixirs.

Although we still do not know precisely what causes this collection of disorders, nor in most cases how to halt its course, modem medicine has an arsenal of treatments available that attempt to make life easier. With better understanding of the immune system's role in the spectrum of arthritis, more treatment options may become available.

Lyme Disease

Bacterial infection was added to the list of causes behind arthritis in 1974, when 30 neighbors in the rural town of Lyme, Conn., came down with a baffling illness. It began with flu-like symptoms and a rash resembling a bull's-eye. This would happen 3 to 32 days following a tick bite, although the person might be unaware of the bite. A few weeks after the initial symptoms, about half of the people developed joint, tendon, muscle, and bone pain, without swelling. In a few, swelling developed, mimicking juvenile rheumatoid arthritis or rheumatoid arthritis.

The first clue that the illness was not juvenile rheumatoid arthritis was, that the cases appeared in clusters. In Lyme and two neighboring towns, 39 youngsters and 12 adults, in a population of 12,000, had the mysterious illness. Normally, juvenile rheumatoid arthritis affects only 1 in 100,000 children. If the illness was juvenile rheumatoid arthritis, the incidence in this area would be 100 times greater than normal. In heavily wooded areas, the incidence was even more striking 1 in 10 children, or 10,000 times greater than normal.

The people with what would become identified as Lyme disease were brought to the attention of Allen Steere, M.D., then a rheumatologist at Yale University in New Haven, Conn., and now affiliated with New England Medical Center in Boston. He eventually put together the pieces to find the culprit a tick. "The initial challenge was to evaluate the clusters of children and adults in Lyme with the unusual form of arthritis. What suggested that it was arthropod [tick] transmitted was the rural setting, the onset in early summer through fall, and the fact that multiple family members were affected yet had onset of symptoms in different years," Steere recalls.

Today we know that Lyme disease is actually caused by a spiral-shaped bacterium (spirochete) harbored in the deer tick, which spends part of its life cycle in mice and deer.

Since its identification, the locations and the number of cases of Lyme disease have continued to increase. In 1983, 48 cases were reported to the national Centers for Disease Control in Atlanta, and by 1986, the number had risen to 439. In 1989, 7,400 cases were reported in 46 states, a 15-fold increase over the incidence in 1982, when national surveillance began.

Antibiotics administered promptly can halt the course of Lyme disease. With later disease and involvement of the heart, brain or joints, antibiotic therapy is not as effective. Once arthritis appears, the joint pain and stiffness can come and go, recurring even years later. Ten percent of those with Lyme disease arthritis are left with permanently stiffened joints. Researchers are optimistic that understanding how joints are affected by Lyme disease may have wide-ranging benefits. "We're hoping that the lessons we learn from Lyme disease will provide helpful clues in studying other types of arthritis," says Steere.

Common Types of Arthritis

The result of any arthritis is painful joints, but the conditions have a variety of symptoms that make them distinguishable from one another.

Osteoarthritis

This most common form of arthritis is also known as degenerative joint disease, or simply the "wear-and-tear" disease, because it tends to affect older people. Even so, osteoarthritis can appear earlier as the result of a metabolic disorder, congenital or hereditary disorders, or injury or trauma. Triathlete Jay Lehr attributes his arthritic knees to old football injuries. However, findings in a variety of studies that relate osteoarthritis to prolonged occupational or sports-related stress have been inconsistent.

In osteoarthritis, the smooth cartilage on facing bone ends wears away, and new bone forms on the exposed ends. This bony overgrowth is a criterion for diagnosis, along with pain when joints move and a grating sensation called "joint crepitus" when the dry, exposed bone ends rub against each other. Osteoarthritis is not usually associated with inflammation.

Darwin J. Prockop, M.D., and his coworkers at Jefferson Medical College in Philadelphia recently uncovered a clue to the underlying cause of osteoarthritis. They examined an extended family of 19, spanning three generations, in which nine members developed osteoarthritis in the fingers, elbows, hips, and knees by their 20s or 30s far younger than the usual onset of the disorder after age 40 or 50.

The researchers zeroed in on a protein called type II pro-collagen. This protein forms coils that intertwine in groups of three to build the cartilage that protects bone ends and reduces the friction in joints. Because of a glitch in the gene that instructs cartilage cells to manufacture collagen, the triple fibrils in the arthritis sufferers in this family unravel after 20 to 30 years. As a result, the cartilage wears down and no longer offers its protective cushion.

Rheumatoid Arthritis

In rheumatoid arthritis, the immune system attacks the joints as if they were an enemy to be vanquished. This autoimmune response is a chain reaction of sorts, for as the synovial joints themselves become inflamed, the swelling weakens ligaments, pushes fingers away from thumbs, and throws muscles out of alignment. This can lead to deformity and disability. Holding a pencil, opening a can or bottle, or even shaking hands become monumental tasks requiring the person to use both hands, often in awkward positions. Rheumatoid arthritis can progressively worsen or stay the same for years before worsening.

Rheumatoid arthritis progresses through five distinct stages.

Stage 1. Stage 1 generally has no symptoms, but deep in certain joints, the cells forming the synovial membrane begin to attract T cells, a specialized type of white blood cell. The T cells and synovial lining cells stick to each other when proteins on their surfaces fit together like interlocking puzzle pieces. Once attached to the joint lining cells, the T cells turn on B cells (another type of white blood cell that makes antibodies that attack the joint) and release small proteins called cytokines. In rheumatoid arthritis, cytokines called interleukin-1, tumor necrosis factor, and gamma interferon are released. Inflammation is detectable by lab results showing elevated numbers of white blood cells in the synovial fluid.

Stage 2. In stage 2, the immune assault gears up. The cytokines attract more white blood cells to the joints, and cause the malaise and fatigue, mild joint stiffness, and swelling that are the earliest signs of the disease. At this stage, more than a billion white blood cells a day collect in a knee joint. The joint capsule begins to fill with scaffolds built of new blood vessels.

Some More Common Forms of Arthritis

Type	Incidence in U.S.
osteoarthritis	15.8 million
rheumatoid arthritis	2.9 million
spondyloarthropathies	2.5 million

Some Less Common Forms of Arthritis

Type	Incidence in U.S.	Age of Onset	Symptoms
gout	1.6 million (85% male)	>40	sudden onset of extreme pain and swelling of a large joint
juvenile rheumatoid arthritis	250,000	<18	joint stiffness, often in knee
scleroderma	300,000	30–50	skin hardens and thickens
systemic lupus erythematosus	300,000 (>90% female)	teens–50s	fever, weakness, upper body rash, joint pain
Kawasaki disease	hundreds of cases in local outbreaks	6 months–11 years	fever, joint pain, red rash on palms and soles, heart complications
strep A infection	100,000	any age	confusion, body aches, shock, low blood pressure, dizziness, arthritis, pneumonia

Table 38.1. *Some more Common Forms of Arthritis. Some less common forms of Arthritis.*

Stage 3. By stage 3, in response to all this activity, the cells forming the synovial membrane begin to proliferate. Symptoms intensify, and drug therapy must start now to prevent irreversible cartilage loss and joint deformity.

Stage 4. In stage 4, the disease process extends to the cartilage, tendons, and, finally, the bone. Joint swelling is far more pronounced. As a result of increased cell numbers and connective tissue, the synovial membrane can weigh 100 times its normal weight. However, the destruction of the cartilage, tendon and bone is by far the most important consequence of the inflammatory process at this stage.

Stage 5. By stage 5, overgrowth of cartilage and destruction of bone are so great that the ligaments surrounding the joint are thrown out of position. The destruction that results is irreversible. The diagnosis of rheumatoid arthritis is based on the presence of all of the following four symptoms, for six or more weeks:

- joint stiffness upon awakening that lasts an hour or longer.
- swelling in specific finger joints or wrist joints
- swelling in the soft tissue around three or more joints
- swelling of both sides of the joint.

The swelling can occur with or without pain. Additional diagnostic signs include x-ray evidence of bone erosion, nodules under the skin, a blood test that reveals a "rheumatoid factor" antibody (found in 80 percent of sufferers), or other key signs of the disease.

Spondyloarthropathies

The spondyloarthropathies are a collection of disorders that tend to affect the spine and include: Reiter's syndrome, psoriatic arthritis, intestinal arthropathy, juvenile ankylosing spondylitis, reactive arthropathy, and the most common type, ankylosing spondylitis, in which the spinal bones fuse. Of the 2.5 million people with these ailments in this country, 75 percent are male.

This particular form of arthritis has been under intense scrutiny since 1973, when researchers in the United States and Great Britain found that 90 percent of patients with ankylosing spondylitis have a protein on their cell surfaces called HLA-B27. The HLA proteins are controlled by a group of genes that oversees immune system function. The HLA protein so common among those with ankylosing spondylitis is found in only 7 percent of the general population, suggesting that there might be a link between HLA-B27 and the arthritis. HLA-B27 is also found in the other spondyloarthropathies to a greater extent than is seen in the general population.

Although the nature of the link between HLA-B27 and the spondyloarthropathies is still elusive, researchers at the Harold C. Simmons Arthritis Research Center at the University of Texas Southwest Medical Center in Dallas recently came a giant step closer to explaining it by introducing into rats through genetic engineering the human HLA-B27 gene. The rats developed symptoms remarkably like their human counterparts persistent diarrhea, skin and hair scaliness, and joint inflammation. The rats with arthritis in their gene will be raised in a germ-free environment from birth. If they fail to develop symptoms, it will mean that an environmental trigger is required to start the disease process.

Commenting on this research, James O. Mason, M.D., assistant secretary for health in the U.S. Department of Health and Human Services, says, "This important work, which could only be performed in animals, holds great promise for helping us to better diagnose and treat these diseases in humans."

— by Ricki Lewis, Ph.D.

Ricki Lewis is the author of Beginnings of Life and teaches biology at SUNY Albany. She was diagnosed as having osteoarthritis while writing this article.

Chapter 39

Unproven Remedies: Hocus Pocus as Applied to Arthritis

You can sit in an abandoned radium mine, hang a Vryllium tube on your lapel, bury yourself up to the neck in horse manure, swill Dr. Fenby's Formula X, or take a dose of "Chuifong Touku-Wan," but you will not be able to cure your arthritis.

It is a distressing fact of life that although there are drugs to relieve the pain and reduce the inflammation of arthritis, there are no cures for most of the more than 100 types of this painful and sometimes crippling disease. Yet many people with arthritis turn to unproven devices and "miracle" cures, such as those mentioned above. They do no good and in some cases can do considerable harm. However, the peddling of these unproven cures is a big business, with more than a billion dollars a year spent on them.

It is not too surprising that this business flourishes. There are plenty of people to prey on, over 37 million Americans suffer from arthritis and related disorders. Arthritis is a chronic condition. Once you develop it, it often stays with you the rest of your life, bringing pain and sometimes disability. Not only are there few cures, but also scientists don't know for sure what causes most types of the disease.

Arthritis apparently has been around as long as man. Bones of the Java Ape Man and Egyptian mummies show signs of arthritic damage. The word arthritis literally means inflammation of a joint. Like many medical words, it is taken from Greek, combining the Greek words *arthron* for joint and *itis* for inflammation. The various types

FDA Consumer Reprint DHHS Pub. No 89-1080.

of arthritis have different causes, symptoms, and types of treatment. Medication, rest, heat or cold, special exercise, and surgery are all used to relieve symptoms. What's best for a person with arthritis depends on an accurate diagnosis of the type of disease that person has. Treatment programs are tailored to fit the individual because the disease varies from person to person, and people themselves vary in the way they react to therapies.

Promoters of unproven remedies don't take such factors into consideration when they peddle their wares. All forms of arthritis are the same to them: One drug or one device cures all. Unfortunately, quacks persist even in this age of enlightenment. In part, that's because arthritis has a way of coming and going unpredictably, an aspect of the disorder known as spontaneous remission. The pain and swelling can simply disappear for days, weeks, months, or even years. People who experience such a remission are easily convinced that whatever they were taking or doing brought relief.

The Food and Drug Administration has long been concerned about fraudulent drugs and devices and has, over the years, taken legal action to get many of them off the market.

One of the earliest gadgets to make its appearance in this country was "Perkins Tractors," two pointed rods about three inches long: one gold-colored, the other silver. A number of conditions—especially gout, pleurisy, rheumatism, violent insanity, "inflammatory tumors" and yellow fever—resulted from a surcharge of an electric fluid in the body, inventor Elisha Perkins claimed. This electricity could be released through drawing the tractors over the affected area. Perkins and his "tractors" were the biggest thing going in 1796.

In the 20th century, people with arthritis have been lured by an astounding variety of quack devices, ranging from simple copper or magnetic bracelets to complex "electronic" mechanisms, such as the Palorator device seized by FDA in 1954. It had two electromagnetic coils that vibrated a couple of knobs on the front of a box. Another was the Gonsertron. Billed as "A New Concept in the Field of Electrotherapy," it was a cabinet filled with various electrical components connected to a chair and, not coincidentally, to the house current. Still another was the Magnetron, a 6,000-volt transformer hooked up to a homemade condenser; the claim was that it provided an adequate and effective treatment for diabetes, tumors, varicose veins, and rheumatoid arthritis. Other such devices are still turning up despite FDA efforts to get them out of circulation.

Things that vibrate—chairs and mattresses for example—also have been "hot" items in the arthritis quack's bag of tricks. The vibrators may produce interesting sensations, but they certainly are not harmless since they could further aggravate already inflamed joints. So too could the Slim-Twist Exerciser, two pieces of wood connected by a ball-bearing swivel joint. Stand on the top piece, pretend to dance the "Twist," and you can lose weight, cure heart and vascular problems, or relieve arthritis, asthma and diabetes, the promoters claimed.

Another popular unproven remedy is uranium. Not only have people sat in abandoned mines to soak up the "curative" powers of this dangerous ore, but they have been hoodwinked into buying mittens, gloves, mattresses, and pads of assorted sizes supposedly filled with radioactive material. What they receive is crushed rock with less radiation than a radium watch dial emits.

According to the Arthritis Foundation, there are some scientific reasons to think that diet affects arthritis, but there is not enough evidence to tell how diet helps or hurts or to recommend any specific diet as a treatment.

Everything from cod liver oil, alfalfa, pokeberries, and blackstrap molasses to a mixture of honey, vinegar, iodine, and kelp have been sold for arthritis diets. At one time "immune milk" was a big item. This supposedly came from cows injected with streptococcus and staphylococcus vaccines. Seawater was highly promoted in the early 1960s by a physician who claimed to have rejuvenated his 97-year-old father with this treatment. Serious complications were reported in cardiac and rheumatic patients who were swept up by what then FDA Commissioner George Larrick called a "nation-wide seawater swindle." FDA went into action in Texas, California, Indiana, Ohio, Pennsylvania, and Michigan to seize about 2,000 bottles of seawater packaged by a Florida laboratory.

Diet cookbooks for arthritics have appeared on the scene, as have special biological health regimens. One book, *There Is a Cure for Arthritis*, recommends a treatment that includes elimination of all drugs, therapeutic fasting, enemas two or three times a day, and a diet heavy in fresh fruits, raw vegetables, herb teas, and other so-called natural or whole-grain foods. Two professors at Rutgers University theorized that arthritis is caused by eating vegetables classed as "nightshades." This includes tomatoes, white potatoes, green peppers, and eggplant. Such treatments have not been studied scientifically.

An offbeat diet might not do too much injury, but an unapproved drug could. Groff's Arthra Tone, Ar-Thry-Go Tablets, Ring's Golden Herb Tonic, Elmore's R'heumative Goutaline, and Dr. Fenby's Formula X are the names of some drugs that FDA and the U.S. Postal Service authorities put a stop to. Many of these "cures" were combinations of herbs, aspirin and alcohol.

Not so innocuous was the Tri-Wonda Treatment, a three-part concoction consisting of one bottle of dilute hydrochloric acid and dilute nitric acid with traces of tartaric and acetic acids; a second bottle containing cream of tartar, senna, sulfur, and phenophthalein, a laxative; and a third bottle containing a 44 percent alcohol solution of fluid extract of Jamaica dogwood, thiamine hydrochloride, and wild cherry flavoring. It took seven years for FDA to get Tri-Wonda off the market, because of legal maneuvering by the manufacturer.

Even more dangerous is Leifcort, a powerful drug and an unapproved arthritis treatment. Leifcort is a hormone compound developed and promoted some 30 years ago by a Dr. Robert Leifmann, who fled to Canada because he was wanted by U.S. marshals for selling a baldness cure. Leifmann prescribed his compound in Montreal until the Canadian Food and Drug Directorate raided his clinic. Charged with marketing an unapproved drug and other violations, Leifmann continued treating his own patients while various appeals were pending.

FDA became concerned about Leifcort after the death of an American woman who went to Canada and came back with a year's supply of the drugs on the strength of a glowing report in a popular magazine. The agency issued press information alerting the public to the danger of this drug.

Leifmann has since died, but his scheme made a comeback a number of years after his death, being sold as "Hormone Balance Treatment," "Holistic Balance Treatment," and "Rheumatril." Whatever the name, Leifcort was sold in clinics often set up in hotel rooms. There the victim got a cursory physical examination and a six-month supply of the drug for $640.

A more recent case of arthritis hocus-pocus involved a "magic wand" type device imported and advertised by a Fort Worth, Texas, firm. Called an Energy Point Stimulator, the device purported to relieve arthritis by applying an electric energy charge to certain "energy points" in the ear. Literature accompanying the device implied that digestive problems could be treated by stimulating the leg, and that migraine headaches responded to stimulation of the lower leg and wrist. A bulk order of the devices seized from Kansas stores was destroyed by court order in June 1988.

Still other recent examples involved unproven arthritis remedies containing drugs or for which drug claims were made. A Phoenix firm agreed to stop distributing two over-the-counter products that contained potent prescription drugs. One, imported from Hong Kong, in tea bag form, was called Chuifong Touku-Wan. In December 1988, the same firm was ordered to pay the government $68,000 in court costs for a newer product called "Earth's Magic" that contained the same two potent drugs.

Drug claims, including arthritis cures, were made for 40 items sold over-the-counter in 1988 by a Utah firm. The items were for treatment of a variety of maladies. The arthritis treatment products were called AR-ALL and ARTHO-Pak. The firm, Nature-All Inc., has agreed to abide by a court injunction against the products.

While no one would consider aspirin an unproven remedy, a number of medical writers have labeled the "glorification" of the more expensive forms of aspirin a kind of medical misrepresentation. Special arthritis-strength formulas are nothing more than plain aspirin with small amounts of caffeine or antacid added. The tablet may be bigger than an ordinary aspirin, but so is the price.

A few years ago, a panel of nongovernment experts evaluating aspirin and other pain relievers for FDA said that terms such as "arthritis strength" or "arthritis pain formula" should not be included in the labels or advertising of aspirin products. Ads suggesting arthritis is a minor disease or that alleviation of pain with "extra strength aspirin" will control the disease could delay proper diagnosis and treatment, the group said.

Arthritis is not a minor disease, but its pain can be relieved and its crippling effects can be prevented in many cases by prompt and proper treatment. People with the disease should be wary of products that offer "special" or "secret" formulas that promise quick or easy cures, and that are promoted by case histories and testimonials. Such products should be shunned or left capped; there are no genies in those bottles, and the products can do more harm than good.

—by Annabel Hecht.

Chapter 40

Nonsteroidal Anti-Inflammatory Drugs

How to Take Your Medicine

How you take a drug can be very important to both its effectiveness and safety. Sometimes it can be almost as important as what you take. Timing, what you eat and when you eat, proper dose, and many other factors can mean the difference between feeling better, staying the same, or even feeling worse. This drug information page is intended to help you make your treatment work as effectively as possible. It is important to note, however, that this is only a guideline. You should talk to your doctor about how and when to take any prescribed drugs.

Generic Names

diclofenac	ketoprofen	phenylbutazone
diflunisal	ketoralac	piroxicam
fenoprofen	Meclofenamate	sulindac
ibuprofen	mefenamic acid	tolmetin
indomethacin	naproxen	

Conditions These Drugs Treat

- symptoms caused by rheumatoid arthritis, osteoarthritis, and other rheumatic conditions, such as redness, warmth, swelling, stiffness, and joint pain

FDA Consumer, June 1990. Nonsteroidal Anti-Inflammatory Drugs.

- menstrual cramps

- pain, especially that associated with dental problems, gout, episiotomy, tendinitis, bursitis, and injuries such as sprains and strains.

NSAIDs are not a cure for diseases such as arthritis. These drugs temporarily relieve pain by blocking the body's production of chemicals known as prostaglandins, which are believed to be associated with the pain and inflammation of injuries and immune reactions.

How to Take

Indomethacin and phenylbutazone should always be taken with food. Meclofenamate may be taken with meals. For other NSAIDs, however, your doctor may tell you to take the first several doses 30 minutes before or two hours after eating. This will help the medicine relieve the symptoms more quickly.

Like food, antacids may prevent an upset stomach when taking NSAIDs. However, both food and some over-the-counter antacids may interfere with an NSAID's effectiveness. Ask your doctor for the best approach for a particular NSAID.

Tablets and capsules should be washed down with eight ounces of water to help prevent the drugs from irritating the delicate lining of the esophagus and stomach. In addition, to let gravity help move the pills along—don't lie down for at least 15 to 30 minutes after each dose.

Be sure to take the right number of tablets or capsules for each dose. Liquid doses are best measured in special spoons available from your pharmacist. Teaspoons or tablespoons from the kitchen drawer are rarely the right dosage size.

Missed Doses

In general, only take a missed dose within two to four hours of its originally scheduled time. However, because the duration of action of NSAIDs varies, contact your doctor for specific advice.

Do not double doses.

Be sure to refill your prescriptions soon enough to avoid missing any doses.

Relief of Symptoms

Most NSAIDs start to relieve pain symptoms in about an hour. However, for long-term inflammation and for severe or continuing arthritis, relief may not come for a week to several weeks.

How long you will need to take the medicine depends on the condition being treated. Make sure you understand your doctor's instructions.

Side Effects and Risks

Common side effects include nausea, cramps, indigestion, and diarrhea or constipation. Other side effects can include increased sensitivity to sunlight, nervousness, confusion, headache, drowsiness, or dizziness. If you have any of these side effects, notify your doctor.

Occasionally, NSAIDs can cause ulcers or bleeding in the stomach or small intestine. Warning signs include severe cramps, pain, or burning in the stomach or abdomen; diarrhea or black tarry stools; severe, continuing nausea, heartburn, or indigestion; or vomiting of blood or material that looks like coffee grounds. If any of these side effects occurs, stop taking the medicine and call your doctor immediately.

Other Serious but Rare Reactions Are:

- **Anaphylaxis**—Signs of this severe allergic reaction are very fast or difficult breathing, difficulty in swallowing, swollen tongue, gasping for breath, wheezing, dizziness, or fainting. A hive-like rash, puffy eyelids, change in face color, or very fast but irregular heartbeat or pulse may also occur. If any of these occurs, get emergency help at once.

- **Sore throat and fever**—With phenylbutazone, sore throat or fever can be early signs that the drug has impaired the bone marrow's ability to produce blood cells. Call your doctor immediately. Because of the seriousness of this side effect, phenylbutazone is usually prescribed as a last resort and then for short periods only.

- **Swelling**—Unusual swelling of the fingers, hands or feet, weight gain, or decreased or painful urination can indicate worsening of an underlying heart or kidney condition. If any of these symptoms occurs, call your doctor.

Precautions and Warnings

- During pregnancy or while breast-feeding, these drugs should not usually be taken.

- People 65 and older are more likely to experience the side effects of NSAIDs and get sicker with those effects than younger adults.

- Alcoholic beverages should be avoided, as they increase the potential for stomach problems while taking NSAIDs.

- Don't take acetaminophen or aspirin or other salicylates with NSAIDs *unless* directed by your doctor. Taking these drugs along with NSAIDs may increase the risk of side effects.

- Tell your physician if you are taking any other medication— prescription or nonprescription.

- Before any surgery or dental work, tell the physician or dentist that you are taking NSAIDs.

- Don't drive or operate machines if the medicine makes you confused, drowsy, dizzy, or lightheaded. Learn how the medicine affects you.

- Increased sensitivity to sunlight can occur in some people. To avoid the risk of a serious burn, stay out of direct sunlight, especially between 10 a.m. and 3 p.m.; wear protective clothing; and apply a sunblock with a skin protection factor of at least 15.

Safety Tips

Don't store drugs in the bathroom medicine cabinet. Heat and humidity may cause the medicine to lose its effectiveness.

Keep all medicines, even those with child-resistant caps, out of the reach of children. Remember, the caps are child-resistant, not child-proof.

Discard medicines that have reached the expiration date.

—by Dori Stehlin

Chapter 41

Corticosteroid Medications

What are corticosteroids?

Corticosteroids are medications often used to treat arthritis and related conditions. These medications are widely used because of their overall effectiveness in reducing inflammation the process that causes the joint pain, warmth, and swelling of arthritis and related conditions. Examples of corticosteroids include cortisone, prednisone, and methylprednisolone.

These medications are related to cortisol, which occurs naturally in the body. Cortisol is a hormone that controls many important body functions. You could not live without cortisol.

Corticosteroids also are hormones, but they are not sex hormones. Sex hormones regulate sexual and reproductive function; corticosteroids do not. Doctors sometimes refer to corticosteroids as steroids. However, corticosteroids are not the same as anabolic steroid drugs that some athletes abuse.

How do corticosteroids work?

Corticosteroids are used in arthritis for two reasons. First, they are anti-inflammatory; that is, they decrease inflammation. Many

---

people who have rheumatic diseases experience a lot of inflammation, which is the process that causes the joint pain, warmth, and swelling of arthritis and related conditions. Inflammation can take place in the joints (rheumatoid arthritis), in the tendons (tendinitis), or in different organs at the same time (lupus). In rheumatic diseases, one of the purposes of therapy is to stop inflammation and the damage it causes. Medications known as nonsteroidal anti-inflammatory drugs (NSAIDs) often are used to stop inflammation, but they may not be strong enough or may have too many side effects. When side effects from NSAIDs present a problem or inflammation is severe and threatens to cause serious damage, your doctor may prescribe corticosteroids to decrease inflammation.

Second, corticosteroids are immunosuppressive. This means that they reduce the activity of your immune system. A healthy immune system helps defend your body against bacteria, viruses, and cancer. However, sometimes the immune system goes out of control and starts attacking the tissues and organs of its own body. This is called autoimmunity, and most doctors feel that with diseases like rheumatoid arthritis, lupus, and vasculitis, the immune system has started attacking the body's own tissues and organs. In these diseases, corticosteroids help by decreasing the harmful autoimmune activity. However, they also decrease the body's helpful immune activity, which can increase susceptibility to infection and interfere with the healing process.

The benefits and the risks of corticosteroid treatment depend upon many factors, including:

- **Dose**. With some forms of arthritis, the treatment may start off with high doses. However, the treatment goal is to find the smallest possible dose that is still effective.

- **Dosage form**.

- **Length of treatment**. This can range from several days to many years.

- **The specific disease being treated**.

- **Individual characteristics**, such as your age, sex, physical activity, and other medications.

Corticosteroid dosage varies from disease to disease and from person to person.

How are corticosteroids taken?

Doctors often prescribe corticosteroids in pill form, but there are other ways of taking them. For osteoarthritis and bursitis, corticosteroids often are injected directly into the joint or bursa; for other conditions, they are injected into a muscle or vein. Doctors may use "pulse" corticosteroids a procedure in which a very high dose of the medication is injected into a vein e.g., when lupus seriously affects the kidneys, nervous system, or brain. Pulse corticosteroid treatment is a serious procedure that involves risks. It should only be used by specialists with appropriate training, preferably in a hospital.

Skin conditions caused by certain forms of arthritis often are treated with corticosteroid creams applied directly to the spot. Certain eye conditions associated with arthritis are treated with corticosteroid eye drops. Some allergies can be treated with nasal sprays. Unlike corticosteroid pills, corticosteroid creams, eye drops, sprays, and injections into joints or bursae are less likely to cause side effects in other parts of the body.

What are the side effects?

When taken as prescribed, corticosteroids can provide welcome relief from pain and inflammation. However, like any other medication, corticosteroids can cause side effects and serious medical problems if not carefully monitored by a doctor. It is very important to understand the differences between safe, proper use and improper use of these powerful drugs.

Most side effects are predictable and related to the dose. Some side effects occur in almost anyone who takes them. Other side effects are unpredictable; they may or may not occur.

Side Effects Associated with Corticosteroid Use

Very Common Side Effects

- **Weight gain**. At first, most of the weight is water retention only, but as time goes by, corticosteroids also may increase your body fat. Corticosteroids also will increase your appetite. Anyone with a history of heart trouble or swelling in the legs should consult his or her doctor, since corticosteroids could affect such conditions.

- **Mood swings**. Some people find that corticosteroids make them feel more positive and uplifted while others feel sad, anxious, or depressed. Nervousness may occur, and difficulty in sleeping is common, especially if a dose is taken later in the day. People with a history of serious mental health problems should consult their doctor about how to deal with these risks.

Common Side Effects (in People Who Take Corticosteroids Continuously for More than a Few Weeks)

- **Mild weakness** in the muscles of arms or legs
- **Blurred vision**
- **Hair growth**: both thinning and excessive growth
- **Easy bruising** of the skin
- **Slow healing** of cuts and wounds
- **Acne**
- **Round face** (moon face)
- **Slowed growth** in children and adolescents
- **Osteoporosis** (loss of bone calcium), especially in women, people with chronic kidney disease, those with a history of osteoporosis in the family, people who smoke, and people who are not physically active

Occasional Side Effects (in People Who Take Corticosteroids for Weeks to Months, Especially at Moderate to High Doses)

- **High blood pressure**
- **Elevated blood sugar**
- **Red or purple stretch marks** on the skin
- **Stomach irritation or stomach ulcers**, especially when also taking aspirin or nonsteroidal anti-inflammatory drugs (NSAIDs)

Corticosteroids can make high blood pressure, diabetes, blood sugar problems, or ulcers suddenly worse.

Less Common Side Effects (in People Whose Corticosteroid Use Is Moderate or Prolonged)

- **Blurred vision** from cataracts
- **Glaucoma**

- **Fractures** due to osteoporosis, most often in the hip and spine
- **Avascular necrosis**, a serious and painful condition that occurs most often in the hip or shoulder when the bone is deprived of circulation
- **Severe weakness** of the muscles (myopathy)
- **Psychosis**, which is a severe disturbance of thinking
- **Serious infections** due to suppression of the immune system

Tips for Taking Corticosteroids

Corticosteroid use is less likely to cause side effects when you take your medication as prescribed and practice healthy habits (exercise regularly, eat nutritious foods, get enough rest).

- Take your corticosteroids and other medications exactly as prescribed.
- Unless told otherwise, take a once-a-day dosage of corticosteroids early in the morning.
- Visit your doctor frequently.
- Contact your doctor if you develop high fevers with chills or shakes, severe pain in a joint or bone, persistent blurred vision, severe muscle weakness or drastic mood changes that affect your behavior.
- Wear a medical identification tag.
- Make sure you eat a healthy diet.
- Exercise to maintain healthy bones and muscles.

Information about Dose Reduction

Stopping corticosteroids can be difficult and dangerous. The patient should follow the doctor's instructions carefully and fully. If the dosage has lasted for only a few days, stopping presents no particular problem. However, after more than a few days, the doctor may prescribe a "tapering schedule" which gradually reduces the dosage and allows the adrenal gland to resume normal production of Cortisol hormones.

If the patient has taken the drug for several weeks or months, stopping will probably trigger "steroid withdrawal syndrome" which involves aching in the muscles, bones, and joints; nausea weight loss; head-ache; and/or fever. Usually these symptoms are not serious and do not last for more than a few weeks. However, if the patient was on a ta-pering schedule and still experiences these symptoms, he or she should consult with the doctor to be sure the disease has not flared up again.

Another method of preparing for withdrawal is the "alternate-day schedule" which uses a higher dose on one day and a lower dose on another. The prepares the body for the withdrawal of the drug while maintaining an effective dosage level averaged over the two days.

A "steroid-sparing agent" supplements the steroid drug during withdrawal. Generally safer than steroids, it still controls the disease and can be supplemented with nonsteroidal anti-inflammatory drugs to control aches and inflammation in joints and muscles. The most common of these steroid-sparing agents are: methotrexate (Rheumatrex®), azathioprine (Imuran®), and hydroxychloroquine (Plaquenil®).

Chapter 42

Methotrexate

What is methotrexate?

Methotrexate is a medicine used to treat rheumatoid arthritis (RA), psoriatic arthritis, dermatomyositis and other conditions. First developed to treat certain types of cancer, methotrexate is routinely used at higher doses as a cancer therapy and is now used at much lower doses to treat rheumatic diseases, like rheumatoid arthritis.

Methotrexate has been studied for more than 25 years in the treatment of rheumatoid arthritis, and in 1988 was approved for this use in adults by the U.S. Food and Drug Administration (FDA). For the purposes of this chapter, the focus will mainly be on the use of methotrexate to treat rheumatoid arthritis.

Methotrexate alters the way your body uses folic acid, which is necessary for cell growth. Methotrexate also decreases inflammation. Scientists suspect that these actions account for methotrexate's beneficial effect on rheumatoid arthritis.

Methotrexate belongs to a group of medicines called second-line therapies or disease-modifying antirheumatic drugs. These drugs may affect the activity of RA to a greater extent than such drugs as aspirin or other nonsteroidal (non-cortisone) anti-inflammatory drugs (NSAIDs). Methotrexate usually is taken along with NSAIDs. It may begin to work as early as three to six weeks after beginning treatment but can take as long as two to three months.

Because methotrexate benefits a high percentage of those who take it and because it is well tolerated, it is a very commonly used second-line therapy. Benefits include a decrease in the number of painful and swollen joints as well as an overall reduction in RA disease activity.

When is methotrexate used?

Methotrexate is used in both children and adults with active or progressive rheumatoid arthritis, although FDA approval is only for adults.

The decision to start methotrexate or any second-line drug is a critical part of the treatment of a child or adult with rheumatoid arthritis. Keep in mind that the decision to begin methotrexate will be based on the opinions of both you and your doctor regarding the progression and activity of your disease. Methotrexate may be prescribed if you do not respond to other second-line therapies, such as anti-malarials or gold salts. If your arthritis is particularly severe, other second-line therapies may be bypassed and methotrexate may be prescribed right away.

How is methotrexate taken?

Methotrexate is taken once a week, either orally (as pills or liquid) or by injection. The tablet strength is 2.5 milligrams, and the starting dose is usually three pills (7.5 milligrams) taken one day a week. The dose may be increased over time to as much as 20 milligrams one day a week if there is no benefit on lower doses. Weekly doses higher than 20 milligrams may occasionally be used.

If taken orally, methotrexate usually is taken all in one dose, although the dose may be split up and taken two or three times over a 24-hour period, once a week. For example, you can either take it all on Monday morning or divide the dose and take a portion of it Monday morning, a portion of it Monday evening and the remainder of it Tuesday morning.

Methotrexate also may be given by injection, either just under the skin, into the muscle or directly into the vein. Injections may be recommended for people who are not responding to oral methotrexate or are developing intestinal side effects such as nausea or stomach upset.

Methotrexate should not be taken more often than one day per week. More frequent administration can be associated with serious side effects. You should take the medicine on the same day each week.

Mark a calendar to remind yourself when to take your dose. If you become confused about when to take the drug, call your doctor to clarify the situation before you take the next dose.

What are the side effects?

Rare but most common:

- upset stomach,
- nausea,
- vomiting,
- loss of appetite,
- diarrhea or
- mouth sores.

Less common

- headaches,
- dizziness,
- mood alterations,
- skin rashes or
- unexplained weight loss
- increased sensitivity to sun
- blood count decrease

  — decrease in the number of white blood cells that help fight infection.

  — decrease in the platelet count or red blood cell count could also occur, which could lead to bruising, bleeding or fatigue. Factors that increase the possibility for these blood cell changes with methotrexate include pre-existing kidney disease, low levels of folic acid, certain infections and the use of certain medications, including an antibiotic called trimethoprim/sulfamethoxazole *(Bactrim, Septra, Cotrim).*

Rare

- lung damage. Call your doctor immediately if you develop a rough, progressive shortness of breath and fever.

- liver damage. Since regular use of alcoholic beverages can increase the risk of liver damage, you are advised to stop drinking alcohol while on methotrexate.

Concerns for Pregnancy and Conception

- birth defects if taken by a woman at the time of conception or during pregnancy.

- lower sperm count in men

Breast-feeding should be avoided while taking methotrexate, because the medicine may be passed to the child through the mother's milk.

Chapter 43

Gold Treatment

What is gold treatment?

Gold treatment includes the use of different forms of gold compounds. Such treatment is beneficial for some types of arthritis and related diseases. Gold treatments are used to help relieve joint pain and stiffness, reduce swelling and joint damage, and reduce the chance of joint deformity and disability. However, taking gold also involves some risks.

When is gold used to treat arthritis?

Many doctors prescribe gold for people with rheumatoid arthritis, juvenile rheumatoid arthritis, or psoriatic arthritis. This type of treatment appears to work best in the early stages of arthritis, but it may be effective in anyone with active joint pain and swelling.

Gold often is used with other medicines such as aspirin and other nonsteroidal anti-inflammatory drugs (NSAIDs) or with cortisone-like drugs, such as prednisone. Doctors frequently prescribe a combination of exercise, physical therapy, and rest along with gold treatment.

Before recommending gold treatment, your doctor or rheumatologist (an arthritis specialist) will consider its risks and benefits and the severity of your condition:

Does gold treatment help everyone?

Gold treatment does not help everyone. Arthritis usually improves in about one-half of all people treated with gold early in the course of the disease. Many people who have had arthritis for a longer period of time also may benefit from gold.

However, two to three of every 10 people do not benefit from gold. Another two to three of 10 people stop taking it for other reasons, such as inconvenience or side effects. It is impossible to predict who will benefit from it and who will not.

How does it work?

It is not known exactly how gold compounds help rheumatoid arthritis. Gold may affect the inflammatory process that causes the joint pain and swelling.

Does it cure arthritis?

Gold does not cure arthritis. However, it does help keep the disease under control. On occasion, some people receiving gold treatment go into remission. However, gold treatment mainly relieves the pain caused by active joint swelling. It also may help prevent future joint damage caused by this swelling.

Gold treatment will not repair or correct existing joint damage or deformities. It will not reduce the disability caused by these problems. Other types of treatment may be available for these problems.

How long does it take to work?

Gold works slowly and gradually. Most people begin to notice a decrease in stiffness, joint pain, and/or swelling two to six months after they start taking it.

How long will you benefit from gold treatment?

The long-term effectiveness of gold treatment varies among different people. In some people, gold continues to be effective for many years; in others, it becomes less effective as time goes on. There is no way to predict how long gold will continue to be beneficial. You should continue to take it as long as your arthritis is under control and you don't have any serious side effects. If you stop taking the medicine while you are feeling better, your arthritis may become active again within several months.

How is it given?

Gold can either be injected into a muscle or taken in capsule form (oral gold). You and your doctor can decide which form is best for you. Oral gold may cause fewer side effects, but may not be as effective as injectable gold.

Injections

Gold sodium thiomalate (brand name, Myochrysine) and aurothio-glucose (brand name, Solganal) are two forms of injectable gold. Injections must be given by a qualified health care professional. This person will give you a small dose to make sure that you won't have a severe reaction to the medicine. Then you'll receive larger doses until the full dose is reached. The frequency of the doses is then adjusted, depending upon how your arthritis improves and whether or not you have any side effects. When things are going well, the periods between injections will be increased, sometimes up to four weeks. Since everyone reacts differently to gold, you may or may not require more frequent injections than others.

You may notice that your arthritis seems worse for a day or two after a gold injection. This does not necessarily mean you must stop taking injections, but you should report these symptoms to your doctor.

Capsule Form

Auranofin (brand name, Ridaura) is an oral form of gold. Doctors usually prescribe two capsules per day. Some doctors prefer to start treatment with a single capsule for the first several weeks. You may be given slightly higher or lower doses from time to time, depending on the side effects and how well your arthritis responds. Never change the dose on your own. Talk with your doctor if you have specific questions about dosage; your pharmacist can answer general questions about the drug.

What are the side effects?

Not everyone taking gold will have side effects. Most side effects are minor, but some can be serious. Side effects can occur at any time during treatment with gold. They may persist for several months after you stop taking it.

Talk to your doctor about the side effects. The benefits of taking the medicine usually outweigh the risks.

Common Side Effects

Contact your doctor right away if you have any of the following side effects:

Rash: This side effect is more frequently associated with injections. The rash usually is itchy, red, and scaly, with bumps. Although it may appear anywhere on the body and can eventually cover the entire body, it usually occurs on the chest, arms, and legs. The rash can be severe and uncomfortable. Generally, however, it is mild and affects only a few spots. It usually goes away on its own within several weeks if gold is stopped. Once the rash has disappeared, your doctor may have you resume gold therapy at a lower dose.

Mouth sores: Similar to canker sores, these painful sores can form inside the mouth.

Metallic taste: This problem often disappears when the dosage of gold is lowered.

Thinning of the hair: Likewise, this problem often disappears when the dosage of gold is lowered.

Diarrhea/loose stools: Diarrhea is a common side effect of oral gold; it occasionally occurs with injectable gold.

This does not mean you'll have to stop taking the medicine. The problem may go away by itself or disappear if the dose is lowered. Taking a bulk-forming laxative may help manage this side effect. If you have diarrhea for more than a few days or if you have severe abdominal pain, bleeding, or other symptoms, contact your doctor as soon as possible.

Nitritoid reactions: These reactions, named because of their resemblance to reactions to nitrites, sometimes occur shortly after an injection of gold sodium thiomalate. You may feel weak, faint, dizzy, or nauseous. Lying down for a few minutes usually helps relieve these symptoms.

Less Common Side Effects

Kidney damage: To detect early signs of kidney problems, urine tests are done regularly during therapy.

Damage to the bone marrow (where the body produces red and white blood cells and platelets): This is uncommon, but can cause serious problems—even death, in rare instances. Your doctor will take regular blood tests to check for this side effect.

Liver, intestinal, and lung damage: These have been reported in people treated with gold, but these reactions are very rare.

If any side effects are severe, your doctor will stop the gold treatment. It takes many months for injectable gold to be eliminated from the body, but complete recovery from the side effect usually occurs much sooner. In the meantime, your doctor may treat serious reactions with cortisone-like drugs or other measures. Some side effects can be relieved by reducing the dosage of gold; others can be relieved by temporarily stopping the gold treatment and later resuming the drug at a lower dose. In either case, a doctor's supervision is necessary.

Drug Monitoring

If you are taking gold, it is important that you visit your doctor on a regular basis. In the beginning, your doctor should obtain a blood and urine sample before each injection or once every four to six weeks if you are taking oral gold. The frequency of such testing usually can be decreased with time. If there are any changes in test results, then the necessary adjustments can be made to the amount of gold you receive.

Chapter 44

Hydroxychloroquine

Hydroxychloroquine (hi-DROCKS-ee-KLOR-oh-kwine) is a medicine sometimes used to treat such rheumatic diseases as arthritis and systemic and discoid lupus erythematosus if other medicines do not work. Sometimes it also is used to treat Sjögren's syndrome and juvenile rheumatoid arthritis. However, it has not yet been approved by the Food and Drug Administration (FDA) for these purposes. It helps relieve inflammation, swelling, stiffness and joint pain. It also is known by the brand name Plaquenil.

Hydroxychloroquine is a disease-modifying antirheumatic drug, or DMARD, available only by prescription. DMARDs are similar to nonsteroidal anti-inflammatory drugs, or NSAIDs (pronounced EN-seds), in that they reduce inflammation. However, DMARDs are slower acting and more powerful anti-inflammatory agents than NSAIDs.

Unlike other disease-modifying drugs used to treat rheumatic disorders, hydroxychloroquine neither increases your risk for infection nor lowers the number of white cells in your blood needed to fight infection.

Dosage is usually once or twice per day but can be once per week. The film coating helps most people digest the pills but they should be taken with food to reduce stomach upset unless otherwise directed by the doctor.

The doctor may prescribe NSAIDs to supplement the hydroxy-chloroquine until it has built up sufficiently in the body to take effect. This can take as long as several months.

When you start taking hydroxychloroquine, tell your doctor about all other medicines you are taking, including prescription and non-prescription products.

Most side effects are minor and short in duration and most people suffer none at all. However, they can occur at any time during treatment or even months after treatment stops. Talk to your pharmacist and your doctor about any side effects that arise.

The following side effects may go away as your body adjusts to the medicine or as the dose is lowered. If they last more than two weeks or if they bother you, call your doctor as soon as possible. Since hydroxychloroquine builds up in the body over time, you can stop taking the drug safely for a few days if necessary to contact the doctor.

- Diarrhea
- Loss of appetite
- Nausea or vomiting
- Headache, dizziness
- Skin rash, itching
- Stomachaches

Rarely, deposits from hydroxychloroquine may form in your cornea. This is the transparent outer covering of the eye. You won't be able to tell the deposits are there, but you may notice a blurry ring around lights. The deposits won't harm your eye. They usually go away six to eight weeks after you stop taking the medicine.

In rare cases that usually follow prolonged or excessive use, hydroxychloroquine may injure the retina, nerves from the back of the eye that enable you to see. Early detection of this unusual occurrence can minimize its damage. Regular visits to an ophthalmic specialist who is familiar with this toxicity help to reduce the slight risk from this medication. Patients who experience visual change while taking hydroxychloroquine should discontinue this medication until the cause of the change can be determined.

If you are pregnant or planning to become pregnant you should discuss the risks of hydroxychloroquine with your doctor. In some cases, the disease may present greater risk than taking the drug and your doctor may suggest a small dose.

Never use hydroxychloroquine when breast-feeding; babies are extremely sensitive to the effects of hydroxychloroquine, and toxic doses in the breast milk can be reached very quickly.

Tips for Taking Medications

To get the most benefit from your medicine, take it as directed. Taking your medicine incorrectly can result in serious side effects:

- Always take the prescribed dose.
  - If you miss a dose, do not double.
  - If you are taking two or more pills per day, only take the missed dose if less than an hour has passed. Otherwise skip the dose and resume your regular schedule.
  - If you are taking one pill per day, take the missed dose as soon as possible and resume your schedule.
  - If you are taking one pill per week, take the missed dose as soon as possible and then resume your schedule.

- Discuss with your doctor any allergies, other drugs—prescription or over-the-counter—and other medical problems especially eye or blood problems, or diseases of the liver, nerves, brain or stomach.

- Keep this medicine away from children.

Chapter 45

Penicillamine

Penicillamine is related to penicillin but has very different effects. (Even if you are allergic to penicillin, you probably can take penicillamine.) Penicillamine is a medication used to treat several conditions, including several kinds of arthritis, Wilson's disease (too much copper in the body), and lead poisoning. It also is used to prevent kidney stones.

Penicillamine is the generic name for this medication available only by prescription in capsule or tablet form; it also is known by the brand names Cuprimine® and Depen®.

This medication is used to treat several forms of arthritis, including rheumatoid arthritis, juvenile rheumatoid arthritis, psoriatic arthritis, and scleroderma. It generally is used if you have active joint pain, swelling, and stiffness or if other medicines do not work for you.

Penicillamine works to produce significant improvement in joint pain, swelling, and stiffness. Unlike aspirin, it is not classified as an anti-inflammatory medicine. Instead, it is considered to be a disease-modifying agent. It is thought to act on the immune system in a way that helps slow down the entire disease process.

However, it takes considerable time to become effective—as much as two to three months. Be sure to continue taking this medicine as prescribed, even if you don't experience any improvement right away.

The dosage is usually once or twice a day and it should be taken on an empty stomach (at least one hour before meals or two hours after meals) and at least one hour before or after any other food, milk, or medication.

You can use other medications for arthritis, but only as your doctor directs. Before you start taking penicillamine, tell your doctor all the supplements and medications you are taking, including:

- vitamins
- minerals, particularly iron
- prescription medications, particularly those containing iron
- over-the-counter (non-prescription) medications, particularly those containing iron

Penicillamine may delay healing so be sure to inform your doctor or dentist you are taking the drug before undergoing any form of surgery.

Caution

Follow the directions for taking penicillamine. Do not stop taking this medication and then restart it without first checking with your doctor. Stopping and restarting your dosage of penicillamine without your doctor's guidance may increase the chance of side effects.

If you forget to take your medicine do not double the dose. Seee the chapter on Gold Treatment for instructions on missed doses.

Side Effects

Penicillamine has several side effects. Some can be serious, so follow your doctor's instructions and visit him or her regularly. Side effects may include:

- Fever, chills and/or a rash that usually occur in the first month or so but may occur later.

- Loss of taste or an odd taste sensation. These symptoms usually will go away even if you continue taking the medication. Sores in the mouth or a sore throat. Sometimes these may disappear if the dose is lowered.

- Upset stomach, heartburn, nausea, poor appetite.

- Protein in the urine, which may lead to swelling of the lower legs. This indicates the kidneys are being affected.

- Muscle weakness. This is rare and usually disappears when penicillamine is stopped.

- Increased number of infections.

- Easy bruising or bleeding.

You'll need to have regular blood and urine tests to be sure that neither your blood nor kidneys are affected. Undergoing these tests regularly helps ensure that no serious side effects have occurred. It may take some time for the side effects to disappear when penicillamine is stopped.

Chapter 46

Surgery

Reasons for and Against Surgery

Arthritis is usually a chronic (lifelong) condition and sometimes can lead to disability and deformity. Most people manage these problems by non-surgical treatment—proper medication, exercise, physical and occupational therapy, rest and joint protection. However, surgery may be necessary if these treatments fail.

Benefits of Surgery

Your doctor and a surgeon will determine if surgery might help you. The decision to have surgery is a major one. It is not a decision to be made quickly. Joint surgery can offer several benefits:

- Improved movement and use of a joint are the most important benefits of joint surgery. Continuous inflammation and the wearing away of bone and cartilage can cause joints, tendons and ligaments to become damaged or pulled out of place. Losing the use of a joint can seriously hamper a person's activities. When this happens, surgery to replace or stabilize the joint may be suggested.

- Relief of pain is also an important benefit of joint surgery. Many people with arthritis have constant pain. Some of this pain can be relieved by rest, heat and cold treatments, exercise, splints and medication. When these therapies don't help, surgery may be considered.

• An improvement in the alignment of deformed joints, especially in the hand, can be expected with some types of surgery. However, this should not be the main reason for surgery.

Your doctor can tell you what to expect from your surgery. In the case of severe joint deformity, you can usually expect to have better range of motion and relief from pain. The joint that was operated on may also look better. However, you won't have a joint as perfect as you did before the damage began.

Before you decide to have surgery, be sure to ask your doctor what all the risks and benefits are of having surgery versus not having surgery.

Risks and Other Things to Consider

As you consider whether or not to have surgery, keep in mind that every person's needs are different. Your doctor may inform you that surgery won't give you the results you want. If your doctor thinks that surgery can help you, there are still many things you need to know.

If you have lung problems or heart disease, the strain of some types of surgery may be too much for you. Before any surgery, it's important to have other health problems under control.

In addition, any type of bacterial infection must be cleared up before surgery. One possible problem after joint surgery is infection, which can spread throughout the body using the bloodstream.

Occasionally people develop blood clots in their legs or arms after surgery. The risk of this may be decreased by using blood-thinning drugs. Discuss this and other potential problems with your surgeon.

Being overweight may put extra stress on the heart and lungs. Also, if the surgery is on a weight-bearing joint (like a hip or knee), recovery of the joint maybe slower. Excess weight puts added strain on the joint and makes it harder to do the exercises needed to make the joint stronger after surgery.

Before you decide on surgery, you must be aware that you have to follow a strict treatment plan after the operation. The operation is only the first step toward restoring joint function.

The amount of work you put into the recovery process often makes the difference between success and failure. Your doctor's orders regarding medication, joint protection, rest, exercise, physical therapy, and the possible use of splints must be followed very carefully. If you don't believe you can follow through on all your prescribed care, then surgery may not be the best treatment for you.

Getting a Second Opinion

If you're not sure about having surgery, ask for a second opinion from another doctor. Ask your doctor to suggest a surgeon with arthritis experience. Sign a release form and ask that your medical records and X-rays be sent to the consulting physician.

Consider the advice of all your doctors carefully.

How Much Will Surgery Cost?

Costs will vary depending on many factors—the surgeon, anesthesiologist, admitting physician, hospital, type of surgery performed, medication, physical therapy requirements, types of implants used and any other special tests or treatments. Check with your doctor, insurance company and (if you qualify) Medicaid or Medicare to find out what your coverage includes. Do this before the surgery so you won't have any unpleasant surprises.

If you've already spent time in the hospital during the year, you should check your insurance policy for benefits coverage during the remainder of the year. You will probably want to check on the managed care requirements of your policy, which may include second surgical opinions and assigned length-of-stay designations.

Types of Surgery

Synovectomy is the removal of diseased synovium. This reduces the pain and swelling of rheumatoid arthritis and prevents or slows down the destruction of joints. However, the synovium often grows back several years after surgery and the problem can happen again.

Osteotomy is the correction of bone deformity by cutting and repositioning the bone, then resetting it in a better position. Osteotomy of the tibia (shinbone) is occasionally performed to correct curvature and weight-bearing position of the lower leg in people with osteoarthritis of the knee.

Resection is the removal of part or all of a bone. This is often done when diseased joints in the foot make walking very painful and difficult.

Resection is also done to remove painful bunions. Resection on part of the wrist, thumb, or elbow can help improve function and relieve pain.

Arthrodesis, or bone fusion, is done to relieve pain, usually in the ankles, wrists, fingers and thumbs. The two bones forming a joint are joined together so that the resulting fused joint loses flexibility. However, a fused joint can bear weight better, is more stable and is no longer painful.

Arthroplasty is the rebuilding of joints. This can be done by resurfacing or relining the ends of bones where cartilage has worn away and bone has been destroyed. It also refers to total joint replacement, where all or part of an arthritic joint is removed and replaced with metal, ceramic and plastic parts.

Total joint replacement has been widely used for many years, and the results are excellent, especially in the hips and knees. Other joints, such as the shoulders, elbows, ankles and knuckles, may also be replaced. With new materials, improved surgical methods and a better understanding of replacement joint function, this procedure has enabled many people who were severely disabled to become more active again.

Arthroscopy is a process chat allows a doctor to see directly into the joint through an instrument called an arthroscope. This is a very thin tube with a light at the end. The arthroscope is connected to closed-circuit television. Arthroscopic surgery can be used to find out what kind of arthritis exists and how much damage is present. Also, the surgeon can perform many other procedures such as biopsy, cutting away a loose piece of tissue that is causing pain, repairing a torn cartilage or smoothing a joint where the surface has become rough. Extensive surgery, such as synovectomy or reconstruction of ligaments, is also performed through an arthroscope.

Arthroscopic surgery does not require as much anesthesia or as much cutting as a standard operation. A person can recover from it much more quickly. The procedure is most often done on the knee or shoulder, but is being used more often on other joints such as the elbow, wrist, hip and ankle.

Preparing for Surgery

Preparing mentally and physically for surgery is an important step toward a successful result. People who understand and are knowledgeable about the process have swifter recoveries and fewer problems.

If you smoke, you should stop prior to surgery. A well-balanced diet is an important factor in general health and becomes especially important in times of stress, such as around the time of surgery. Daily multivitamins may be necessary if you feel your diet is deficient. Vitamin C intake may entrance the healing process after surgery.

Do not take aspirin or aspirin-like medications for three days before surgery. These medications interfere with blood clotting. If you take cortisone, prednisone or any steroid medication, you must tell your surgeon before the operation. These medications should not be stopped before or after surgery.

After Surgery

Depending on the type of surgery, your doctor will usually prescribe a period of rest, physical therapy and limited activity. Before you decide on surgery, make sure your household can be arranged so that your full recovery is possible. You may need days or weeks of rest. In addition, you may need to use splints, a cane, a walker, a wheelchair or crutches before you are able to perform your usual tasks. Talk with your doctor about any short-term limitations and what you can expect during the recovery period. You may also be referred to an occupational therapist for advice on how to do your daily activities in ways that are safe for your joints.

If your surgery involved your hand(s) or arm(s), you will most likely be able to get up the first day after the operation. If it involved one or both legs, how soon you are allowed out of bed will depend on the surgery. You may be able to get up the first day after surgery. Once your doctor has given permission for you to get up, you will begin to feel better the more you move around.

As soon as you're able and depending on the type of surgery you've had, you will begin physical therapy. Be prepared to work hard. If you don't, your repaired joint may be less useful than it could be.

Some pain is common during the early stages of physical therapy. This pain usually comes from the muscles, not the joint. Some of your muscles have not been used much or may have been working in abnormal ways to protect a sore joint. Some muscles may have been cut and stitched during surgery. It is important to realize that muscles strengthen in response to exercise. An exercise that hurts today may hurt a little less tomorrow. You will see improvements in range of motion, along with decreased pain, as you continue therapy.

You will have to work hard for the first few weeks after surgery to achieve range of motion, and a little less so for several months after that to regain strength. Keeping up with your physical therapy requires dedication. You may become bored with the exercises and be tempted to slack off. Don't! Remember it takes time, but the rewards can be great. You should start to see some encouraging results, such as the ability to perform a task that was too painful to do before surgery.

A Final Word about Surgery

Joint surgery is not for everybody. Even if your doctor and surgeon determine your condition would be improved by surgery, the decision to operate is up to you. You need to weigh your options and understand what the surgery will involve—before, during and after surgery, and over the months of physical therapy. Your commitment is the key ingredient in the success of joint surgery.

Chapter 47

Arthroscopic Surgery

The medical technique of arthroscopy produces a clear image of tissue located inside skeletal joints. The arthroscope, derived from Greek roots meaning "to look at joints," allows a surgeon to see within a damaged knee, shoulder or other joint so that repairs can be made with miniature surgical tools. Its advantages include reduced discomfort for the patient, a shorter postoperative recovery and often a better surgical outcome.

A Japanese physician, Kenji Takagi, pioneered the technique in the early 1930s, but it remained a curiosity until one of Takagi's students, Masaki Watanabe, developed the first modern arthroscope more than 35 years ago. Although crude by current standards, it still produced a good image of knee joints. Orthopedists began to take up the procedure widely in the 1970s, when optical fibers made the use of scopes more practical. Today surgeons perform more than 1.5 million arthroscopies every year in the U.S.—and the technique has transformed the discipline of sports medicine.

The procedure begins when a surgeon makes a six-millimeter incision in the knee or other joint. The joint is inflated with a saline solution to provide a working space for the instruments. The surgeon then introduces the arthroscope, a four-millimeter-diameter telescope attached to a miniature color camera. Light channeled through optical fibers in the scope illuminates damaged cartilage. Lenses create an image that is relayed by a camera to a television screen that the orthopedist observes while the operation is in progress. Miniaturized cutting and grasping tools are inserted through other similarly small incisions.

A motorized cutting device, for example, might remove torn cartilage in the knee during a procedure known as a meniscectomy. Before the advent of arthroscopic surgery, a meniscectomy involved a many-centimeter-long incision along the side of the knee, with a recovery period that could last months. An arthroscopic operation requires a recovery period of only a few days. The technique has given meaning to the notion of minimally invasive surgery.

— by Michael A. Pierce

Michael A. Pierce is vice president of business development for Stryker Endoscopy in Santa Clara, Calif.

Chapter 48

Total Hip Replacement

Introduction

More than 120,000 artificial hip joints are being implanted annually in the United States. Successful replacement of deteriorated, arthritic, and severely injured hips have contributed to enhanced mobility and comfortable, independent living for many people who would otherwise be substantially disabled. New technology involving prosthetic devices for replacement of the hip, along with advances in surgical techniques, have diminished the risks associated with the operation and improved the immediate and long-term outcome of hip replacement surgery.

Questions remain, however, concerning which prosthetic designs and materials are most effective for specific groups of patients and which surgical techniques and rehabilitation approaches yield the best long-term outcomes. Issues also exist regarding the best indications and approaches for revision surgery.

As a follow-up to the National Institutes of Health (NIH) Consensus Development Conference (CDC) on Total Hip Joint Replacement held in 1982, the National Institute of Arthritis and Musculoskeletal and Skin Diseases, together with the Office of Medical Applications of Research of the NIH, convened a second CDC on Total Hip Replacement on September 12-14, 1994. The conference was cosponsored by the National Institute on Aging, the National Institute of Child Health

NIH Publication Volume 12, Number 5. Sept. 1994. NIH Consensus Statement.

and Human Development, and the Office of Research on Women's Health. After 1-1/2 days of presentations by experts in the relevant fields and discussion by a knowledgeable audience, an independent, non-Federal consensus panel composed of specialists from the fields of orthopedic surgery, epidemiology, rehabilitation and physical medicine, biomechanics and biomaterials, geriatrics, rheumatology, as well as a public representative, weighed the scientific evidence and formulated a consensus statement in response to the following six previously stated questions:

1. What are the current indications for total hip replacement?

2. What are the design and surgical considerations relating to a replacement prosthesis?

3. What are the responses of the biological environment?

4. What are the expected outcomes?

5. What are the accepted approaches and outcomes for revision of a total hip replacement?

6. What are the most productive directions for future research?

This consensus statement reflects a synthesis of generally accepted observations and recommendations derived from the scientific presentations as well as a general review of current literature by the consensus panel. This panel also identified areas of limited information where further research would be most productive.

What are the current indications for total hip replacement?

Primary total hip replacement (THR) is most commonly used for hip joint failure caused by osteoarthritis; other indications include, but are not limited to, rheumatoid arthritis, avascular necrosis, traumatic arthritis, certain hip fractures, benign and malignant bone tumors, the arthritis associated with Paget's disease, ankylosing spondylitis, and juvenile rheumatoid arthritis. The aims of THR are relief of pain and improvement in function. Candidates for elective THR should have radiographic evidence of joint damage and moderate to severe persistent pain or disability, or both, that is not substantially relieved by an extended course of nonsurgical management. These measures usually include trials of analgesic and nonsteroidal anti-inflammatory drugs (NSAIDs), physical therapy, the use of walking aids, and reduction in physical activities that provoke discomfort.

In certain conditions such as rheumatoid arthritis and Paget's disease, additional disease-specific therapies may be appropriate. The patient's goals and expectations should be ascertained before THR to determine whether they are realistic and attainable by the recommended therapeutic approach. Any discrepancies between the patient's expectations and the likely outcome should be discussed in detail with the patient and family members before surgery.

In the past, patients between 60 and 75 years of age were considered to be among the best candidates for THR. Over the last decade, however, the age range has been broadened to include more elderly patients, many of whom have a higher level of comorbidities, as well as younger patients, whose implants may be exposed to greater mechanical stresses over an extended time course. In patients less than 55 years of age, alternative surgical procedures such as fusion and osteotomy deserve consideration. However, there are no data showing that the outcomes of these procedures are as good or better than those from THR when performed for similar indications. Advanced age alone is not a contraindication for THR; poor outcomes appear to be related to comorbidities rather than to age. There are few contraindications to THR other than active local or systemic infection and other medical conditions that substantially increase the risk of serious perioperative complications or death. Obesity has been considered a relative contraindication because of a reported higher mechanical failure rate in heavier patients; however, the prospect of substantial long-term reduction in pain and disability for heavier patients appears to be similar to that for the population in general.

Thus, although the clinical conditions and circumstances leading to THR are broadly defined, several issues regarding indications remained unresolved. For example, data are insufficient on the associations between potential risk factors (e.g., age, weight, smoking, medications) and outcomes to guide treatment of the individual patient. Moreover, indications are not clear for use of the various surgical approaches and types of prostheses in individual patients. Finally, standardized instruments to measure levels of pain, physical disability, and quality of life as perceived by the patient need to be used to guide clinical decision-making and choice of surgery.

What are the design and surgical considerations relating to a replacement prosthesis?

At the NIH CDC on Total Hip Joint Replacement held in 1982, aseptic loosening was identified as a major problem with THR. It was especially prevalent in young, active patients and after revision surgery. Because it appeared with increasing frequency over time, it was feared that a much larger problem would emerge. Newer fixation (cement and cementless) techniques had been introduced, but their long-term efficacy was unknown. Cobalt-, titanium-, and iron-based alloys, higher molecular weight polyethylene, and autocuring polymethyl-methacrylate (PMMA) bone cement were the materials used in most implants. Chemical modifications and altered processing of the alloys had been introduced to deal with the problem of fractured stems.

As of 1994, state of the art pertaining to THR has changed substantially. For example, changes have been made in fixation (cement and cementless), device designs, and some materials (see the THR schematic drawing shown in Figure 48.1). Concerns remain about the in vivo durability of femoral and acetabular components of the implants, but the procedure has a more predictable outcome. The newer cementing techniques have proven to be more successful than the original ones on the femoral side. Improved techniques include the use of a medullary plug, a cement gun, lavage of the canal, pressurization, centralization of the stem, and reduction in porosity in the cement. However, the optimum cement-metal interface has yet to be identified. These newer procedures minimize defects and localized stress concentrations in the cement. Their current success indicates

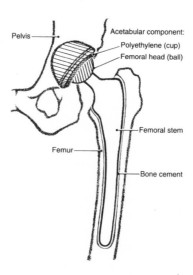

Figure 48.1.

that previously observed aseptic loosening within the first 10 years following implantation was primarily a mechanical process and that steps to reduce stresses in the materials and improve strength of the interfaces are reasonable to reduce loosening. Further optimization of the bone implant interface constitutes an important opportunity for future research.

Another important change in fixation has been the introduction and widespread use of noncemented components that rely on bone growth into porous or onto roughened surfaces for fixation. In the femur, selected cementless components have exhibited clinical success, although with shorter follow-up, similar to that of cemented components installed with the newer cementing techniques. There is evidence that bone changes (osteolysis or bone resorption) can occur as well with some of the cementless components. Numerous reports document resorption, and although it has not usually become symptomatic during early stages of follow-up, concerns nevertheless exist about progressive osteolysis and consequent aseptic loosening or fracture.

On the acetabular side, the cementless components have demonstrated less aseptic loosening compared with the cemented components over the short term, although long-term results are not yet available. The prospective and retrospective studies conducted have been specific to device design and technique, and any general comparison of cemented and noncemented systems should be viewed with caution.

The implants themselves have undergone multiple changes. As a result of improved alloys and designs, fracture of femoral stems is no longer a significant problem. Stem cross-sections have been rounded to avoid high stresses in the cement. There is still controversy over the appropriate length of uncemented stems and the extent and location of porous or roughened regions. Metal backing of cemented acetabular components has not been associated with a high degree of success and is now used infrequently. Metal-backed acetabular components with porous coatings have demonstrated good to excellent results in regard to loosening noted at 5- to 7-year follow-up and continue to be followed. Modular components have been introduced and are widely used, but it is recognized that in vivo disassembly, fretting and corrosion, and wear between components can be a source of debris and may contribute to osteolysis and isolated implant fractures. Given the potential problems, routine use of modular components needs to be evaluated specific to particular applications. There appears to be little justification for modularity or customization of femoral stems below the head-neck junction in primary THR, although the modular stem components for revisions may be useful.

Revision rates for cemented femoral components, using modern techniques, have been reported to be less than 5 percent at 10-year follow-up; revision rates for uncemented acetabular components are approximately 2 percent at 5-year follow-up. To be deemed efficacious, new design features should be shown to have a mechanical failure rate equal to or lower than these figures.

As in 1982, the primary implant materials are cobalt- and titanium-based alloys, PMMA bone cement, and ultra-high molecular weight polyethylene. These continue to demonstrate biocompatibility in bulk, but particles of these materials, particularly the polyethylene, are suspected to have a role in bone resorption and potential implant loosening. Osteolysis that can occur with both cemented and cementless components on both the femoral and acetabular sides is thought to be due to an inflammatory process brought on by particulate matter. The articulating surfaces between the femoral and acetabular components are now recognized as a major source of debris, which has been shown to be important in this pathologic tissue response. Most components for femoral heads have polished cobalt alloy, which articulates with polyethylene sockets. Longitudinal research continues on smoothness and ion implantation of the articulating surfaces, ceramic-polymer, ceramic-ceramic, and alloy-alloy components, although the in vivo data remain limited at this time. Efforts to alter or replace the polyethylene are under way, but no new materials with reduced clinical wear rates are routinely available.

Several factors have been suggested to minimize the production of wear debris. Polyethylene acetabular cups with minimum wall thickness of 6 mm and femoral heads with diameters of 28 mm are important design considerations associated with reduced wear. Where metallic shells are used to contain the polyethylene cup, the interior of the shell should be smooth with a minimum number of openings for screws, and the polyethylene liner should be highly conforming and mechanically stable. Polyethylene of the highest quality is strongly advised for the manufacture of the components. Femoral heads with highly polished cobalt alloy, or polished ceramics as some data suggest, may be advantageous to minimize effects of wear on the polyethylene surface.

Studies also continue on surface modifications of implants to provide direct attachment to bone. For example, several types of calcium phosphate ceramics (CPC) (often called hydroxylapatite) have been added as coatings to THR surfaces to enhance fixation of non-ingrowth implants to bone. Concerns have been expressed about the longer term in vivo fatigue strengths of the substrate to coating interfaces, biodegradation, and the potential for generating ceramic particulates, although so far data addressing implant performance are comparable to those from other device designs at the same follow-up times. Research and development on the enhancement of bone growth into porous biomaterials using CPC has also shown promise, although longitudinal data are incomplete at this time. Long-term data are needed on the benefit-to-risk ratio of clinical outcomes for these types of surface modifications.

Although there are in vitro tests for evaluating implant design features and material characteristics, as well as animal testing regimens, the relevance of these tests to in vivo human performance are often unknown and additional approaches are necessary. Long-term clinical studies are the only accepted method for evaluating the efficacy of the design and materials in human use, particularly with regard to patient-defined outcome measures. Since these take many years and are very expensive, few implant design features are supported by well-designed studies.

Adaptive bone remodeling around the prosthesis continues to be a concern, but there is little evidence that it is a significant clinical problem during the first 10 years of follow-up. Joint forces are known with better confidence than in 1982, but it is still unknown which elements of force, magnitude, and time are relevant to implant failures. Detailed analysis of stress distribution is still limited by imprecise data on joint forces, viscoelastic properties, and failure modes of the materials and tissues.

In 1994, the main problems of concern related to implant design are long-term fixation of the acetabular component, osteolysis due to particulate materials, biologic response to particles of implant materials, and the less favorable results of revision surgery.

What are the responses of the biological environment?

Since the NIH CDC on Total Hip Joint Replacement held in 1982, bone resorption, or osteolysis, has emerged as the major concern with regard to the long-term survival of total hip arthroplasty. Significant resorption and massive osteolysis as well as more limited areas of bone destruction had been associated with cemented components and attributed to cement debris. Subsequent findings confirm that similar problems can be associated with cementless prosthetic implants, and some degree of osteolysis may be present in up to 30-40 percent of cases within 10 years of surgery. Both acetabular and femoral components may be affected. Components may remain well fixed in the presence of significant bone loss, but indications are that once osteolysis appears it tends to progress and may ultimately lead to implant failure. This bone loss is now considered to be a reaction to particulate matter derived from the implanted prosthetic components as well as the cement when used. Because osteolysis is an important contributor to failure of hip arthroplasties and may occur in the absence of clinical symptoms, it is important that patients with implants be followed and evaluated at regular intervals throughout life to ensure timely operative intervention, if necessary.

Quantitatively, the material causing the most tissue reaction appears to be particulate polyethylene. These particles have been recovered in significant quantities from periprosthetic tissues, including sites remote from the source. Particle size varies, but the majority recovered are approximately 0.5 micron, with 90 percent less than 1.0 micron. It has been estimated that the average rate of wear for cobalt alloy-to-polyethylene interface is 0.1-0.2 mm/year. The volume of wear debris may increase with larger femoral head size.

Metallic debris has also been identified in significant quantities. The source may be related to stem-bone fretting, particularly in loose prostheses and in more distal portions of proximally fixed prostheses where significant motion between stem and bone may persist. With the use of modular prostheses, corrosion and/or fretting have been identified in up to 35 percent of some retrieved specimens, and these connections could serve as a source of metallic particles. Fretting and corrosion are not limited to the interface between dissimilar alloys. Interactions have also been identified with cobalt-cobalt and titanium-titanium as well as titanium-cobalt alloy junctions. Reactions at the head-neck junctions have been studied in depth. Corrosion and wear debris products can also form at the interfaces between screws and acetabular shells and at modular collars for adapting proximal femoral stems. Some of the metallic particles generated may be larger than the polyethylene debris. The major effect of these larger metallic debris may relate to promoting third body wear of the polyethylene, with the derivative polyethylene particles of submicron size triggering the cellular response. However, smaller metal particles and ions have been demonstrated to be active in direct stimulation of biologic processes.

The leading hypothesis to explain the development of massive osteolysis is that particulate matter derived from prosthetic components and cement stimulates an inflammatory response. Phagocytosis of the particles by macrophage and foreign-body giant cells (arising from the macrophage) appears to be the initial biologic response to particulate matter. The presence of intracellular particles is associated with the release of cytokines and other mediators of inflammation. These factors initiate a focal bone resorptive process largely mediated by osteoclasts. These osteoclasts do not contain debris particles.

Thus, the long-term threat to component failure from a biologic standpoint appears to be wear-debris-associated periprosthetic osteolysis as a result of osteoclastic activity. This is stimulated by cytokines such as tumor necrosis factor, interleukins, and prostaglandins released by macrophages and possibly other cells including fibroblasts. The critical initiating sequence involves the interaction between small particulate materials and responding cells. The process is affected by the number, size, distribution, and type of particulate material, as well as responsiveness of the ingesting cells.

The debris may be distributed beyond the hip joint. Material has been identified in distant lymph nodes, but no systemic consequences are documented up to this time. Since it is now recognized that both cobalt- and titanium-based alloys release soluble products in patients, long-term surveillance to assess possible systemic and remote side effects after THR is advisable.

Adaptive bone remodeling occurs in the proximal femur in response to an altered mechanical environment following hip replacement. This process is commonly referred to as "stress shielding" or stress transfer. Stem rigidity or elasticity plays a major role. Bone resorption in unstressed areas is a common observation, but it has not been shown to be related to loosening. Nevertheless, it presents an important concern in terms of long-term stability and effect on revision surgery.

Factors influencing adaptive bone remodeling have been considered in determining the location and extent of porous coating on uncemented stems. Finite element analysis suggests that proximally coated porous stems are associated with less cortical bone stress shielding than fully coated stems, but the extent of coating on most currently used prosthetic stems is still greater than that calculated necessary to significantly reduce the stress-shielding effect on the proximal femur. Decreasing porous coating to reduce stress shielding must be weighed against providing sufficient coating to ensure fixation. Efforts to reduce stem stiffness have been shown to lessen proximal cortical atrophy under experimental conditions.

What are the expected outcomes?

The success of THR in most patients is strongly supported by nearly 30 years of follow-up data. There appears to be immediate and substantial improvement in the patient's pain, functional status, and overall health-related quality of life. Promising data suggest that these immediate improvements persist in the long term. Over the last two decades, complications associated with THR have declined significantly. Prophylactic antibiotic therapy has helped to prevent infection. Use of anticoagulants in the perioperative period has reduced deep venous thrombosis and pulmonary emboli. The incidence of mechanical loosening has decreased with the introduction of improved fixation techniques. More than 90 percent of all artificial joints are never revised. Rates of revision are decreasing with improved surgical techniques.

The important questions of today are not whether THR is effective compared with no treatment but rather which technology and methodology used for THR are best for a particular patient. For example, the various total hip designs, fixation methods, and surgical techniques need to be rigorously compared with one another. Surgeon's experience and hospital environment should be investigated for possible independent effects. Various rehabilitation interventions, including long-term therapeutic exercise, should be evaluated for effectiveness. Similarly, little is known about patient-level predictors of outcome, e.g., patient expectations, quality of the individual patient's bone stock, demographic characteristics, comorbidities, obesity, and activity level.

Since length of acute hospital stay has become progressively shorter, more emphasis must be given to determining the role of preadmission educational programs, appropriate physical therapy, and rehabilitation during the acute stay and following discharge. Home health programs when indicated may be more effective than prolonged hospitalization. The benefits of a long-term therapeutic exercise program for patients who have undergone THR have not been clearly demonstrated to improve mobility or hip stability. There appears to be insufficient appreciation for the role of exercise in THR rehabilitation; however, there is evidence that hip weakness persists up to 2 years after surgery in the presence of a normal gait. Multiple studies have demonstrated that weakness in the lower extremities is a major risk factor for falls in the geriatric age group. Thus, further studies are needed to assess the relationship between muscle function following THR, mobility, and risk for falls, as well as the role of therapeutic exercise in improving muscle function, with enhancement of mobility and stability.

Outcome assessment in THR has been limited by the lack of standardized terminology and by the use of various scales that have traditionally relied on the surgeon's assessment of the patient's pain, range of motion, muscle strength, and mobility. Most of these measures have not been adequately characterized in terms of validity, reliability, and responsiveness to change. The traditional assessments have not included patient-oriented evaluation of function or satisfaction. There is no consensus on the standard definitions of endpoints with respect to prosthesis failure. The American Academy of Orthopaedic Surgeons has developed recommendations for data to be collected, and this approach should be endorsed for use in clinical practice. The patient's functional status should be further assessed in follow-up by standardized, patient-reported, disease-specific measures and by at least one global outcome measure. Finally, the radiographic and clinical criteria for prosthesis failure should be defined.

Long-term follow-up is essential to determining outcomes and pathological processes (e.g., failures related to osteolysis and particulate debris). These complications were not emphasized in the 1982 CDC on Total Hip Joint Replacement. The problems have been identified only by long-term follow-up of patients.

Methodological issues that have limited THR outcomes assessment include lack of randomized trials and other well-controlled studies, lack of well-characterized patient cohorts for prospective observational studies, and insufficient sample sizes followed for prolonged periods of time.

THR is performed more than 120,000 times per year in the United States. This represents a 64-percent increase in the number of THR procedures per year in the United States since the 1982 CDC. Analysis of Medicare claims data demonstrates significant variations in the rates of performance of THR with respect to geography, age, gender, and race. The highest rates of THR are in the Midwest and Northwest and the lowest rates in the South and East. A fourfold difference exists between the State with the highest rate of THR (Utah) and the State with the lowest rate (Wyoming). A previous study demonstrated a 50-percent higher rate of THR in Boston, Massachusetts, compared with New Haven, Connecticut. Other procedures such as hip fracture repair have very low variation from one geographical area to another. In today's era of cost-containment and outcomes research, it is important to understand the factors contributing to these wide area variations as well as which rate of THR is most appropriate.

Sixty-two percent of all THR procedures in the United States are performed in women. Furthermore, women have significantly worse preoperative functional status than do men and are 35 percent more likely to report the use of a walking aid at the time of surgery. These differences persist even after adjustment for other demographic and clinical characteristics. These data suggest that, compared with men, women are being operated on at a more advanced stage of the disease. Two-thirds of all THR procedures are performed in individuals who are older than 65 years of age. The rate of THR increases for patients up to 75 years of age and then declines. The highest age-specific incidence rates of THR are between 65 and 74 years of age for men and 75 and 84 years of age for women. Recent comparisons of rates of THR reveal that more are being done in the young and in the oldest patients. Among the older patients, there has been an increase in THR in patients with more comorbidities.

Most THR procedures are performed in whites. The prevalence rate of hip implants (fixation devices and artificial joints) was 4.2 per 1,000 in whites compared with 1.7 per 1,000 in African-Americans. The disparity by race increases markedly with age. These findings were confirmed by an analysis of Medicare claims data that focused solely on THR. Observed differences in the rate of THR by race may reflect a disparity in access or referral for care for African-Americans. Additionally, individuals with higher income were 22 percent more likely to undergo THR than were individuals with low income. Health care providers and patients must be cognizant of the variations in the THR rate. It is important to carefully consider the potential influence of access to care, treatment selection biases, and patient knowledge and preferences on these variations in rates.

In this era of cost-containment and managed care, the ultimate selection of a THR system should be based on individualized patient needs, safety, and efficacy. There is consensus that the THR patient requires periodic follow-up including appropriate x-ray examination throughout life. Periodic follow-up, perhaps at 5-year intervals after the first 5 years, could allow identification of osteolysis and other indicators of impending failure in their earliest forms and permits institution of treatment before catastrophic failure.

What are the accepted approaches and outcomes for revision of a total hip replacement?

As more primary THRs occur on a cumulative basis, as indications extend to more conditions and to older and younger individuals, and as the population ages, the absolute number of revision hip replacements will increase, even if the frequency of failures in primary procedures continues to decrease. Revision surgery is highly complex and costly and requires considerable scientific and technical expertise, an array of expensive technological options, a supportive health care

410

environment, and a skilled health care team. Consequently, issues such as the surgeon's experience, the hospital characteristics, the related health care costs, and appropriateness of current hospital reimbursements associated with revision should be carefully examined.

Currently, the results of revision THR are inferior to those of primary procedures. It remains important to refine the indications for revision and to do so on the basis of the best available outcome data. Not all "failed" primary THRs require revision. The decision to revise, as is true of decisions regarding primary procedures, must consider such circumstances as the presence of disabling pain, stiffness, and functional impairment unrelieved by appropriate medical management and lifestyle changes. In addition, radiographic evidence of bone loss or loosening of one or both components should be present. Indeed, evidence of progressive bone loss alone provides sufficient reason to consider revision in advance of catastrophic failure. Fracture, dislocation, malposition of components, and infection involving the implant are other reasons to consider revision.

A number of options must be considered in planning a revision operation. The selection of specific technology is currently a judgment of the surgeon and depends on the amount and quality of the bone stock, the age and functional demands of the patient, and the reason for failure of the primary procedure. The weight of clinical experience suggests that a loose acetabular component, either cemented or porous coated, can be reliably replaced by a porous-coated component in the presence of adequate bone stock. In one study using this approach, 91 percent of implants were radiographically stable and 9 percent required re-revision (for dislocation and infection rather than aseptic loosening) between 8 and 11 years after revision. In elderly patients with lower functional demands and those with osteogenic bone, cemented implants have also provided satisfactory results. To achieve prosthetic stability in the absence of sufficient bone stock, deficits can be filled with morselized or structural bone grafts (either autografts or allografts obtained from accredited tissue banks), customized metal components, or, under some circumstances, bone cement.

The approach to revision of the femoral component must be based on the nature of the remaining bone stock in the proximal femur, and clinical judgment usually takes into account the age and functional demands of the patient. Under many circumstances, revision of the femoral component with a cemented stem is possible using modern cementing techniques. The re-revision rate for this approach is between 10 and 18 percent at 10- to 11-year follow-up.

An acceptable alternative approach to revision of femoral components when there is substantial residual bone stock has been the use of noncemented implants, particularly the extensively coated components. This approach has resulted in 90-percent stem survivorship at a 9-year follow-up.

Morselized bone graft can be used successfully to fill defects in the femoral canal with or without the use of bone cement, and cortical bone can be augmented with only grafts as necessary. Under exceptional circumstances, it may be necessary to use large structural allografts when the proximal femoral bone stock deficiency is substantial. If this is done, the implant should be cemented into the graft.

Both the diagnosis and the treatment of infected implants remain challenging. The infection rates of the past have been dramatically reduced. Current infection rates of less than 1 percent at one year after primary THR are now being reported. Nonetheless, infection remains a devastating complication, and treatment alternatives remain controversial. Recovery of the infecting organism is essential to the selection of appropriate antibiotics and the planning of surgical approaches. For organisms highly susceptible to multiple antibiotics, one-stage surgical approaches that combine extensive debridement and an ensuing exchange of implants are associated with a 77- to 94-percent success rate. Two-stage revisions that include at least four weeks of appropriate antibiotic treatment following implant removal and wound debridement and a variable period of time before reinsertion determined by the characteristics of the organism have resulted in a success rate greater than 80 percent. In young people, there may be value to a third, intermediate stage in which the bone stock is augmented in anticipation of later reimplantation.

What are the most productive directions for future research?

THR is acknowledged as a highly successful procedure that has provided relief of pain, increased mobility, and improved tolerance for activity for thousands of people. Despite the advances made in the past decade, obvious deficiencies in knowledge remain regarding treatment alternatives, patient characteristics, and environmental issues. To address these concerns most effectively, it is important to identify those avenues of investigation that will lead to decreased morbidity and enhanced quality of life for the population at large affected by debilitating hip disease.

Standardized instruments for assessing outcomes need to be developed, validated, and introduced into clinical use. These may also be useful in developing guidelines for surgery and in making physicians aware of their patients' physical capabilities and expectations.

The issues of age, sex, weight, activity level, and comorbidities have been implicated for their effects on the outcome of THR and need to be studied in relation to the indications for surgery and timing of the procedure.

Serious questions have been raised concerning the disparate rates for THR between racial groups and geographic locations that seem to have no direct relationship to incidence of disease. In-depth analysis of rate differential can lead to an identification of underlying reasons. In this way, the benefits of THR can be extended to an appropriate segment of the population that appears to have limited access.

Materials currently used for the manufacture of THR implants have been improved with regard to design and finish. Wear debris, however, remains a factor that affects the durability of the implants and their fixation. Research is ongoing and support is needed to expand investigations of new materials and to create a better understanding of wear processes that can prolong the life of the implant and reduce the wear and wear products.

One of the necessary approaches for evaluating implant failure modes is an organized, ongoing analysis of in situ prostheses retrieved from cadavers. Such a program should be national in scope and supported by grant monies. As part of this effort, it is anticipated that significant data could be obtained concerning wear processes involving the articular surfaces under circumstances where the implant did not fail. At the same time, this avenue of research would further clarify the device and tissue interactions that are characteristic of the cemented and noncemented types of devices.

Randomized clinical trials are needed to determine the efficacy of implant designs and surgical approaches, including the effect of coatings that encourage appositional or interpositional bone growth for fixation.

The contribution of prehospital, inhospital, and posthospital education and rehabilitation programs to the eventual outcome of the surgical procedure deserves an organized, in-depth study to determine optimum regimen, duration of treatment, and expected outcomes. Clinical data suggest that potential capabilities of the patients are not being fully developed.

The biologic interface between the implant and the host bone has been recognized as a source of potential failure. Basic research efforts into the mechanisms by which these changes occur are providing some clues, but much more needs to be known about specific cellular mechanisms associated with osteolysis, suggested immunologic or inflammatory responses, and the reactions to varying stresses encountered by the bone. In addition, further investigation should be encouraged into the ways by which the local inflammatory response to particulate matter could be modified by regional or systemic interventions.

As the indications for THR are extended into the younger age group, patients with THR will be exposed to more rigorous environmental demands, both occupational and recreational. Investigations are needed into the environmental modifications, activity limitations, or types of physical effort that contribute to extended prosthesis survival. Physical conditioning activities—muscle development, improvement in coordination, and exercises that enhance bone integrity without affecting fixation—need to be studied as they relate to the anticipated lifestyle and occupational objectives of the patient.

Outcomes of revision hip surgery are less reliable and satisfactory than those of primary procedures. Those biologic, biomechanical, and rehabilitation factors that influence these results need to be explored and solutions developed.

Regional or national registries should be established to capture a minimum data set on all THR and revision procedures. The goals of this registry should be to better define the natural history and epidemiology of THR in the U.S. population as a whole and to identify risk factors for poor outcomes that relate to the implant, procedure, and patient characteristics.

Conclusions

- THR is an option for nearly all patients with diseases of the hip that cause chronic discomfort and significant functional impairment.

- In the aggregate, THR is a highly successful treatment for pain and disability. Most patients have an excellent prognosis for long-term improvement in symptoms and physical function.

- Perioperative complications such as infection and deep venous thrombosis have been significantly reduced because of use of prophylactic antibiotics and anticoagulants and early mobilization.

- The predominant mode of long-term prosthetic failure appears to be related to generation of particulate matter, which in turn causes an inflammatory reaction and subsequent bone resorption around the prosthesis.

- Revision of THR is indicated when mechanical failure occurs. The surgery is technically more difficult and the long-term prognosis is generally not as good as for primary THR. The optimal surgical techniques for THR revision vary considerably depending on the conditions encountered. Continued periodic follow-up is necessary to identify early evidence of impending failure so as to permit remedial actions before a catastrophic event.

- Improved methods for evaluating existing technology should be developed and implemented, especially with respect to patient-defined outcomes.

- Future research should focus on refining indications for surgery; defining reasons for differences in procedure rates by age, race, gender, and geographic region; developing surgical techniques, materials, and designs that will be clearly superior to current practices; understanding the inflammatory response to particulate material and how to modify it; determining optimal short- and long-term rehabilitation strategies; and elucidating risk factors that may lead to accelerated prosthetic failure.

Statement Availability

Preparation and distribution of this statement are the responsibility of the Office of Medical Applications of Research of the National Institutes of Health. Free copies of this statement as well as all other available NIH Consensus Statements and NIH Technology Assessment Statements may be obtained from the following resources:

NIH Consensus Program Information Service
P.O. Box 2577
Kensington, MD 20891
Telephone 1-800-NIH-OMAR (644-6627)
Fax (301) 816-2494

NIH Office of Medical Applications of Research
Federal Building,
Room 618
7550 Wisconsin Avenue MSC
9120 Bethesda, MD 20892-9120

Full-text versions of statements are also available online through an electronic bulletin board system and through the Internet.

NIH Information Center BBS (301) 480-5144

Internet Gopher://gopher.nih.gov/Health and Clinical Information.

World Wide Web http://text.nim.nih.gov

ftp://public.nim.nih.gov/hstat/nihcdcs

Part Seven

Living with Arthritis

Chapter 49

Coping with Arthritis in Its Many Forms

It may begin as a slight morning stiffness. For the lucky person with arthritis, that's as far as it goes. But for millions of others, arthritis can become a disabling, even crippling, disease. Roman Emperor Diocletian exempted citizens with severe arthritis from paying taxes, no doubt realizing that the disease itself can be taxing enough.

One in seven Americans—nearly 40 million—have some form of arthritis. That number will climb as the baby boomers age. By 2020, about 60 million Americans will have arthritis, according to The National Arthritis Data Workgroup of the National Institute of Arthritis and Musculo-skeletal and Skin Diseases. The disease is physical, but also exacts a mental, emotional and economic toll.

"Chronic illness impacts a person's entire lifestyle—work, family and recreation," says Gail Wright, Ph.D., a rehabilitation psychologist at the University of Missouri, Columbia. To improve quality of life, doctors and health educators increasingly advise combining drug treatment with education, social support, and moderate forms of exercise.

Arthritis means joint inflammation. In a normal joint, where two bones meet, the ends are coated with cartilage, a smooth, slippery cushion that protects the bone and reduces friction during movement. A tough capsule lined with synovial membrane seals the joint and produces a lubricating fluid. Ligaments surround and support each joint, connecting the bones and preventing excessive movement.

FDA Consumer, March 1996.

Muscles attach to bone by tendons on each side of a joint. Inflammation can affect any of these tissues.

Inflammation is a complex process that causes swelling, redness, warmth, and pain. It's the body's natural response to injury and plays an important role in healing and fighting infection. Joint injury can be caused by trauma or by the wear and tear of aging. But in many forms of arthritis, injury is caused by the uncontrolled inflammation of autoimmune disease, in which the immune system attacks the body's own tissues. In severe cases, all joint tissues, even bone, can be damaged.

The general term arthritis includes over 100 kinds of rheumatic diseases, most of which last for life. Rheumatic diseases are those affecting joints, muscle, and connective tissue, which makes up or supports various structures of the body, including tendons, cartilage, blood vessels, and internal organs. The Food and Drug Administration has approved a wide variety of drugs to treat the many forms of arthritis.

The most common type of arthritis is Osteoarthritis, affecting more than 16 million Americans. This degenerative joint disease is common in people over 65, but may appear decades earlier. It begins when cartilage breaks down, sometimes eroding entirely to leave a bone-on-bone joint in extreme cases. Any joint can be affected, but the feet, knees, hips, and fingers are most common. It may appear in one or two joints and spread no further. Painful and knobby bone growths in the fingers are common, but usually not crippling. The disease is often mild, but can be quite severe.

Second most common is rheumatoid arthritis, which affects 2.5 million Americans. It can strike at any age, but usually appears between ages 20 and 50. The hands are most commonly affected, but it can affect most joints of the body. Inflammation begins in the synovial lining and can spread to the entire joint. Highly variable and difficult to control, the disease can severely deform joints. Some people become bedridden. Others continue to run marathons.

An autoimmune disease affecting the whole body, rheumatoid arthritis can also cause weakness, fatigue, loss of appetite, muscle pain, and weight loss. Blood tests may reveal anemia and the presence of an antibody called rheumatoid factor (RF). However, some people with RF never develop rheumatoid arthritis, and some people with the disease never have RF. In about one in six, the disease becomes severe and can shorten life. Researchers hope to find ways to predict which patients should be treated more aggressively.

Ups and Downs

With so many kinds of arthritis, which can appear and progress unpredictably, diagnosis and treatment can be trying for both physician and patient. Diagnosis depends on integrating a host of factors, including the possibility that a person may have two forms of the disease.

The normal ups and downs of chronic, painful disease further complicate matters. "Just about any painful condition will wax and wane on its own," says rheumatologist Dennis Boulware, M.D., University of Alabama, Birmingham.

A worsening or reappearance of the disease is called a flare. Remissions bring welcome relief, but can also obscure whether symptoms decreased on their own or due to treatment.

Proper treatment depends on correct diagnosis of the specific disease, and varies with severity and location, as well as from person to person. But treatment need not wait for a final diagnosis because initial treatment options, such as anti-inflammatory drugs and exercise, are similar for many forms of the disease. Treatment should begin early to reduce joint damage.

The drugs used for treating most types of arthritis are drawn from many categories, but can be thought of in a few broad groups, such as anti-inflammatory drugs and disease-modifying drugs. For treating gout, there are also drugs that reduce the amount of uric acid in the blood. More than one medication may be required for treating arthritis.

Anti-inflammatory agents generally work by slowing the body's production of prostaglandins, substances that play a role in inflammation. Many have an analgesic, or painkilling, effect at low doses. Usually, higher, sustained doses are required to see sufficient anti-inflammatory activity for treating arthritis. The most familiar anti-inflammatory agent is aspirin, often a good arthritis treatment. Like aspirin, nonsteroidal anti-inflammatory drugs (NSAIDs) fight pain and inflammation. More than a dozen NSAIDs are available, most by prescription only. At press time, FDA was considering whether labeling changes to prescription-strength NSAIDs are necessary, due to gastrointestinal side effects.

FDA has approved three NSAIDs for over-the-counter (OTC) marketing: ibuprofen (marketed as Advil, Nuprin, Motrin, and others), naproxen sodium (sold as Aleve), and ketoprofen (marketed as Actron and Orudis). Although these drugs are available OTC, a doctor should be consulted before taking any medication for arthritis symptoms.

"People shouldn't be mixing medications," says Linda Katz, M.D., of FDA's pilot drug evaluation staff, and anyone regularly taking NSAIDs should carefully read the labels of OTC products to make sure they don't contain similar drugs. For example, many cough and cold preparations contain analgesics such as aspirin, acetaminophen or ibuprofen.

The most potent anti-inflammatories are corticosteroids, synthetic versions of the hormone cortisone. Like prednisone and dexamethasone, the generic names often end in "-one." They're usually reserved for short periods of use during intense flares or when other drugs don't control unrelenting disease. Relief can be dramatic, but long-term use causes side effects, such as weight gain, high blood pressure, and thinning of bones and skin. Usually given orally, they can also be injected directly into a joint to reduce side effects.

Disease modifiers slow the disease process in autoimmune diseases such as rheumatoid arthritis or systemic lupus erythematosus. Patients taking these drugs are closely monitored. It may take weeks or months to learn if a drug works. During that wait, it's important to keep taking other medications such as NSAIDs. Cold salts have been used to treat rheumatoid arthritis for 60 years, although nobody knows why this treatment works. Penicillamine, methotrexate, and antimalarials such as hydroxychloroquine are also used. Doctors usually reserve other powerful drugs that suppress the immune system for extremely serious disease.

Most people with arthritis never need surgery, but when all else fails, it can dramatically improve independence and quality of life by reducing pain and improving mobility. The surgeon may remove damaged or chronically inflamed tissue, or replace the joint entirely. Artificial replacements are available for all of the most commonly affected joints.

Use it or Lose it

In the past, doctors often advised arthritis patients to rest and avoid exercise. Rest remains important, especially during flares. But doing nothing results in weak muscles, stiff joints, reduced mobility, and lost vitality. Now, rheumatologists routinely advise a balance of physical activity and rest. Exercise offers physical and psychological benefits that include improved overall fitness and well-being, increased mobility, and better sleep.

For example, twice a week for three years, Elsie Sequeira, 81, of Concord, Calif., has attended a water-based exercise class sponsored by the Arthritis Foundation. "It's helped me a lot," she says. Sequeira has rheumatoid arthritis in her shoulders and legs. She had also had a mild stroke and got to her first classes with the help of a walker and an attendant.

A few weeks passed before she saw any improvement, but within a few months she no longer needed either the walker or the attendant. "The warm water is very soothing and we can do things in the water that we couldn't do on land," Sequeira says. She enjoys the social contact, and feels better able to take care of herself. "I don't feel so hamstrung," she says.

Joints require motion to stay healthy. That's why doctors advise arthritis patients to do range-of-motion, or flexibility, exercises every day—even during flares. Painful or swollen joints should be moved gently, however.

Strengthening and endurance activities are also recommended, but should be limited or avoided during flares. Arthritis patients should consult their doctors before starting an exercise program, and begin gradually. Exercises must be individualized to work the right muscles while avoiding overstressing affected joints. Doctors or physical therapists can teach proper ways to move.

Muscle strength is especially important because strong muscles better support and protect joints. "Several studies show that if you improve muscle strength, you decrease pain," Boulware says. Joints will probably hurt during exercise, but shouldn't still hurt several hours later.

"There's a fine line between doing too much and too little," says rheumatologist William Ginsburg, M.D., of the Mayo Clinic, Jacksonville, Fla. "Sometimes people have to be reminded to slow down and listen to their disease."

Support groups and arthritis education can help people learn how to listen to their disease, and cope with it. "The psychological aspects are very important because that's what changes people's lives," Ginsburg says.

Participants learn practical things, such as how to: get up off the floor after a fall, protect joints with careful use and assistive devices, drive a car, get comfortable sleep, use heat and cold treatments, talk with their doctors, and cope with emotional aspects of pain and disability. They may also learn to acquire and maintain what health experts have long touted—a positive attitude.

Health education not only improves quality of life, but also lowers health-care costs, and the benefits are lasting, according to studies at Stanford University, Palo Alto, Calif. Four years after a short Arthritis Self-Management Program, participants still reported significantly less pain and made fewer physician visits, even though disability increased. The benefits came, not from the specifics taught, but from improved ability to cope with the consequences of arthritis—in other words, confidence. "It's the same thing that any good coach tries to instill," says Halsted R. Holman, M.D., Stanford University.

Avoiding Fraud

Learning to understand their disease can also help make people less likely to fall victim to fraud. Because they have a painful, incurable condition, people with arthritis are among the prime targets for fraud and spend nearly a billion dollars annually on unproved remedies, largely diets and supplements.

A claim describing the relationship between a nutrient or dietary ingredient and a disease, such as arthritis, cannot be made on the label or in labeling of a dietary supplement unless the claim is authorized by FDA. In order for FDA to consider authorizing the use of a health claim, there must be significant agreement among qualified experts that the health claim is scientifically valid. Frequently, however, dietary supplements are found on the market labeled in violation of these requirements.

"If the claim sounds too good to be true, it probably is. Talk to your doctor or other health professional," says Peggy Binzer, a consumer safety officer in FDA's Center for Food Safety and Applied Nutrition.

Consumers who have questions or who wish to report a company for falsely labeling its products should call FDA's Office of Consumer Affairs at (301) 443-3170 from 1 p.m. to 3:30 p.m. Eastern time. Consumers who have suffered from a serious adverse effect associated with the use of a dietary supplement should report the effect to their health care professional or to *Medwatch* at (1-800) FDA-1088.

Some remedies, such as vinegar and honey or copper bracelets, seem harmless. But they can become harmful if they cause people to abandon conventional therapy. Others, such as the solvent dimethyl sulfoxide (DMSO), can be outright dangerous.

It's tempting to conclude that arthritis pain gets better or worse because of what was added or eliminated from the diet the day or week before. However, gout is the only rheumatic disease known to be helped by avoiding certain foods. The unpredictable ups and downs of arthritis make it hard to establish a relationship between diet and disease. Scientists have only recently begun to study nutritional therapy for arthritis, and the American College of Rheumatology (ACR) urges continued research.

The ACR Position Statement on Diet and Arthritis advises, "Until more data are available, patients should continue to follow balanced and healthy diets, be skeptical of 'miraculous' claims and avoid elimination diets and fad nutritional practices."

Research under Way

New treatments are likely to stem from better understanding of the underlying causes and destructive processes of the disease. Overuse, injury and obesity are contributing factors in osteoarthritis, and researchers have implicated a faulty gene in the breakdown of cartilage. Heredity plays a role in other forms of arthritis, too, increasing susceptibility in some people. Potential genetic therapy approaches are still far off, however.

Increased knowledge of immunology and the inflammatory process offers more immediate promise. Researchers have developed a drug that blocks the effects of TNF—alpha, an inflammatory protein responsible for reactions resulting in joint damage. In short-term preliminary trials, the drug significantly reduced symptoms in rheumatoid arthritis patients.

Such results are encouraging, but the ultimate goal is to understand what starts the immune response in the first place. "Until you know the real cause, you're not going to have the right drug," Ginsburg says.

That quest continues and offers hope. But short of a cure, enlightened coping may be the most promising avenue to a less taxing life for people with arthritis. Emperor Diocletian would be pleased.

Normal Joint

In a normal joint (where two bones come together), the muscle, bursa and tendon support the bone and aid movement. The synovial membrane (an inner lining) releases a slippery fluid into the joint space. Cartilage covers the bone ends, absorbing shocks and keeping the bones from rubbing together when the joint moves.

Osteoarthritis

In osteoarthritis, cartilage breaks down and the bones rub together. The joint then loses shape and alignment. Bone ends thicken, forming spurs (bony growths). Bits of cartilage or bone float in the joint space.

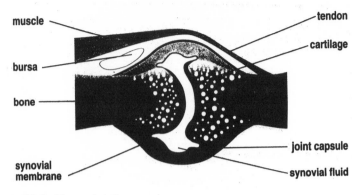

Figure 49.1. *Normal Joint*

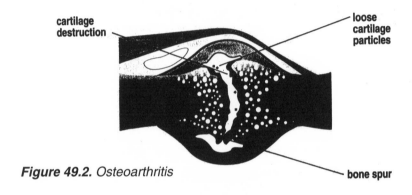

Figure 49.2. *Osteoarthritis*

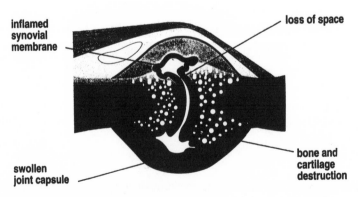

Figure 49.3. *Rheumatoid Arthritis*

Rheumatoid Arthritis

In rheumatoid arthritis, inflammation accompanies thickening of the synovial membrane or joint lining, causing the whole joint to look swollen due to swelling in the joint capsule. The inflamed joint lining enters and damages bone and cartilage, and inflammatory cells release an enzyme that gradually digests bone and cartilage. Space between joints diminishes, and the joint loses shape and alignment.

Common Types of Arthritis

Of more than 100 different kinds of arthritis, these are the most common:

- **Osteoarthritis**—Also called degenerative arthritis. Occurs when the cushioning cartilage in a joint breaks down. Commonly affects feet, knees, hips, and fingers. Affects 16 million Americans, mostly 45 and older. About half of those 65 and older have this form.

- **Rheumatoid Arthritis**—Immune system attacks the lining, or synovial membrane, of the joints. Joint damage can become severe and deforming. Involves the whole body, and may also cause fatigue, weight loss and anemia, and affect the lungs, heart and eyes. Affects about 2.1 million Americans, three times more women than men.

- **Gout**—Causes sudden, severe attacks, usually in the big toe, but any joint can be affected. A metabolic disorder in which uric acid builds up in the blood and crystals form in joints and other places. Drugs and attention to diet can control gout. Affects about one million Americans (70 to 80 percent men), with first attack starting between 40 and 50 years of age.

- **Ankylosing Spondylitis**—A chronic inflammatory disease of the spine that can result in fused vertebrae and rigid spine. Often milder and harder to diagnose in women. Most people with the disease also have a genetic marker known as HLA-B27. Affects about 318,000 Americans, usually men between the ages of 16 and 35.

- **Juvenile Arthritis**—The most common form is juvenile rheumatoid arthritis. Arthritis diagnosis, treatment, and disease characteristics are different in children and adults. Some children recover completely; others remain affected throughout their lives. Affects about 200,000 Americans.

- **Psoriatic Arthritis**—Bone and other joint tissues become inflamed, and, like rheumatoid arthritis, it can affect the whole body. Affects about 5 percent of people with psoriasis, a chronic skin disease. Likely to affect fingers or spine. Symptoms are mild in most people but can be quite severe. Affects about 160,000 Americans.

- **Systemic Lupus Erythematosus**—Involves skin, joints, muscles, and sometimes internal organs. Symptoms usually appear in women of childbearing age but can occur in anyone at any age. Also called lupus or SLE, it can be mild or life threatening. Affects at least 131,000 Americans nine to ten times as many women as men.

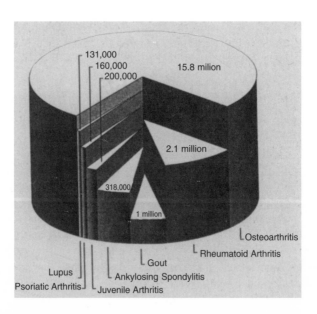

Figure 49.4. *Here are some of the more common of the 100 forms of Arthritis and their approximate number of cases in the United States. (Source: Arthritis Foundation)*

428

- **Other forms**—Arthritis can develop as a result of an infection. For example, bacteria that cause gonorrhea or Lyme disease can cause arthritis. Infectious arthritis can cause serious damage, but usually clears up completely with antibiotics. Scleroderma is a systemic disease that involves the skin, but may include problems with blood vessels, joints, and internal organs. Fibromyalgia syndrome is a soft-tissue rheumatism that doesn't lead to joint deformity, but affects an estimated five million Americans, mostly women.

—by Carolyn J. Strange

Carolyn J. Strange is a science and medical writer in Saratoga, California.

Chapter 50

Managing Your Pain

Questions and Answers about Arthritis Pain

What is arthritis?

The word arthritis literally means joint inflammation, but is often used to refer to a group of more than 100 rheumatic diseases that can cause pain, stiffness, and swelling in the joints. These diseases may affect not only the joints but also other parts of the body, including important supporting structures such as muscles, bones, tendons, and ligaments, as well as some internal organs. This chapter focuses on pain caused by two of the most common forms of arthritis: osteoarthritis and rheumatoid arthritis.

What is pain?

Pain is the body's warning system, alerting you that something is wrong. The International Association for the Study of Pain defines it as an unpleasant experience associated with actual or potential tissue damage to a person's body. Specialized nervous system cells (neurons) that transmit pain signals are found throughout the skin and other body tissues. These cells respond to things such as injury or tissue damage. For example, when a harmful agent such as a sharp knife comes in contact with your skin, chemical signals travel from neurons in the skin

NIH Web Document. National Institute of Arthritis and Musculoskeletal and Skin Diseases. Office of Scientific and Health Communications. [http://www.nih/niams/healthinfo].

431

through nerves in the spinal cord to your brain, where they are interpreted as pain. See Omnigraphics' *Pain Sourcebook* for a more detailed discussion of pain and its treatment.

Most forms of arthritis are associated with pain that can be divided into two general categories: acute and chronic. Acute pain is temporary. It can last a few seconds or longer but wanes as healing occurs. Some examples of things that cause acute pain include burns, cuts, and fractures. Chronic pain, such as that seen in people with osteoarthritis and rheumatoid arthritis, ranges from mild to severe and can last a lifetime.

How many Americans suffer from arthritis pain?

Chronic pain is a major health problem in the United States and is one of the most weakening effects of arthritis. More than 40 million Americans suffer from some form of arthritis, and many have chronic pain that limits daily activity. Osteoarthritis is by far the most common form of arthritis, affecting about 16 million Americans, while rheumatoid arthritis, which affects about 2.1 million Americans, is the most crippling form of the disease.

What causes arthritis pain? Why is it so variable?

The pain of arthritis may come from different sources. These may include inflammation of the synovial membrane (tissue that lines the joints), the tendons, or the ligaments; muscle strain; and fatigue. A combination of these factors contributes to the intensity of the pain.

The pain of arthritis varies greatly from person to person, for reasons that doctors do not yet understand completely. Factors that contribute to the pain include swelling within the joint, the amount of heat or redness present, or damage that has occurred within the joint. In addition, activities affect pain differently so that some patients note pain in their joints after first getting out of bed in the morning whereas others develop pain after prolonged use of the joint. Each individual has a different threshold and tolerance for pain, often affected by both physical and emotional factors. These can include depression, anxiety, and even hypersensitivity at the affected sites due to inflammation and tissue injury. This increased sensitivity appears to affect the amount of pain perceived by the individual.

How do doctors measure arthritis pain?

Pain is a private, unique experience that cannot be seen. The most common way to measure pain is for the doctor to ask you, the patient, about your problems. For example, the doctor may ask you to describe the level of pain you feel on a scale of 1 to 10. You may use words like aching, burning, stinging, or throbbing. These words will give the doctor a clearer picture of the pain you are experiencing.

Since doctors rely on your description of pain to help guide treatment, you may want to keep a pain diary to record your pain sensations. On a daily basis, you can describe the situations that cause or alter the intensity of your pain, the sensations and severity of your pain, and your reactions to the pain. For example: "On Monday night, sharp pains in my knees produced by housework interfered with my sleep; on Tuesday morning, because of the pain, I had a hard time getting out bed. However, I coped with the pain by taking my medication and applying ice to my knees." The diary will give the doctor some insight into your pain and may play a critical role in the management of your disease.

What will happen when you first visit a doctor for your arthritis pain?

The doctor will usually do the following:

- Take your medical history and ask questions such as:
    - How long have you had this problem?
    - How intense is the pain?
    - How often does it occur?
    - What causes it to get worse?
    - What causes it to get better?

- Review the medications you are using

- Conduct a physical examination

- Take blood and/or urine samples and request necessary laboratory work

- Ask you to get x-rays taken or undergo other imaging procedures such as a CAT scan (computerized axial tomography) or MRI (magnetic resonance imaging).

Once the doctor has done these things and reviewed the results of any tests or procedures, he or she will discuss the findings with you and design a comprehensive management approach for the pain caused by your osteoarthritis or rheumatoid arthritis.

433

Who can treat arthritis pain?

A number of different specialists may be involved in the care of an arthritis patients. Often a team approach is used. The team may include doctors who treat people with arthritis (rheumatologists), surgeons (orthopaedists), and physical and occupational therapists. Their goal is to treat all aspects of arthritis pain and help you learn to manage your pain. The physician, other health-care professionals, and you, the patient, all play an active role in the management of arthritis pain.

How is arthritis pain treated?

There is no single treatment that applies to all people with arthritis, but rather the doctor will develop a management plan designed to minimize your specific pain and improve the function of your joints. A number of treatments can provide short-term pain relief.

Short-term Relief

Medications: Because people with osteoarthritis have very little inflammation, pain relievers such as acetaminophen (Tylenol*) may be effective. Patients with rheumatoid arthritis generally have pain caused by inflammation and often benefit from aspirin or other non-steroidal anti-inflammatory drugs (NSAIDs) such as ibuprofen (Motrin or Advil).

Heat and cold: The decision to use either heat or cold for arthritis pain depends on the type of arthritis and should be discussed with your doctor or physical therapist. Moist heat, such as a warm bath or shower, or dry heat, such as a heating pad, placed on the painful area of the joint for about 15 minutes may relieve the pain. An ice pack (or a bag of frozen vegetables) wrapped in a towel and placed on the sore area for about 15 minutes may help to reduce swelling and stop the pain. If you have poor circulation, do not use cold packs.

Joint Protection: Using a splint or a brace to allow joints to rest and protect them from injury can be helpful. Your physician or physical therapist can make recommendations.

Transcutaneous electrical nerve stimulation (TENS): A small TENS device that directs mild electric pulses to nerve endings that lie beneath the skin in the painful area may relieve some arthritis pain. TENS seems to work by blocking pain messages to the brain and by modifying pain perception.

Massage: In this pain-relief approach, a massage therapist will lightly stroke and/or knead the painful muscle. This may increase blood flow and bring warmth to a stressed area. However, arthritis-stressed joints are very sensitive so the therapist must be very familiar with the problems of the disease.

Acupuncture: This procedure should only be done by a licensed acupuncture therapist. In acupuncture, thin needles are inserted at specific points in the body. Scientists think that this stimulates the release of natural, pain-relieving chemicals produced by the brain or the nervous system.

Osteoarthritis and rheumatoid arthritis are chronic diseases that may last a lifetime. Learning how to manage your pain over the long term is an important factor in controlling the disease and maintaining a good quality of life. Following are some sources of long-term pain relief.

Long-term Relief

Medications

Nonsteroidal anti-inflammatory drugs (NSAIDs): These are a class of drugs including aspirin and ibuprofen that are used to reduce pain and inflammation and may be used for both short-term and long-term relief in people with osteoarthritis and rheumatoid arthritis.

Disease-modifying anti-rheumatic drugs (DMARDS): These are drugs used to treat people with rheumatoid arthritis who have not responded to NSAIDs. Some of these include methotrexate, hydroxychloroquine, penicillamine, and gold injections. These drugs are thought to influence and correct abnormalities of the immune system responsible for a disease like rheumatoid arthritis. Treatment with these medications requires careful monitoring by the physician to avoid side effects.

Corticosteroids: These are hormones that are very effective in treating arthritis. Corticosteroids can be taken by mouth or given by injection. Prednisone is the corticosteroid most often given by mouth to reduce the inflammation of rheumatoid arthritis. In both rheumatoid arthritis and osteoarthritis, the doctor also may inject a corticosteroid into the affected joint to stop pain. Because frequent injections may cause damage to the cartilage, they should only be done once or twice a year.

Weight reduction: Excess pounds put extra stress on weight-bearing joints such as the knees or hips. Studies have shown that overweight women who lost an average of 11 pounds substantially reduced the development of osteoarthritis in their knees. In addition, if osteoarthritis has already affected one knee, weight reduction will reduce the chance of it occurring in the other knee.

Exercise: Swimming, walking, low-impact aerobic exercise, and range-of-motion exercises may reduce joint pain and stiffness. In addition, stretching exercises are helpful. A physical therapist can help plan an exercise program that will give you the most benefit. (The National Arthritis and Musculoskeletal and Skin Diseases Information Clearinghouse has a fact sheet on arthritis and exercise which has been reprinted in this sourcebook as chapter 53. See the end of this chapter and the sourcebook for contact information.)

Surgery: In select patients with arthritis, surgery may be necessary. The surgeon may perform an operation to remove the synovium (synovectomy), realign the joint (osteotomy), or in advanced cases replace the damaged joint with an artificial one. Total joint replacement has provided not only dramatic relief from pain but also improvement in motion for many people with arthritis.

What alternative therapies may relieve arthritis pain?

Many people seek other ways of treating their disease, such as special diets or supplements. Although these methods may not be harmful in and of themselves, no research to date shows that they help. Nonetheless, some alternative or complementary approaches may help you to cope or reduce some of the stress of living with a chronic illness. If the doctor feels the approach has value and will not harm you, it can be incorporated into your treatment plan. However, it is important not to neglect your regular health care or treatment of serious symptoms.

How can you cope with arthritis pain?

The long-term goal of pain management is to help you cope with a chronic, often disabling disease. You may be caught in a cycle of pain, depression, and stress. To break out of this cycle, you need to be an active participant with the doctor and other health care professionals in managing your pain. This may include physical therapy, cognitive-behavioral therapy, occupational therapy, biofeedback, relaxation techniques (for example, deep breathing and meditation), and family counseling therapy.

Another technique is to substitute distraction for pain. Focus your attention on things that you enjoy. Imagine a peaceful setting and wonderful physical sensations. Thinking about something that is enjoyable can help you relax and become less stressed. Find something that will make you laugh: a cartoon, a funny movie, or even a new joke. Try to put some joy back into your life. Even a small change in your mental image may break the pain cycle and provide relief.

The Multipurpose Arthritis and Musculoskeletal Diseases Center at Stanford University, supported by the National Institute of Arthritis and Musculoskeletal and Skin Diseases (NIAMS), has developed an Arthritis Self-Help Course that teaches people with arthritis how to take a more active part in their arthritis care. The Arthritis Self-Help Course is taught by the Arthritis Foundation and consists of a 12- to 15-hour program that includes lectures on osteoarthritis and rheumatoid arthritis, exercise, pain management, nutrition, medication, doctor-patient relationships, and nontraditional treatment.

You may want to contact some of the organizations listed at the end of this chapter for additional information on the Arthritis Self-Help Course and on coping with pain, as well as for information on support groups in your area.

Things You Can Do to Manage Arthritis Pain

- Eat a healthy diet
- Get 8 to 10 hours of sleep at night.
- Keep a daily diary of pain and mood changes to share with your physician.
- Choose a caring physician.
- Join a support group
- Stay informed about new research on managing arthritis pain.

What research is being conducted on arthritis pain?

NIAMS, part of the National Institutes of Health, is sponsoring research that will increase understanding of the specific ways to diagnose, treat, and possibly prevent arthritis pain.

Recent NIAMS studies show that levels of several neuropeptides (compounds produced by cells of the nervous system), such as substance P, are increased in arthritic joints. Substance P is involved in the transmission of pain signals via the nervous system. At the University of Missouri-Kansas City, researchers are studying effects of substance P in the spines of animals with chronic arthritis. Findings from this study may be used to develop specific drugs for chronic pain such as that associated with arthritis.

NIAMS studies are also looking at other aspects of pain. At the Specialized Center of Research in Osteoarthritis at Rush-Presbyterian-St Luke's Medical Center in Chicago, Illinois, researchers are studying the human knee and analyzing how injury in one joint may affect other joints. In addition, they are analyzing the effect of pain and analgesics on gait (walking) and comparing pain and gait before and after surgical treatment of knee osteoarthritis.

At the University of Maryland Pain Center in Baltimore, NIAMS researchers are evaluating the use of acupuncture on patients with osteoarthritis of the knee. Preliminary findings suggest that traditional Chinese acupuncture is both safe and effective as an additional therapy for osteoarthritis, and it significantly reduces pain and improves physical function.

At Duke University in Durham, North Carolina, NIAMS researchers have developed cognitive-behavioral therapy (CBT) involving both patients and their spouses. The goal of CBT for arthritis pain is to help patients cope more effectively with the long-term demands of a chronic and potentially disabling disease. Researchers are studying whether aerobic fitness, coping abilities, and spousal responses to pain behaviors diminish the patient's pain and disability.

NIAMS-supported research on arthritis pain also includes projects in the Institute's Multipurpose Arthritis and Musculoskeletal Diseases Centers. At the University of California in San Francisco, researchers are studying stress factors, including pain, that are associated with rheumatoid arthritis. Findings from this study will be used to develop patient education programs that will improve a person's ability to deal with rheumatoid arthritis and enhance their quality of life. At the Indiana University School of Medicine in Indianapolis, health care professionals are monitoring joint pain in patients with osteoarthritis and documenting this information. The goal of the project is to improve doctor-patient communication about pain management and increase patient satisfaction.

Where can you find more information on arthritis pain?

Arthritis Foundation
1330 West Peachtree Street
Atlanta, GA 30309
404/872-7100 or call your local chapter, (listed in the telephone directory)
800/283-7800
World Wide Web address: http://www.arthritis.org

This is the major voluntary organization devoted to arthritis. The Foundation publishes a free brochure, Coping With Pain, and a monthly magazine for members that provides up-to-date information on all forms of arthritis. The Foundation also can provide addresses and phone numbers for their local chapters and physician and clinic referrals.

American Chronic Pain Association
P.O. Box 850
Rocklin, CA 95677
916/632-0922

The Association provides information on positive ways to deal with chronic pain, and can provide guidelines on selecting a pain management center.

American Pain Society
4700 West Lake Avenue
Glenview, IL 60025-1485
847/375-4715

The Society provides general information to the public and maintains a directory of resources, including referrals to pain centers.

National Chronic Pain Outreach Association, Inc.
P.O. Box 274
Millboro, VA 24460
540/997-5004

The Association operates an information clearinghouse offering publications and cassette tapes for people with pain. They also publish a newsletter that includes information on pain management techniques, coping strategies, book reviews, and support groups.

NAMSIC
National Institutes of Health
1 AMS Circle
Bethesda, MD 20892-3675
301/495-4484
Fax: 301/587-4352
TTY: 301/565-2966
World Wide Web address: http://www.nih.gov/niams/
NIAMS Fast Facts: 301/881-2731 (information 24 hours a day by fax)

* Brand names included in this chapter are provided as examples only and their inclusion does not mean that these products are endorsed by the National Institutes of Health or any other Government agency. Also, if a particular brand name is not mentioned, this does not mean or imply that the product is unsatisfactory.

Acknowledgments

The NIAMS gratefully acknowledges the assistance of John H. Klippel, M.D., Clinical Director, National Institute of Arthritis and Musculoskeletal and Skin Diseases; Brian M. Berman, M.D., Director of the Complementary Medicine Program, University of Maryland, School of Medicine; and Laurence A. Bradley, Ph.D., Professor of Medicine/Rheumatology, University of Alabama at Birmingham.

The National Arthritis and Musculoskeletal and Skin Diseases Information Clearinghouse (NAMSIC) is a public service sponsored by the NIAMS that provides health information and information sources, including additional information on arthritis. The NIAMS, a part of the National Institutes of Health (NIH), leads the Federal medical research effort in arthritis and musculoskeletal and skin diseases. The NIAMS sponsors research and research training throughout the United States as well as on the NIH campus in Bethesda, Maryland, and disseminates health and research information.

Chapter 51

Managing Your Fatigue

What is fatigue?

Fatigue is the feeling of extreme tiredness or exhaustion, often involving muscle weakness, that can make it difficult for you to perform tasks. It has been compared with the tired and achy feeling you often have with the flu.

Fatigue is a frequent and troubling symptom of many types of arthritis and other rheumatic diseases, such as lupus and fibromyalgia. Many things may cause fatigue illness, depression, joint and muscle pain, stress, overextending yourself, poor sleep, anemia or a lack of physical activity.

The symptoms of fatigue vary from person to person. They may last a long time or a short time. They may strike at random or may be predictable. However often you have fatigue, you can learn how to decrease its effects. Knowing how it affects you will help you manage it better.

How does fatigue make you feel?

Fatigue affects everyone differently. You may have different feelings at different times. For instance, fatigue may make you feel:

- Very tired with no energy
- Increased pain

- A loss of control
- A loss of concentration
- Irritable

What causes fatigue?

There are many causes of fatigue. Causes are different from person to person. Fatigue may be caused by one thing or it may be caused by several things.

How can you manage your fatigue?

Just as there are many causes of fatigue, there are many approaches to managing it. You may need to use more than one of the following suggestions to cope with your fatigue.

Save Your Energy.

Listen to your body and pace yourself to keep from becoming too tired. Try these ideas to save your energy:

Be Aware of Your Body Positions

- Change the way you do activities so you don't put too much stress on your joints.

- Maintain good posture. Poor posture (slouching) can stress your muscles and lead to fatigue.

Balance Rest and Activity

- Learn your body's signals that it is getting tired. Take breaks during or between tasks, before these signals begin.

- Pace yourself during the day. Switch between doing heavy tasks and light tasks. Do the most difficult things when you're feeling your best. If you pace yourself you probably can do more work than if you work straight through until you're worn out.

- Pace yourself from day to day. Allow plenty of time to finish the things you start so you won't feel rushed. Don't try to do too much at one time.

- When your disease is more active, take longer and more frequent rest breaks. Eliminate energy-draining activities when possible.

- Actively manage the stress of your arthritis. Stress overload can contribute to feelings of fatigue and exhaustion.

Make Your Work Easier

- Plan ahead. Look at all the things you do at home and at work during a normal day and week. Eliminate the ones that are not necessary. Delegate some of the others. Make a schedule for each day. Think about the amount of time each task requires and how tiring it is. Plan your day with this in mind. Schedule rest breaks before you begin.

- Combine chores and errands so you can get more done with less effort. Create shortcuts for yourself You can save time and energy by preparing several meals in advance. Try saving errands until you have several things to do. Then do them all at once, instead of making many trips.

- Sit when you work, if you can. If you can't, take short rest breaks as often as possible.

- Use labor-saving devices, such as an electric garage door opener, a microwave oven or a food processor.

- Use self-help devices, such as tools with enlarged handles or jar openers. These reduce stress on your joints and can make difficult tasks easier.

- Organize work areas so you can get more done with less energy. Keep items needed for a particular task together in one area. As a general rule, keep items you use most often nearest to your work area and place less-used items further away.

Saving your energy may seem like a juggling act, but you soon will discover that it can be done.

Get Enough Sleep

Getting a good night's sleep restores your energy and helps you cope with pain. It also gives your joints a chance to rest. Only you know how much sleep your body needs. Get into the habit of listening to your body. A nap during the day may be all you need to restore your energy and lift your spirits.

If you have trouble sleeping, talk with your doctor. When sleep disturbance is treated, fatigue usually improves.

Exercise

Some people think exercising will reduce their energy, but just the opposite is true. The right type and right amount of exercise helps keep your muscles strong, bones healthy and joints usable. A good exercise program also helps you keep or restore joint flexibility.

Exercise can improve your sense of well being and may result in overall increased energy.

Keep in mind that when you first start exercising, your heart will beat faster, you'll breathe faster and your muscles may feel tense. You may feel more tired at night, but awake feeling refreshed in the morning. These are normal reactions to exercise that mean your body is adapting and getting into shape. You'll know you've done too much if you have joint or muscle pain that continues for more than two hours after exercising or if your pain or fatigue is worse the next day. Next time, decrease the number of times you do each exercise, or do them more gently. If this doesn't help, ask your physical therapist about changing the exercise.

Your exercise program should include range-of-motion, strengthening and endurance exercises. Follow a program designed by your health-care provider.

Follow Your Treatment Plan

Fatigue may be a sign of increased disease activity or inflammation. Be sure to follow the treatment plan you and your health-care provider have designed. Don't skip medications or exercises on days you feel good. This can backfire and lead to increased symptoms. Report any increasing fatigue or changes in general health to your health-care provider so appropriate measures can be taken.

Ask for Help

Don't be afraid to ask for help when you need it. Be honest about your limitations. Talk with your family and friends about your fatigue, your need to rest and how they can help. Family, friends and co-workers would rather help you than have you overextend yourself, trigger a flare and be confined to bed.

Have Fun

Enjoying a fun and relaxing activity can decrease stress and help take your mind off your fatigue. Get involved in activities you enjoy.

Read a good book. Begin a new hobby. Participate in volunteer activities. Make it a habit to schedule some fun into every day.

Use a Fatigue Care Chart

What adds to your fatigue? At what time of day does your fatigue start? What helps decrease your fatigue? Once you know the answers to these questions, you can develop and use a Fatigue Care Chart. There are two parts to this chart. In the left column, list the causes of your fatigue. In the right column, list ways to handle it.

Chapter 52

Managing Your Activities

Why does it hurt to move?

If you do not move a joint regularly, the muscles around it weaken and/or become tight. The joint can stiffen or even freeze. Then when you do try to move, the joint and muscles hurt because they have been still for so long.

Pain may be caused by swelling, joint damage, muscle tightness or spasm. Muscles hurt after doing exercise or activities you aren't used to; sometimes when the joint is damaged, simple activities stress the joint. Using your body wisely can reduce stress on joints, providing you with less pain, easier movement, and even more energy.

- **Use Good Posture.** Good posture is putting your body in the most efficient and least stressful position. Using good posture protects your neck, back, hips and knees.

- **Distribute Your load.** Use your large, strong joints and muscles, and spread the load over stronger joints or larger surface areas.

- **Use Body Leverage.** Lift things close to your body.

- **Move or Change Positions often.** Keeping muscles and joints in the same position adds to stiffness and pain.

- **Control Your Weight.** Extra pounds put more stress on your hips, knees, back and feet. This extra stress can lead to further joint pain and damage.

- **Balance Rest and Activity.** Take short breaks and alternate heavy and light activities during the day. Pace yourself by learning to balance periods of work with rest breaks so you don't place too much stress on your joints or get too tired.

- **Organize.** Organize your work and storage areas. Keep all equipment and tools within easy reach and at a comfortable level. Use a Lazy Susan or plastic bins to keep things close by.

- **Use Self-Help Devices.** Self-help devices can take stress off your joints, but always try to use your own range of motion and strength first. Self-help devices can make tasks easier and more efficient, especially when you're tired, stiff or in a hurry.

- **Ask for Help.**

Make Daily Activities Easier

There are many ways to conserve your energy and use your joints wisely. The following items are not for everyone and can be harmful if used improperly. Remember to use your available joints and muscles in the least stressful way before using these aids.

Cooking and Cleanup

- Plan meals ahead to lessen last-minute tasks.

- Use electric appliances such as can openers, mixers, crock pots, microwave ovens and dishwashers to get the job done with less energy and stress on your joints.

- Use disposable aluminum baking pans for easier cleanup. Spray a non-stick product on pans or line with foil before baking or frying.

- Place a mixing bowl in the sink while stirring. A damp cloth underneath will help keep it from slipping. Hold the mixing spoon like a dagger to take stress off your hands.

- Hammer rust-proof nails through a cutting board to secure vegetables while cutting.

- Use a French chef's knife, which keeps hands in good position for cutting, slicing and chopping.

- Use lightweight baking dishes, plates, pots and pans, and serve from them.

- Use a wheeled cart to move heavy items from place to place.

- Sit on a high stool while cooking or washing dishes.

- Store appliances within easy reach.

- Use long-handled reachers.

Laundry and Housecleaning

- Use separate laundry baskets to sort clothes. After the clothes come out of the dryer, sort them into different baskets for each family member to put away.

- Sit to sort, fold and iron clothes.

- Use a sponge mop with an easy squeezer, a "janitor's pail" with a wringer or a pail on a wooden dolly.

- Use a long-handled feather duster.

- Dust with a mitt, using circular motions with your hand open.

- Store clearing supplies wherever they are used, or keep them on a cart you can wheel from room to room.

- Use an automatic toilet bowl cleaner and spray-on mildew remover so you won't need to scrub.

- Just do one major cleaning task a day, such as washing clothes or cleaning the bathroom.

- Put casters on furniture.

- Do only the tasks that are really necessary. For example, buy permanent-press items that don't need ironing.

In the Bathroom

- Sit on a bath stool in the shower or tub.

- Wash with a bath mitt or long-handled brush.

- Extend or build up handles on brushes and combs with rulers, pink-foam hair curlers or PVC pipe insulation tubing.

- Install lever-type faucets that can be controlled with your palm, or build up faucet handles or use a non-skid pad.

- Squeeze a toothpaste tube between your palms or put a wash-cloth under the tube and lean on it.

- Use an electric toothbrush or one with a built-up handle.

- Use a free-standing mirror to put on your makeup, so you don't have to lean over the sink and strain your back.

- Use a raised toilet seat if you have trouble sitting or rising from the toilet.

- Keep towels within easy reach.

- Put grab bars around the tub and toilet. Use a rubber suction mat or non-skid strips in the tub or shower.

In the Bedroom

- Wear loose-fitting clothes with larger neck and arm holes.

- Use long-handled shoe horns and sock aids. Wear pre-tied neckties

- If possible, replace buttons with Velcro or use a button hook.

- Use a zipper pull or add a loop, chain or large paper clip to make a zipper easier to grasp.

- When making the bed, finish one side at a time.

- Wear shoes with *Velcro* closures.

- Keep shelving and storage within easy reach.

- Sit to dress.

- Keep a rolling laundry cart in your closet.

Leisure

- Wear good walking shoes that fit and provide good support.

- Elastic shoelaces or *Velcro* closures make putting on shoes easier.

- Use a card rack or holder or a brush to hold playing cards.

- Lay newspapers or books open on a table to read; use a book stand.

- Use felt-tippers, which require less pressure, or large-barrel pens, which are easier to grip.

- Use a push-button phone or a pen tip to dial. Get a headset so you don't have to hold the receiver.

- Use specially-made, lightweight tools with built-up or extended handles for gardening and other yard work.

- Break up long shopping trips into several shorter ones.

- Use a three-wheeled bike for greater stability.

In the Workplace

- Sit in a chair that can be easily adjusted.

- Use a footrest.

- Keep files and supplies within easy reach.

- Use vertical files on your desk for current work.

- Install work assist arms or wrist rests at your keyboard.

- Use a glare screen and paper holder on your monitor.

- Use lateral file cabinets for easier access.

In Your Car

- Have power steering, brakes, windows and seat controls.

- Build up tops of keys or use key holders to make turning easier.

- Use a lever-type car door opener to reduce stress on your hands.

- Use a wide-angled mirror if you have trouble turning your neck.

Chapter 53

Exercise and Your Arthritis

Questions and Answers about Arthritis and Exercise

This chapter answers general questions about arthritis and exercise. The amount and form of exercise recommended for each individual will vary depending on which joints are involved, the amount of inflammation, how stable the joints are, and whether a joint replacement procedure has been done. A skilled physician who is knowledgeable about the medical and rehabilitation needs of people with arthritis, working with a physical therapist also familiar with the needs of people with arthritis, can design an exercise plan for each patient.

What is arthritis?

Arthritis is a general term that refers to many rheumatic diseases that can cause pain, stiffness, and swelling in joints and other connective tissues. These diseases can affect supporting structures such as muscles, tendons, and ligaments and may also affect other parts of the body. Some common types of arthritis are osteoarthritis, rheumatoid arthritis, systemic lupus erythematosus, gout, juvenile rheumatoid arthritis, ankylosing spondylitis, and psoriatic arthritis. Osteoarthritis is the most common.

NIAMS Web Publication 2/97. National Institute of Arthritis and Musculoskeletal and Skin Diseases. [http://www.nih/niams/healthinfo].

Should people with arthritis exercise?

Yes. Studies have shown that exercise helps people with arthritis in many ways. Exercise reduces joint pain and stiffness and increases flexibility, muscle strength, and endurance. It also helps with weight reduction and contributes to an improved sense of well-being.

How does exercise fit into a treatment plan for people with arthritis?

Exercise is one part of a comprehensive arthritis treatment plan. Treatment plans also may include rest and relaxation, proper diet, medication, and instruction about proper use of joints and ways to conserve energy (that is, not waste motion) as well as the use of pain relief methods.

What types of exercise are most suitable for someone with arthritis?

Three types of exercise are best for people with arthritis:

1. **Range-of-motion** exercises help maintain normal joint movement and relieve stiffness. This type of exercise helps maintain or increase flexibility.

2. **Strengthening** exercises help keep or increase muscle strength. Strong muscles help support and protect joints affected by arthritis.

3. **Aerobic or endurance** exercises improve cardiovascular fitness, help control weight, and improve overall function. Weight control can be important to people who have arthritis because extra weight puts extra pressure on many joints. Some studies show that aerobic exercise can reduce inflammation in some joints.

How does a person with arthritis start an exercise program?

People with arthritis should discuss exercise options with their doctors. Most doctors recommend exercise for their patients. Many people with arthritis begin with easy, range-of-motion exercises and low-impact aerobics. People with arthritis can participate in a variety of, but not all, sports and exercise programs. The doctor will know which, if any, sports are off-limits.

The doctor may have suggestions about how to get started or may refer the patient to a physical therapist. It is best to find a physical therapist who has experience working with people who have arthritis. The therapist will design an appropriate home exercise program and teach clients about pain-relief methods, proper body mechanics (placement of the body for a given task, such as lifting a heavy box), joint protection, and conserving energy.

Step up to Exercise: How to Get Started

- Discuss exercise plans with your doctor.

- Start with supervision from a physical therapist or qualified athletic trainer.

- Apply heat to sore joints (optional; many people with arthritis start their exercise program this way).

- Stretch and warm up with range-of-motion exercises.

- Start strengthening exercises slowly with small weights (a 1 or 2 pound weight can make a big difference).

- Progress slowly.

- Use cold packs after exercising (optional; many people with arthritis complete their exercise routine this way).

- Add aerobic exercise.

- Consider appropriate recreational exercise (after doing range-of-motion, strengthening, and aerobic exercise). Fewer injuries to arthritic joints occur during recreational exercise if it is preceded by range-of-motion, strengthening, and aerobic exercise that gets your body in the best condition possible.

- Ease off if joints become painful, inflamed, or red and work with your doctor to find the cause and eliminate it.

- Choose the exercise program you enjoy most and make it a habit.

What are some pain relief methods?

There are known methods to stop pain for short periods of time. This temporary relief can make it easier for people who have arthritis to exercise. The doctor or physical therapist can suggest a method that is best for each patient. The following methods have worked for many people:

- **Moist heat** supplied by warm towels, hot packs, a bath, or a shower can be used at home for 15 to 20 minutes three times a day to relieve symptoms. A health professional can use short waves, microwaves, and ultrasound to deliver deep heat to non-inflamed joint areas. Deep heat is not recommended for patients with acutely inflamed joints. Deep heat is often used around the shoulder to relax tight tendons prior to stretching exercises.

- **Cold** supplied by a bag of ice or frozen vegetables wrapped in a towel helps to stop pain and reduce swelling when used for 10 to 15 minutes at a time. It is often used for acutely inflamed joints. People who have Raynaud's phenomenon should not use this method.

- **Hydrotherapy** (water therapy) can decrease pain and stiffness. Exercising in a large pool may be easier because water takes some weight off painful joints. Community centers, YMCAs, and YWCAs have water exercise classes developed for people with arthritis. Some patients also find relief from the heat and movement provided by a whirlpool.

- **Mobilization therapies** include traction (gentle, steady pulling), massage, and manipulation (using the hands to restore normal movement to stiff joints). When done by a trained professional, these methods can help control pain and increase joint motion and muscle and tendon flexibility.

- **TENS**(transcutaneous electrical nerve stimulation) and biofeedback are two additional methods that may provide some pain relief, but many patients find that they cost too much money and take too much time. TENS machines cost between $80 and $800. The inexpensive units are fine. Patients can wear them during the day and turn them off and on as needed for pain control.

- **Relaxation therapy** also helps reduce pain. Patients can learn to release the tension in their muscles to relieve pain. Physical therapists may be able to teach relaxation techniques. The Arthritis Foundation has a self-help course that includes relaxation therapy and also sells relaxation tapes. Health spas and vacation resorts sometimes have special relaxation courses.

- **Acupuncture** is a traditional Chinese method of pain relief. A medically qualified acupuncturist places needles in certain sites. Researchers believe that the needles stimulate deep sensory nerves that tell the brain to release natural painkillers (endorphins). Acupressure is similar to acupuncture, but pressure is applied to the acupuncture sites instead of using needles.

How often should people with arthritis exercise?

- **Range-of-motion** exercises can be done daily and should be done at least every other day.

- **Strengthening** exercises also can be done daily and should be done at least every other day unless you have severe pain or swelling in your joints.

- **Endurance** exercises should be done for 20 to 30 minutes three times a week unless you have severe pain or swelling in your joints.

What type of strengthening program is best?

This varies depending on personal preference, the type of arthritis involved, and how active the inflammation is. Strengthening one's muscles can help take the burden off painful joints. Strength training can be done with small free weights, exercise machines, isometrics, elastic bands, and resistive water exercises. Correct positioning is critical, because if done incorrectly, strengthening exercises can cause muscle tears, more pain, and more joint swelling.

Are there different exercises for people with different types of arthritis?

There are many types of arthritis. Experienced doctors, physical therapists, and occupational therapists can recommend exercises that are particularly helpful for a specific type of arthritis. Doctors and therapists also know specific exercises for particularly painful joints. There may be exercises that are off-limits for people with a particular type of arthritis or when joints are swollen and inflamed. People with arthritis should discuss their exercise plans with a doctor. Doctors who treat people with arthritis include rheumatologists, general practitioners, family doctors, internists, and rehabilitation specialists (physiatrists).

How much exercise is too much?

Most experts agree that if exercise causes pain that lasts for more than one hour, it is too much. People with arthritis should work with their physical therapist or doctor to adjust their exercise program when they notice any of the following signs of too much exercise:

- Unusual or persistent fatigue
- Increased weakness
- Decreased range of motion
- Increased joint swelling
- Continuing pain (pain that lasts more than one hour after exercising)

Should someone with rheumatoid arthritis continue to exercise during a general flare? How about during a local joint flare?

It is appropriate to put joints gently through their full range of motion once a day, with periods of rest, during acute systemic flares or local joint flares. Patients can talk to their doctor about how much rest is best during general or joint flares.

Are researchers studying exercise and arthritis?

Researchers are comparing the development of musculoskeletal disabilities, including arthritis, in long-distance runners and non-runners. Preliminary results show that running does not increase the likelihood of developing osteoarthritis.

Researchers also are looking at the effects of muscle strength on the development of osteoarthritis. Other researchers continue to look for and find benefits from exercise to patients with rheumatoid arthritis, spondyloarthropathies, systemic lupus erythematosus, and polymyositis.

Where can people find more information on arthritis and exercise?

Arthritis Foundation
1330 West Peachtree Street
Atlanta, GA 30309
404/872-7100 or call your local chapter (listed in the telephone directory)
800/283-7800
World Wide Web address: **http://www.arthritis.org**

This is the major voluntary organization devoted to arthritis. The Foundation publishes a free pamphlet on exercise and arthritis and a monthly magazine for members that provides up-to-date information on all forms of arthritis. Local chapters organize exercise programs for people who have arthritis, including People with Arthritis Can Exercise (PACE) and an aquatic exercise program held in swimming pools. The Foundation also can provide physician and clinic referrals.

PACE Catalog Center
Arthritis Foundation
P.O. Box 9020
Pittsfield, MA 01202-9945
800/PACE-236 (722-3236)

This center sells PACE exercise videotapes at two levels, basic and advanced. Each videotape is approximately 30 minutes long and includes a warm-up section, a gentle or moderate exercise routine, and a rhythmic movement sequence to help improve endurance. The videotapes are available for $19.50 per tape, plus shipping charges.

Spondylitis Association of America (SAA)
P.O. Box 5872
Sherman Oaks, CA 91413
818/981-1616
800/777-8189
World Wide Web address: **http://www.spondylitis.org**

This nonprofit, voluntary organization helps people who have ankylosing spondylitis and related conditions. SAA sells books, posters, videotapes, and audiotapes about exercises for people who have arthritis of the spine.

American College of Rheumatology/Association of Rheumatology
Health Professionals
60 Executive Park South, Suite 150
Atlanta, GA 30329
404/633-3777
Fax: 404/633-1870
World Wide Web address: **http://www.rheumatology.org**

This association provides referrals to physical therapists who have
experience designing exercise programs for people with arthritis. The
organization also provides exercise guidelines developed by the American College of Rheumatology.

Acknowledgments

The NIAMS gratefully acknowledges the assistance of Jeanne
Hicks, M.D., and Naomi Lynn Gerber, M.D., both of the Rehabilitation Medicine Department, and Stanley R. Pillemer, M.D., Office of
the Director, NIAMS, at the National Institutes of Health, in the
preparation and review of the text for this chapter.
The National Arthritis and Musculoskeletal and Skin Diseases
Information Clearinghouse (NAMSIC) is a public service sponsored
by the NIAMS that provides health information and information
sources. The NIAMS, a part of the National Institutes of Health (NIH),
leads the Federal medical research effort in arthritis and musculoskeletal and skin diseases. The NIAMS sponsors research and research
training throughout the United States as well as on the NIH campus
in Bethesda, MD, and disseminates health and research information.

Chapter 54

Arthritis on the Job: You Can Work with It

Legal Rights

What Legal Rights Do I Have?

Federal laws have made the playing field more level for people with arthritis and other disabling conditions who wish to remain employed. Between them, the Americans with Disabilities Act of 1990 and its "ancestor," the Rehabilitation Act of 1973, give important protections to workers in the private sector and the federal government. The new Family and Medical Leave Act also provides relief to workers faced with lengthy absences because of illness.

Your state also may have laws that protect people with disabilities from discrimination.

The Americans with Disabilities Act

The Americans with Disabilities Act (ADA), passed by Congress in 1990, is the most extensive bill of rights for people with disabilities ever signed into law. It bans discrimination against people with disabilities in many areas, including hiring and employment. At the same time, it protects employers from having to make changes that are unreasonable or expensive.

While the ADA gives people with disabilities specific rights, the exact meaning of many of its terms such as unreasonable, undue, or essential probably will be decided by the courts.

The ADA and Employment

The ADA applies to companies employing 15 or more people. It bans discrimination against qualified individuals with disabilities by private employers, state and local governments, employment agencies, and labor unions. It applies to all aspects of employment, including hiring, job assignments, training, promotion, pay, benefits, and company-sponsored social events.

For you to be considered an individual with a disability, arthritis must "substantially limit" a major life activity such as walking, performing manual tasks, or working. To be considered qualified you must:

- have the education, skills, and experience the employer requires

- be able to perform the essential functions of the job—those that might be listed in an advertised job description—with or without reasonable accommodation. Reasonable accommodation means any changes in a job or workplace needed to enable an individual to:

- apply for a job

- perform the essential functions of the job

- enjoy all the benefits and privileges of employment.

Examples of reasonable accommodation are:

- part-time or adjusted work schedules

- job restructuring—for example, changing your job to cut out non-essential activities that you have trouble doing

- providing assistive equipment or devices

- providing an access ramp or making the workplace more accessible

- changing the height of a desk

Changes that would put undue hardship, defined as significant difficulty or expense, on an employer are not considered reasonable accommodations. If accommodations are needed, the employer cannot ask you to pay for them, and he cannot pay you less to cover the cost of the accommodations. If the cost of the accommodation is an undue hardship for the employer, he must give you the choice of providing it for yourself or of sharing in the cost. Keep in mind that an employer is not required to place you in a particular job if he believes that doing so would put you or others at increased risk.

Must My Employer Offer Me Health Insurance?

Your employer must offer you the same health insurance benefits he offers other employees. For this reason, he can offer health insurance policies that do not cover pre-existing conditions like arthritis. He does not have to offer you extra benefits to cover your particular medical condition.

Does the ADA Help Me Get Around?

The ADA says that state and local government services and "public accommodations" must be accessible to, or easily entered and used by, people with disabilities. Public accommodations include places like restaurants, doctors' offices, and private schools and colleges.

Public bus and train systems also must be made accessible to people with disabilities, and so must private bus and van companies.

How Can I Make the ADA Work for Me?

The ADA and the legal rights it creates give you the tools to be an effective advocate for yourself and to work with your employer for your mutual benefit.

If you still feel you have not been treated fairly, the ADA allows you to file complaints with the Equal Employment Opportunity Commission (EEOC) and other federal agencies. However, the ADA also encourages other ways of settling disagreements, such as negotiation, mediation, mini-trials, and arbitration. This makes good sense, since litigation may be time-consuming and costly and may not achieve your goal.

If you wish to file a formal complaint, you should contact the field office of the EEOC within 180 days of the time the incident happened. Ask your employer to give you a copy of all letters and reports regarding your situation. Keep them together in a safe place so that it will be easier for you to prove your case, if necessary. If your complaint is upheld, you are entitled to a remedy that will place you in the position you would have been in if the discrimination had never occurred. You may be entitled to hiring, promotion, reinstatement, back pay, or reasonable accommodation, including reassignment to a different job. You may also be entitled to attorney's fees.

The Rehabilitation Act of 1973

The Rehabilitation Act of 1973 was the model for the ADA and contains many of the same protections for people with disabilities. It applies to the federal government and all its agencies, to companies that do business with the federal government, and to institutions that receive federal financial assistance.

The Family and Medical Leave Act

The Family and Medical Leave Act (FMLA), which went into effect in August 1993, includes a provision that allows employees to take up to three months unpaid medical leave per year if they are unable to work because of a serious health condition. You can take FMLA leave all at one time, intermittently (at different periods), or by working part-time. For example, you could use FMLA leave to receive "continuing treatment," such as physical therapy, from a health care provider.

The FMLA applies to companies that employ 50 or more workers within a 75-mile radius. To be eligible for family leave, you must have worked for your employer for 1,250 hours in the previous 12 months. Whenever possible, you should provide advance leave notice and medical certification.

How Could the FMLA Help Me?

Your employer must allow you to take unpaid leave to care for:

- a newborn, adopted, or foster child
- a spouse, child, or parent who has a serious health condition
- your own serious health condition.

You may take "intermittent leave" or work a reduced leave schedule (fewer hours per day) with employer approval. When you return to work (except in certain cases), you must be restored to your original or equivalent positions with equivalent pay, benefits, and other terms of employment. Your medical insurance benefits must be continued on the same terms.

It is against the law for your employer to interfere with or deny rights granted under the FMLA. All employers are required to post notices of rights under the FMLA.

How Do I Handle Work Relationships?

In spite of the protection offered by the ADA, many people are reluctant to mention their arthritis for fear they will be denied promotions or other opportunities. However, if arthritis begins to interfere with your work, you will have to decide whether and how to tell your employer and co-workers about it.

Co-workers who don't know about your arthritis can become resentful if they feel you are not pulling your share of the load. They may get annoyed if they are often asked to help out or to make up for you on days missed if they do not know the reason. Even people who do know about your arthritis may think of it as "just aches and pains." They may feel you are making a fuss about nothing and getting special treatment you don't deserve. These attitudes can trigger anger on both sides.

You, on the other hand, may worry that you will be treated differently or denied opportunities for promotion if people know that you have arthritis. You may be tempted to ignore your body's warnings. In fact, you may work extra hard to cover up the fact that you have arthritis.

How Do I Tell My Employer?

If you decide to disclose your arthritis, plan carefully how and when to discuss the subject of arthritis with your co-workers or supervisors. Research carefully all the changes that could be made to make your work as productive as possible.

Schedule a meeting with your supervisor at a time when neither one of you is under pressure. It may also be helpful to find an opportunity to talk informally with your co-workers or a personnel officer about ways to make things go more smoothly.

In the meetings, describe as simply as possible the ways arthritis may affect your work. Make it plain that you are not looking for sympathy, but for ways to resolve the problem that will benefit both the company (or your coworkers) and yourself. The goal of these meetings should be to generate a supportive atmosphere in which everyone works together as part of a team.

Be prepared to help your employer. You are the expert on what you need to work efficiently. Offer suggestions for changes that could be

465

made, based on the research you have done before the meeting. Chances are any changes you may need will not cost much.

It is a good idea to be as well informed as possible about the ADA, assistive devices you may need and their cost, and resources to help employers. In fact, there may be tax deductions and/or tax credits available to certain employers who provide accommodations and/or jobs for people with disabilities. Excellent sources of information on these topics are listed in the Resources section.

However, realize that subtle discrimination in some companies may still exist, especially when it comes to promotions. Also, some unions may have a problem with allowing workers with disabilities to take jobs that traditionally have been reserved as rewards for workers with seniority. To prevent problems, your company's personnel manager may ask the union's help in working out a solution when an accommodation such as a job change or job restructuring is needed.

What If Arthritis Forces Change?

There are times when, in spite of all your doctor's efforts and in spite of all your own efforts, arthritis makes it impossible for you to continue in your present job.

This does not mean you will have to stop working altogether. With the help of the ADA and vocational rehabilitation services, you may be able to continue working for many years. However, you may have to change jobs, work fewer hours, or consider self-employment.

If your job involves physical labor, it may be helpful to have your doctor refer you to an occupational or physical therapist or a state vocational rehabilitation agency for a physical work performance evaluation or functional capacity evaluation. Such a test will determine exactly how much you can lift, carry, push, pull, and perform fine motor skills.

There are three ways to continue working if arthritis prevents you from doing your present job. They are: reasonable accommodations, vocational rehabilitation, or working from home.

Reasonable Accommodations

The ADA says your employer must make reasonable job accommodations to assist you. These might include:

- restructuring (changing the duties of) your job to cut out tasks you have difficulty doing

- allowing you to work on a flexible schedule or part-time

- placing you in a different job.

Vocational Rehabilitation (VR)

VR is another road to employment if the ADA can't help you. The goal of VR is to help people with disabilities develop job skills and find and keep employment. It has been found to have a 50-percent success rate in helping people with arthritis find employment. Vocational rehabilitation services vary from state to state but usually include:

- counseling and guidance about possible careers

- help in getting transportation and assistive devices such as wheelchairs

- tools, equipment, supplies, and licenses needed to help you work job training and job placement services

- personal assistance services.

For more information on VR, see the Arthritis Foundation's free brochure, *Arthritis and Vocational Rehabilitation*. It also lists the VR agencies in each state. Vocational rehabilitation may also be provided by private non-profit organizations such as Goodwill Industries. For information on agencies in your area, contact your local Arthritis Foundation chapter.

Working from Home

You may work from home by starting your own business or by working at home for an employer. If you are independent, self-disciplined, and like to plan your own hours, then a home business may be right for you.

But before you begin, consider the following questions: Do you have the self-discipline you need to focus on work? Will you miss socializing with others? Will you miss getting out? Will you be able to successfully develop and run a business?

If you feel confident that you can deal with these issues, contact the Small Business Administration Office (SBA) in your area. The SBA's Handicapped Assistance Loan (HAL-2) program provides direct loans and loan guarantees to qualified individuals with disabilities to set up their own businesses. The agency also provides individual guidance and a variety of classes for people starting out in their own business. Many college and community adult education programs offer similar classes.

Some companies will allow you to work for them out of your home. They often provide you with the equipment you will need. Jobs that can be done largely on computers or by telephone are best suited for this arrangement. To find such companies, check with your local chamber of commerce, businesses in your area, classified advertisements, vocational rehabilitation agencies, and friends.

Work Disability: What Next?

If you become disabled because of arthritis and are unable to return to work, you may be eligible for Social Security disability benefits. The Social Security Administration considers you disabled if you are unable to do any kind of work for which you are suited, if your inability to work is expected to last at least one year or to result in death.

There are two kinds of benefits: Social Security Disability Insurance (SSDI) and Supplemental Security Income (SSI). Both offer specific incentives to encourage people receiving these benefits to return to work. For more information on these programs, see the Resources section.

If you have bought private disability insurance, your benefits will be governed by the terms of the policy.

Other Resources

ABLEDATA, A National Database of Assistive Technology Information
8455 Colesville Road,
Suite 935
Silver Spring, MD 20910-3319
(800) 227-0216

Center for Computer Assistance to the Disabled (C-CAD)
1950 Stemmons Freeway,
Suite 4041
Dallas TX 75207-3109
(214) 746-4217

Equal Employment Opportunity Commission
1801 L Street NW
Washington, D.C. 20507
(202) 663-4264

Job Accommodation Network
P.O. Box 6080
Morgantown, WV 26506-6080
(800) 526-7234

**President's Committee on
Employment of People with Disabilities**
1331 F Street NW
Washington, D.C. 20004
(202) 376-6200

Chapter 55

Arthritis and Pregnancy

What to Consider Before Becoming Pregnant

If you have arthritis and are pregnant or are thinking about having children, you may have asked yourself these questions:

Am I Ready?

Any couple who is thinking of having a baby will have certain physical, emotional, and financial issues to consider before conceiving the child. As a woman with arthritis, you have particular concerns related to your arthritis about strength and endurance.

- Can you lift a 10 lb. bag of potatoes (a close approximation of the weight and bulk of a new-born baby) from the bed?

- Can you hold a 10 lb. bag of potatoes in one arm while sitting for at least 10 minutes?

- Can you go up and down stairs easily while carrying a 10 lb. bag of potatoes?

- Can you walk around the house carrying the 10 lb. bag of potatoes for up to 10 minutes?

- Do you get more pain in my hips, knees and/or feet when carrying the 10 lb. bag of potatoes?

- Can you screw on and off the top to a baby bottle?

- Can you push a diaper pin through a thick diaper?

- Can you get through my average day without taking a nap?

- Can you bend your neck (chin to chest) to see the baby if you were holding it close?

Why and Why Now?

It's not uncommon for some women to choose pregnancy when they are feeling lonely and depressed, thinking that a new baby will change things for them. You might want to ask yourself the following questions when thinking about how you feel about having a baby:

- Am I expecting a new baby to fill a void in my life?

- Do I want to get pregnant only to try to relieve some of the pain I'm having from my arthritis?

- Are there people around me who can help me when I'm not feeling well?

- Is this a good time to have a baby, personally, emotionally and financially?

If you're not sure how you feel about some of these questions, discuss your feelings with your family and friends. You might also find it helpful to talk to your doctor or other health team members. These people can also refer you to a counselor or someone specially trained to help with these issues, or to other women in similar situations.

Will My Arthritis Go Away?

In some cases, pregnancy may cause some forms of arthritis, especially rheumatoid arthritis, to improve for a time. However, this does not always happen during pregnancy and should never be your reason for becoming pregnant.

Rheumatoid arthritis: some improvement common by end of fourth month, swelling may reduce, but joint pain and stiffness may persist.

Lupus: may stay the same, improve, or flare (get worse) during pregnancy. Lupus should be in remission for at least six months before pregnancy begins to decrease chances of flares.

Scleroderma and other types of arthritis: some studies report that scleroderma flares, while others report that it improves.

Flares: Illness may flare two to eight weeks after your baby is born.

Abortion: Having an abortion will not prevent a flare. Any type of delivery whether from a spontaneous abortion, a therapeutic abortion, or a stillbirth could cause a flare.

Will My Child Inherit Arthritis?

Probably not. Scientists have found certain genetic markers that may indicate if some people have a higher risk for getting some types of arthritis. However, the relationship between these markers and the actual development of arthritis is still unclear and does not mean you will pass arthritis on to your child. Generally, there is no way to tell if your child will ever have arthritis in the future.

How Will Arthritis Affect My Pregnancy?

Arthritis does not affect the actual course of pregnancy in most women. However, if you have a form of arthritis for example, lupus which affects your internal organs, such as your kidneys or heart, then it may cause some problems during the pregnancy. High blood pressure should be monitored and treated quickly.

Problems That May Occur in Women with Other Rheumatic Diseases

Pregnancy can be life-threatening for women who have lupus, scleroderma, or other rheumatic diseases, especially if the disease has caused kidney problems and/or high blood pressure.

Women with lupus may be at greater risk for:

Toxemia—a condition that may cause high blood pressure, fluid retention, and possibly seizures.
Spontaneous abortion.
Stillbirth—this may happen in a small number of women with lupus.

Neonatal lupus—a very rare condition that may cause a lupus-like rash in some newborns. It usually goes away within six to twelve months after birth. Some babies may also develop congenital heart block. This is a malfunction in the electrical system of the heart, which causes a slow heartbeat. If this problem is severe, a pacemaker may be inserted in the baby. In most cases, these infants do well and have no further problems.

Slowed growth of the fetus—a common problem that your doctor will monitor. If this problem becomes severe, you may have to deliver your baby earlier than planned.

Your doctor may perform the following blood tests to assist him or her in planning the frequency and type of evaluations you may need during your pregnancy.

- **Anti-cardiolipin (AN-tie car-dee-oh-LE-pin) antibody test:** a test associated with an increased risk for miscarriage.

- **Anti-Ro (SS-A) and Anti-la (SS-B) antibody tests:** tests associated with an increased risk for congenital heart block in the baby.

- **Lupus anticoagulant (AN-tie-koe-AGG-you-lant):** a test associated with an increased risk for spontaneous abortion.

If you have kidney problems, such as with lupus or scleroderma, your doctor will monitor these problems and perform tests more frequently during your pregnancy. Sometimes it is difficult to tell the difference between kidney problems caused by the illness or pre-eclampsia (toxemia) caused by the pregnancy. If there is a chance that your kidney problems may improve or go away, your doctor may ask you to delay your pregnancy until these changes occur.

How Will Pregnancy Affect My Arthritis

The physical changes that normally occur during pregnancy may affect your joints and muscles in the following ways:

1. Joints may become looser and less stable. This may cause you to "waddle" when you walk.

2. Knee problems may become worse due to your increased weight, or because the muscles along the side of the knee become weaker. This might cause knee pain, especially while going up or down stairs or when straightening your knee.

3. As your uterus grows, your spine curves slightly to support it. This can lead to muscle spasms in your back. Sometimes this can also cause pain, numbness and tingling in your legs.

4. Much more blood flows through your body during pregnancy, so it is important that your heart is functioning normally. If your heart is functioning normally, you shouldn't have any problems. If you have any heart problems such as pericarditis (pare-ih-card-EYE-tiss) inflammation of the sac surrounding the heart or myocarditis (my-oh-card-EYE-tis) inflammation of the heart muscle your doctor may ask you to delay pregnancy until these problems are under control.

5. Water weight gain may increase stiffness, especially in your weight-bearing joints (hips, knees, ankles, and feet). It may also cause problems with carpal tunnel syndrome a condition that causes pain, numbness, and tingling in the thumb, index, and middle finger. This usually goes away after delivery. Report all water gain to your obstetrician during your office visit. Report any unusual water gain (any beyond the lower legs, such as in the thighs or face) to your doctor right away.

6. Breathing. Your breathing muscles will move upward due to the growing baby. This may cause only mild shortness of breath. If you have significant shortness of breath or a change in your breathing, contact your doctor right away.

What to Do Once You've Decided to Have a Baby

To feel your best during your pregnancy and after your baby is born, try to get your arthritis under the best possible control before you become pregnant. This means keeping in close touch with your doctors and following your treatment program carefully before, during, and after pregnancy. Here are some ways to do this:

Visit your health care team: doctor (preferably a rheumatologist AND an obstetrician), Maternal fetal specialist, Rheumatology nurse, Nutritionist or dietitian, Occupational therapist, Physical therapist, and Social Worker.

Follow your treatment plan: As a pregnant woman with arthritis, your plan should include:

1. Arthritis Medicines—know what arthritis medicines you're taking and how they will affect your baby

Table 55.1. Arthritis Medicines That May Be Used Cautiously During Pregnancy

Medicine	Brand-Name Examples
aspirin	Anacin, Bayer, Bufferin, Ecotrin
prednisone	Deltasone, Meticorten, Orasone, Panasol

Discuss any medicines you use either prescription or over-the-counter with your doctor(s). If you must take medicines during your pregnancy, your doctor will give you the lowest possible dose and will monitor the effect of the medicine on you and the baby. Do not start or stop taking any prescription or over-the-counter medicines without first contacting your doctor.

Any medicines you take may be passed to your baby through breast milk. Here are some tips to consider if you intend to breast feed:

- Talk to your doctors and to your baby's doctor about your medicines and their possible effects on your baby.

- Never take any prescription or over-the-counter medicines without first checking with your doctor or pharmacist.

- Take your medicines after the baby's morning feeding, so less medicine will be passed through your milk.

2. **Exercise**—to keep your muscles strong and your joints flexible Discuss your exercise program with your doctors before you begin, especially if you have:

- heart problems
- phlebitis inflammation of the veins, usually in the legs
- a serious infection
- severe high blood pressure
- high risk for premature labor
- incompetent cervix a problem that could cause your baby to be born prematurely
- any bleeding from the uterus
- any problems with the fetus

Talk to your obstetrician about the types and amount of muscle strengthening (isometric) exercise you should do. Too much of the wrong type of exercise could reduce the amount of blood flowing to the baby, which can cause problems. Try walking or swimming. These are general exercises that help keep your muscles strong, increase your endurance, and are generally safe for pregnant women.

3. Diet—eat a balanced diet. Good nutrition is very important for your health and for your baby's health. You should eat a balanced diet and practice good eating habits before, during, and after your pregnancy, especially if you are breast-feeding. A dietitian, nutritionist, or other health care worker can help you plan a balanced diet. The following are some common eating problems:

Weight gain or weight loss: Your obstetrician or dietitian can help you plan a diet to make sure you get enough vitamins and minerals.

Nausea and vomiting:

- Eat small, frequent meals.
- Eat slowly and chew food thoroughly.
- Avoid greasy, fried foods.
- Eat toast or crackers when you get up in the morning.
- Avoid drinks that might upset your stomach, such as coffee and fruit juices.
- Talk to your doctor about your arthritis medicines and how they might be affecting your nausea.

Heartburn: Talk to your doctor about this and how your arthritis medicines might be affecting you heartburn. To reduce heartburn:

- Eat small, frequent meals.
- Decrease caffeine in your diet.
- Avoid fried, fatty, and spicy foods.
- Avoid carbonated drinks, such as soda.
- Raise the head of your bed by placing 6" blocks beneath it.
- If you use antacid, choose one which is low in sodium.

Constipation: Bowels may slow down during pregnancy and cause constipation. Some forms of arthritis, such as scleroderma, also cause bowel changes. Contact your doctor immediately if you are having bloating, gas, diarrhea, or constipation problems beyond what your doctor thinks is normal for you. To relieve constipation:

- Eat high-fiber foods (whole-grain breads, fresh fruits and vegetables, cereals with bran, beans such as kidney and pinto).

- Drink 6 8 glasses of water daily.

- Exercise (such as walking or swimming).

- Try a high fiber laxative, such as Metamucil®.

4. Joint protection—learn ways to ease joint pain and to reduce stress on your joints. The extra weight of pregnancy may make your joints hurt more. To avoid further damage to your joints, it's important to learn ways to protect your joints from extra stress and strain. Here are some ways to do this. To relieve joint pain:

- Avoid pain-relief medicines, when possible.

- Use hot or cold packs on your joints.

- Use splints. They may be especially helpful for your hands and knees.

- Rest whenever possible.

- Try relaxation exercises, such as biofeedback or visual imagery.

- Wear comfortable shoes (such as jogging shoes) that give you good support. Shoes should have a 1" to 1 1/2" heel, good arch support, roomy toe box, and firm heel-counter. Lace-up or Velcro-closure shoes provide the most support.

- Practice good posture and gait at all times.

- Sleep on a firm, supportive mattress to reduce muscle spasms.

- Ask your obstetrician about using support hosiery to reduce fluid retention in your legs, ankles, and feet.

- Notify your doctor of any increased pain in joints and muscles and of any numbness or tingling in your hands or feet.

- Exercise to keep your joints flexible and your muscles strong.

- If you need joint surgery, it could affect your ability to care for your baby. Consider having the surgery before you become pregnant so that you'll be able to recover before you have to care for your baby.

- Do not drink alcohol to control or ease pain. Alcohol may harm your unborn baby.

5. Stress Management—to help ease the emotional ups and downs of pregnancy. The emotional changes that ordinarily occur during pregnancy should be no different for a woman with arthritis. Your moods may range from anxiety to elation, and may be very temperamental and erratic. Discuss these emotions with your doctor, especially if they interfere with your ability to carry out your regular activities. Since some types of arthritis, such as lupus, can also cause psychological changes, your doctor should be aware of how you and your family perceive your behavior. The following issues may also be of particular concern during your pregnancy:

- **Sexuality:** The fatigue, nausea, and emotional changes of pregnancy often cause sexual desire and the frequency of intercourse to decrease during your first three months. Desire often increases during the second trimester, but may decrease again during the third trimester when you may feel uncomfortable and/or unattractive. Fatigue or fear of another pregnancy may decrease sexual desire after your baby is born. The additional pain and fatigue of arthritis may make these problems worse. If these changes are a problem for you, talk openly with your partner about them. Often, open communication can help solve many of these problems.

- **Self-esteem:** If joint problems, pain, or fatigue decrease your ability to care for your baby, you may feel you're an inadequate mother. This can be especially true when the arthritis flares. It's important to remember that you are capable of caring for your child, but that you may need a little more help than other people. Accepting help does not make you less of a mother it simply means you're accepting responsibility for your well-being and your baby's well-being. If you are troubled by such thoughts, it may be helpful to talk to someone who specializes in these problems.

Will I Have Difficulty with Labor and Delivery?

Probably not, but you'll want to find a comfortable position during the labor and delivery process. You probably can deliver your baby as most women do: vaginally, lying on your back. If this position is uncomfortable, you may want to lie on your side or sit in a rocking chair or birthing chair. Even if you have had a hip replacement, you may be able to deliver your baby vaginally, without complications.

As with any pregnant woman, you may need monitoring and certain blood tests during labor and delivery. However, the amount of monitoring you may need will depend on how active your disease is. If you have lupus or scleroderma, your fetus probably will be monitored throughout labor. In some cases, it may be necessary to check the fetus' blood during labor to determine if there are any problems that might require the baby to be born by cesarean section rather than vaginally.

Chapter 56

Travel Tips for People with Arthritis

Planning Your Trip

Plan Ahead

The key to successful travel is advance planning. The first step includes making realistic plans—ones that fit your capabilities and interests. For example, a hiking trip may be unreasonable for a person with hip and knee limitations; instead, a week at the beach may be a better choice. Plans must also be flexible, allowing people with arthritis to set their own pace. You might consider spending one or two days or afternoons alone if other family or group members plan more strenuous activities or extensive sightseeing. While alone, occupy your time with a good book, craft item, letter writing, or better yet, use that time to catch up on your rest. Frequent rest periods may be the most important ingredient for an enjoyable trip.

Travel Agents

Some people prefer to make all their travel arrangements themselves, while others find it more convenient to work with a travel agent. Travel agents do not charge for their services and can often save you money, as well as time.

Choosing a Travel Agent

Selecting a good travel agent is relatively easy. Ask for referrals from friends and relatives or call various agencies and ask about their experience arranging trips for people with illnesses or physical limitations. Be sure to select an agent with whom you feel comfortable discussing your special needs, and make sure he or she is willing to spend the extra time necessary to work out your particular arrangements.

Don't assume anything. For example, not all travel agents are familiar with the terms "accessible" or "disabled accommodations." Be specific about your requirements. Keep in mind that the travel agent cannot and should not make all the decisions for you. You will be more satisfied if you work with the agent to select the arrangements that suit your needs and interests.

Travel plans should be made at least four to six months in advance, especially for trips to popular holiday spots. The more time you give an agent, the better the chances he or she will be able to make any special arrangements for you.

Group Tours

Group tours may not be for everyone, although many people find them an enjoyable way to travel. Either you or your travel agent can reserve space on a group tour. Be careful, however, about joining "budget" tours. They may not provide arrangements for special access or accommodations. They also work on a tight, fast-paced schedule which may not be appropriate for you.

Tours for people with limited mobility may be more suited to your needs. These are moderately paced and designed to meet the special requirements of the group. They include hotel lodging, transportation, sights, and restaurants that are suitable and accessible for people with limited mobility. Individuals are generally expected to make their own arrangements for nursing or attendant care if needed. If provided by the tour agency, additional payment is required for the attendant's travel costs and escort services. Most often, families and friends are also welcome to join these tours.

Many travel agents and tour agencies also arrange special tours for senior citizens. These tours are generally slower-paced and provide luggage-carrying assistance. Tours for senior citizens are often advertised in the travel section of newspapers or as part of senior citizen clubs' membership activities.

You might consider arranging your own tour with a group of friends or members from your arthritis club or self-help group. Whichever tour you select, study the details carefully.

Hotel Accommodations

Hotel arrangements can make your trip pleasant and enjoyable or totally unbearable. Therefore, keep your needs in mind when selecting hotels. Many of the better hotel chains have specially designed rooms available at no extra charge for people who have disabilities. Many also publish free directories describing their features and any special accommodations. Make sure to specify any special arrangements you will need well in advance and get written confirmation of any guaranteed accommodations. Organizations such as the Society for the Advancement of Travel for the Handicapped (SATH) and the Association for Specialized Services Involving Special Travelers (ASSIST) provide hotel and other travel information for people with disabilities.

Find out about the Following Accommodations

Before making hotel reservations, ask about any of the following accommodations that pertain to you.

- Walking distance and amount of stairs to the room, restaurant, pool, beach, gift shop or other areas of interest.

- Whether telephones are placed conveniently beside the bed and in the bathroom.

- Location of the elevators.

- Availability of hotel-provided transportation to and from the airport which can easily be used by someone with mobility limitations or a wheelchair.

- Accessibility and availability of heated pools for exercise and relaxation.

- Whether hand rails are located beside toilet and tub.

- Availability of levers instead of round knobs for doors, faucets, and shower/ bathtub controls.

- Availability of room service where food and laundry services are inaccessible.

- Distance from the lobby to your room.

- Lowered light and thermostat switches or closet bars.

- Low pile carpet.

- Raised toilet seat.

- Bathroom accessibility.

- Sinks and vanity tops which allow space for wheelchairs.

- Trapeze bar above the bed to aid with transfer to and from the wheelchair. (Consider bringing your own trapeze bar.)

- Ramp to entrance door.

- Disabled parking.

- Fire exits for the disabled or first floor rooms in case of fire.

Travel Insurance

Illness of any kind can interrupt travel plans, yet most airline and hotel reservations are made well in advance. While some deposits can be refunded, others cannot. You may receive full or partial refunds if cancellations are due to illness and if refund requests are accompanied by a doctor's statement. Nonetheless, some people prefer to purchase trip cancellation insurance which reimburses portions of your deposit for hotel, holiday package, and airfare. It can be purchased from a travel or insurance agent.

Some people purchase medical insurance for travelers called "trip or travel insurance." This type of insurance provides payment for medical services received during a trip. Some policies have a clause that exempts coverage of any pre-existing condition (treated 60-90 days prior to purchase or travel date), so be sure to understand the policy and what it covers. Also find out about the policy's maximum payouts, age restrictions, and types of services covered.

The cost of trip medical insurance for a two-week stay may range from $50 for a single person to $200 for a family. The American Automobile Association (AAA) has low-cost trip insurance available to nonmembers. NEAR Services, a travel services company, provides insurance coverage for illness expenses incurred during a trip, as well as expenses to get you home if necessary. NEAR also provides members with other trip services such as lost and found, physician referral, and meet and assist airline arrangements. For more information about NEAR Services call (800) 654-6700.

Before purchasing medical trip insurance, find out what provisions your own health insurance has for covering medical care during travel.

Medical Considerations

Medical Care

- Wear a medic-alert bracelet at all times in order to get appropriate medical care in case of an emergency. This is especially important for people who take steroids, or who have allergies, heart disease, diabetes, or other special medical conditions or requirements.

- Discuss your travel plans with your doctor. Ask if you need any special tests, treatment, or travel precautions. Also ask your doctor what to do in case symptoms worsen during the trip.

- Complete any necessary lab studies or medication injections before you leave.

- If you anticipate stomach or motion sickness, ask your doctor to recommend appropriate medication.

- Eat lightly before and during travel.

- Obtain the name of a physician or clinic at your destination from your doctor or someone familiar with your destination. Bring along a summary of your medical history.

- If you have arthritis in your neck or neck pain, support your neck in an upright position with a soft cervical collar or horseshoe pillow. This will protect your head from bobbing if you should fall asleep.

- Should you become ill, most hotels employ a doctor or can refer you to a clinic.

Medications

- Always carry medications with you in your carry-on bag or purse; luggage may get lost or over-heated.

- Take medications with you when sightseeing so you can stay on schedule. You never know when you may be delayed.

- Bring enough medications to last the length of the trip plus an extra refill in case of spills or delays.

- Take along current prescriptions in case medications get lost.

- Keep medications in labelled plastic containers.

- Containers with liquid medications should only be 3/4 full. Keep these in plastic bags in case of leakage.

- Carry snacks with you if you need to take food with your medications.

Items to Bring along

- Name and phone number of your doctor

- Prescriptions

- Insurance forms and insurance group or policy number

- Sunblock for people whose medications promote burning

- Any arthritis aids you absolutely need such as:
  - built-up eating utensils
  - rubber lever door handle for hotel rooms
  - portable, raised toilet seat
  - long-handled comb or brush
  - special pillows for neck or back
  - device for manipulating hotel key
  - reacher for picking up items
  - heating pad
  - folding cane

- Sunscreen, hat, and protective clothing for people with Systemic Lupus Erythematosus (SLE)

Saving Your Joints and Your Energy

General Tips for Travel and Sightseeing

- Begin a trip or outing well rested.

- Set aside time to rest at your destination before beginning activities.

- Prevent stiffness with simple range-of-motion exercises such as:
  - ankle circles
  - shoulder circles
  - wrist and hand exercises

— leg lifts
— moving legs in a jogging or walking motion to stimulate circulation
— getting up and moving around if possible.

- Accept help and special services when needed.

- Ask tour guides how much walking is required.

- If walking is difficult for you or if you tend to tire easily, consider requesting a wheelchair or motorized cart, even if you usually do not require one. It may allow you to enjoy activities which might otherwise be painful or impossible. (Some recreational facilities provide wheelchairs.)

- Don't let yourself get overtired.

  — Set priorities for activities.
  — Don't expect to do everything—especially in one day
  — Alternate active periods with restful ones.
  — Schedule rest periods for yourself, as well as your family. Traveling may be tiring for them also.

- Anticipate how you will spend time by yourself in case you are unable to join or keep up with the group's activities. (For example, browse through a book store or enjoy a snack at a corner cafe while others shop more extensively.)

Luggage and Packing Tips

- Use light-weight luggage with shoulder straps or wheels.

- Ask porters to carry your luggage whenever possible.

- Use luggage carts when assistance is unavailable.

- Carry dollar bills for tips—a few extra dollars spent for luggage assistance may be well worth the cost.

- Pack lightly—most hotels have laundry facilities.

- Take comfortable clothing that is easy to get on.

- Check weather conditions ahead of time to decide what type of clothing to bring. Clothes that can be layered allow you to adapt more easily to changes in the weather.

- Bring a sweater for air-conditioned buildings, transportation, or cooler days.

- Travel in low-heeled shoes with good support.

Travel Options

Tips for Air Travel

- Request any special services at the time you book your reservation.

- Reserve seats ahead of time to avoid standing in lines.

- If you will need special assistance, arrive at least one hour before the normal check-in time and allow extra time to get to the airport and through the terminal to the departing gate.

- If you have difficulty walking, request an airport wheelchair or motorized cart to save energy. Such requests should be made in advance.

- Ask skycaps to carry your luggage.

- Curbside check-in saves on luggage carrying and standing in lines.

- Check all luggage through to your final destination, especially if you have connecting flights.

- Prevent stiffness during a flight with simple range-of-motion exercises or by getting up and moving around if possible.

Tips for Car Travel

Keep the following items in the car:

- All medications (if left in the trunk, they may spoil from the heat).

- Snacks and beverages (especially if you need to eat when taking your medications).

- Hand-held lighted magnifying glass for reading detailed maps.

- Emergency Kit (including tire pump, jumper cable, jug of water for radiator leaks, flashlight, emergency flares, change for phone calls).

- First Aid Kit (including bandages and tape, Band-Aids, bee sting ointment, mosquito repellent and salve, burn/sunburn cream, tweezers, alcohol pads, chemically activated ice packs, antiseptic cream).

- Consider installing a CB radio to obtain current traffic or weather conditions, or to secure help in an emergency.

Joint protection devices for a more comfortable ride:

- Special inflatable horseshoe pillow for head and neck support.

- Cervical collar for neck pain.

- Cushioned seat belt to minimize shoulder discomfort.

- Back cushion to provide additional back support.

- Sheepskin steering wheel cover to protect hand joints by allowing a looser grip and also protecting hands from a hot or cold steering wheel.

- Wide-angled side and rear-view mirrors.

Tips for Train Travel

- Make reservations early.

- Request assistance with the special service desk.

- Request a wheelchair if you anticipate difficulty walking.

- Reserve a seat in the food service car if you anticipate difficulty walking through the train.

- Find out whether Amtrak personnel will be available to accompany wheelchair passengers to and from the train and assist with boarding and exiting.

- Make advance reservations for the special swivel seat for wheelchair travelers.

- Request that a wheelchair be available at each scheduled stop.

- Ask whether restrooms, bedrooms, and train aisles are accessible.

Tips for Bus Travelers

- Ask what kind of assistance is available.

- Take snacks or lunch on board if you anticipate difficulty getting on and off the bus at food stops or if you will need food with your medications.

- Try to schedule your trip during midweek and non-holiday times when fewer people are traveling.

- Avoid too many bus or terminal transfers.

- Bring a small pillow or cervical collar for naps.

- Do range-of-motion exercises on the bus and at rest stops to prevent stiffness.

- If traveling with an aide, ask about the two-for-one fare. Present the necessary doctor's statement when you purchase your ticket.

- Determine services and accessibility at each scheduled stop.

- Ask whether wheelchairs must be collapsible for storage.

- Obtain an advance travel schedule and make any necessary hotel accommodations.

Tips for Ship Travel

- Choose a cabin near the elevator and reserve a table near the entrance of the dining room if you anticipate difficulty walking.

- Confirm that special requests have been passed on to the crew.

- Choose a cruise with fewer stops if you anticipate difficulty getting on or off the ship.

- Take along motion sickness medication prescribed by your doctor.

- Make sure the ship is accessible to wheelchairs.

- Ask whether it is necessary to bring a ramp or wheelchair narrowing device.

- Be sure wheelchair brakes are in good working order.

- Determine in advance whether any ports of call will require a license for a motorized wheelchair.

- If required, present a medical statement stating that the disabled person is physically able to travel by cruise.

Health Tips for Overseas Travel

- **Immunizations:** Get all required vaccines before leaving the U.S. Information is available from your doctor, state health department, or the Center for Disease Control (CDC)—Division of Quarantine (404) 329-3311.

- **Infections:**

  — Avoid areas with unsanitary or contaminated food or drinking water

  — Prevent mosquito and insect bites with the use of nets and repellents. (Some insect bites in other countries can cause mild to serious illnesses.)

  — Avoid swimming or wading in fresh water where snails are common, as these may harbor infectious bacteria.

  — See your doctor soon after arriving home from a developing country to be examined for any infectious diseases you may have acquired. Bring a copy of your itinerary

- **Medical Care:**

  — If you require medical care while you are overseas, attempt to call your doctor at home for a second opinion.

  — Obtain names of English-speaking doctors at your destination before leaving on your trip. A listing for 450 cities and 120 countries can be obtained from the International Association for Medical Assistance to Travelers (IAMAT), 417 Center Street, Lewiston, New York, 14092 (716) 754-4883, or contact the American Embassy, Consulate, Military or Missionary Hospitals in each country.

Medication Tips for Overseas Travel

- Do not take Chloromycetin for upper respiratory infections or Enterovioform for diarrhea. Both are commonly prescribed abroad in spite of serious side effects.

- Ask your doctor for a prescription of medications to bring along in case of an upper respiratory infection or diarrhea (the two most common travel illnesses).

- Bring enough medication and necessary syringes to last the trip, plus an additional refill in case of delays or spills.

- Foreign pharmacists generally do not accept prescriptions from doctors in other countries. If they do, beware that drugs in other countries are distributed in different strengths and with different names.

- Customs officials are especially suspicious of capsules or syringes they may find during baggage inspections. To avoid problems, provide a written list of medications with a doctor's statement describing your need for taking them.

Chapter 57

When Your Student Has Arthritis

If you are surprised that arthritis affects children, you are not alone. Most people think of it as a disease limited to old age. However, an estimated 285,000 infants, youngsters and teenagers in the U.S. have arthritis.

When one of your students has arthritis, it is important that you know about the disease and its potential effects on the child in classroom activities. Because the severity and pattern of the disease are different for each child, this chapter can provide only general information and guidelines to help you help your student.

Before or soon after the school term begins, you the teacher, (and perhaps the principal, physical education teacher and school nurse) should meet with the child's parents to discuss the student's health. You need to be alerted to any problems that could affect the child's performance and attitude. Throughout the school year, you and the parents should inform each other about significant changes in the child's physical and emotional health. It might be helpful to share this chapter with other school staff so everyone who will have contact with the student will be aware of her abilities and needs.

The parents of a child with arthritis, like other parents, are very concerned about school activities. They are eager to work with you and other school staff to help ensure the best environment for their youngster's academic and social development.

Symptoms of Arthritis May Not Be Apparent

Childhood arthritis may be a "hidden" handicap—the damage and pain are inside the body. Therefore, your student may show few outward signs of the disease. Swollen joints often are not noticeable except when the disease has caused deformities in the wrists and fingers. A child may not complain of pain, but only show the effect of stiffness in the difficulty of performing certain tasks. Because the damage is not visible it may be hard to understand that the pain is genuine and the limitations are legitimate. One sign to watch for is fatigue, sometimes extreme a common symptom of arthritis and other rheumatic diseases.

Another deceptive and misunderstood aspect of childhood arthritis is the erratic and unpredictable change from day to day, and even from morning to afternoon. Fatigue, joint stiffness and pain may be so mild one day that the child shows no signs of illness. The next day, these symptoms may be so severe that the child cannot move without painful difficulty. On such bad days, your student may be very slow, uncoordinated and irritable, and barely able to walk or raise her hand to ask a question. Trying to do normal activities may cause severe fatigue. On the other hand, many children with arthritis want so much to be like the other youngsters that they try to ignore or conceal their stiffness and pain.

At these times, emotional support from parents, other family members, classmates, and you is essential to your student's well-being.

Treatment

Your student's treatment program is individualized according to age, disease activity and affected joints. Typically it will include medication, a proper balance of rest and special exercises, splints worn at certain times, heat or cold therapy and possible surgery. There are still no cures for any of the common forms of arthritis in children, so treatment is aimed at keeping the disease under control. That means relief of pain, control of inflammation, and prevention of the deformities and other consequences of the condition. When possible, children are encouraged to learn the skills necessary to manage their own care as they grow and become independent. For example, an older child may be encouraged to keep her own medications timetable while the teacher provides supervision.

Medication

Medication is used to suppress and control joint inflammation and pain. The most commonly prescribed drugs are aspirin or related drugs such as ibuprofen. These drugs are often taken in high daily doses. This means that they must be taken frequently and consistently on a strict daily schedule as prescribed by the doctor. If these drugs cannot be tolerated or are not effective, other medications are usually given.

How Can You Help?

Know the child's medication schedule: Your student will probably have to take medications during the school day often with meals or snacks to prevent stomach upset. The child's parents should outline the schedule for you and the school nurse.

Eliminate roadblocks: Since your student may have to take pills during school hours, it should be routine and simple, without roadblocks. Taking medication on time can be critically important to the child's well-being. Be sure the arrangements and responsibilities are clear and consistent, and are understood by the child as well as the parents. Each school district's rules vary—strict procedures may be in order to avoid possible legal difficulties.

Learn medication side effects: The medication your student takes may cause side effects, such as a headache, stomach ache, or mood changes, that may affect her behavior in class. You should be aware of and review any side effects with the parents, the principal, and the school nurse.

Work with the child: Your student may be embarrassed to take medication in front of classmates because it calls attention to her condition. A child of any age may hide, "forget" or throw away the pills. You may have to subtly supervise your pupil, in order to allow her to take the required medication unobtrusively. For instance, establish a routine whereby you casually check with your student once or twice a day to make sure she has taken the medicine.

Occupational Therapy/Physical Therapy

Your student may have to practice special exercises that help improve joint mobility and function, as well as prevent or minimize disabilities. Sometimes the exercises are done at home in the mornings and evenings. Exercise or therapy may also have to be provided in school through the school system. You and the parents may need to discuss a plan for this therapy. Although you are not responsible for supervising this therapy, you should be aware of its potential effects on the student at school. Joint stiffness typically varies from one day to the next. Usually the most severe discomfort is experienced in the mornings, upon awakening. To allow time to loosen up and get going, your student must start the day one or two hours earlier than her classmates. A 10-15 minute warm bath is usually followed by special exercises that move the affected joints through their full range of motion. The time needed for this therapy varies, depending on the extent of stiffness and pain on a given morning or on a given day. The length of morning stiffness can be an indicator of disease activity. The longer morning stiffness lasts, the more active the disease, and the greater the need for rest.

How Can You Help?

Understand that the child may be late from time to time: On particularly bad days during disease flare-ups, or when the child has a doctor's appointment, she may miss some school time. You need to appreciate that such tardiness or absence is necessary. Children with arthritis are very sensitive about being tardy or anything else that calls attention to their condition and sets them apart from their classmates. By being aware and understanding of this, you can help keep it from being an added problem.

Help the child complete missed work: You, the child, and the child's parents should see that missed work is completed. You might try instituting a buddy system. When the student misses class, she can telephone her buddy and find out about assignments. Another method is to write out assignments ahead of time so that the child with arthritis knows what is planned and can keep up.

Splints/Braces

Occasionally, your student may wear a plastic or leather splint, particularly on her arm, wrist or hand. They are usually worn at night. However, sometimes they must be worn during the day and removed during exercise. Splints reduce pain, rest inflamed joints, keep them in proper position, and help to prevent or correct deformities. Children who have severe deformities, joint damage or muscle weakness in their legs may have to wear metal or plastic leg braces.

If arthritis has affected your student's cervical spine, she may have to wear a cervical collar (neck brace) to maintain proper alignment and reduce pain.

How Can You Help?

Know the child's splint schedule: Just as you know your student's medication schedule, know when she must wear and remove her splint, and encourage her to do so.

Surgery

Most children with arthritis will not need surgery. However, a few with severe arthritis require surgery to relieve pain, correct joint deformity and repair damage caused by the disease. These children may have to miss days or weeks of school. Corrective surgery may also be needed at a later stage to alter the effects of growing up with arthritis.

How Can You Help?

Help the student keep up with work: For long absences, make arrangements before surgery with the hospital tutor or homebound teacher to help the student keep up with assignments. Help the student stay in touch with classmates: Work out a plan to help your student keep up to date with school friends and activities so that she continues to feel part of the class.

Activity: How Much and When?

Your student's physical ability to participate in classroom, playground or gym activities should follow guidelines developed by the doctor, the child's parents and you. Proper exercise and activity are necessary to lessen and prevent joint stiffness and loss of range of motion. It can also give the child a psychological boost by helping her feel like a member of the group. Everyone concerned, though, should be careful that she doesn't overdo it.

How Can You Help?

Be aware of the child's limitations: Your student may have certain physical limitations. To please you and gain acceptance from classmates, she may overextend herself by participating in strenuous activities. She should not be forced or pressured to participate in physical education or other activities which are prohibited by her doctor or therapist. As a general rule, if her joints are painful and swollen, she should rest them and only move them gently. Remember that although pain does not show, it can be disabling. At the same time, she should not be excluded from activities in which she is able to participate. She may also be able to participate in a different way, e.g., as a scorekeeper.

Know if the child is in pain: If your pupil is very young, her parents will rely heavily on your judgment of her condition to guide her participation in school activities. The child may not obviously hurt, but if you closely observe her facial expression, way of walking, and general behavior, you usually can learn to detect signals that she is not feeling well. Many schoolage children are able to talk about their pain. If you ask them how much hurt or pain they are having on a scale of 0-10 (where 0 is no hurt and 10 is the worst possible hurt), most can tell you what their pain level is.

Allow the child to move around: Sitting in one position for too long can cause stiffness and pain. Allow your student to move around frequently in the classroom.

Discuss activity guidelines with parents: You and the student's parents should discuss physical activity guidelines and make sure that the child understands them. For example, adapted physical education activities that put less stress on inflamed joints may be necessary. Some examples may include swimming, walking, tossing a beach ball, or dancing without jumping. These types of activities have less impact on joints than sports such as football, track, or soccer. Some activities may be fine for one child, but too intense for another. In general, the child should be encouraged to set her own limits on activity at school, and to let you know when she isn't feeling well.

Keeping up at School

Arthritis and the medication and therapy used to treat it do not affect your student's mental ability. However, she may be physically slow or awkward, become fatigued very quickly, or have to go at a slightly different pace than the rest of the class in performing certain tasks. If she is unable to walk, to grasp or hold objects as quickly and easily as other students, or has been advised by the medical team not to do certain activities, she may have some problems with everyday activities that the other students do without a thought. Some examples are:

- carrying school books and lunch trays
- turning door handles
- taking off her coat and boots and changing clothes
- standing in line for a long time
- sitting on the floor cross-legged
- rehearsing fire drills
- walking from one class to another in the short time allowed
- opening lockers
- walking up or down stairs
- flushing toilets
- fuming water faucets
- using regular pens or pencils
- writing fast enough to take notes or complete tests during allotted time
- completing homework
- writing on a blackboard
- raising her hand to ask a question or participate in class discussions
- participating in a regular PE class.

Educational Rights

If such limitations affect your student's ability to learn and to benefit from her education, then the school district is required by federal law to supply the accommodations and/or services needed to allow her to fully benefit from the educational process. Consult the following laws for the specific requirements:

P.L. 94-142, Education for All Handicapped Act, reauthorized and renamed in 1990 by PL 101-476 the Individuals with Disabilities Education Act (IDEA) mandates free and appropriate education to all children regardless of disability. Parents can request eligibility for special services including:

- **An Individualized Education Plan (IEP)** which must be developed collaboratively and approved each year by parents.

- **Special related services** including school health services, occupational therapy, physical therapy, or adaptive learning experiences or assistive devices and classroom accommodations.

- **Transition services** for every student age 16 and over to assess the student's future educational, vocational, and community living needs and provide smooth transition to adult services.

Section 504 of P.L. 93-112, Rehabilitation Act of 1973 and amendments in the Americans with Disabilities Act (ADA): These are civil rights laws which protect a student's rights in school, employment, public accommodations, transportation, and telecommunications.

P.L. 94-482, Vocational Education Act of 1976 stipulates that children with special health care needs must have equal access to the full range of vocational education programs, including the development of an individual vocational education plan (IVEP), similar to an IEP, for every eligible child.

P.L. 99457, The "Early Intervention" law of 1986 extends the age of eligibility for school-based special education and related services to children three years of age and older, and allows states to provide early intervention services for children with special needs from birth to age three.

Part Eight

Additional Help and Information

Chapter 58

Glossary

A

Aerobic exercise: Exercise that requires continuous, rhythmic motion of large muscle groups such as the quadriceps. Swimming, running, and walking are examples of aerobic exercise. Aerobic exercise also improves the ability to perform activities of daily living.

Ankylosing spondylitis: See Spondyloarthropathies.

Antibody: A special protein produced by the body's immune system that recognizes and helps fight infectious agents and other foreign substances that invade the body.

Antinuclear antibody (ANA) test: A blood test done to find out if the body is producing antinuclear antibodies.

Antinuclear antibody: Abnormal antibodies that are often present in people who have connective tissue diseases or other autoimmune disorders. These antibodies target material in the nucleus (the "command center") of healthy cells instead of fighting specific disease-causing agents.

NIH Web Publications, "Arthritis and Exercise Keywords," "Polymyalgia Rheumatica and Giant Cell Arteritis Glossary," "Psoriasis Glossary," and "Raynaud's Phenomenon Keywords." Office of Scientific and Health Communications. [http://www.nih.gov/niams/healthinfo]

Arteries: Large blood vessels that carry blood and oxygen from the heart to all parts of the body.

Arterioles: Small blood vessels that branch off from arteries and connect to capillaries.

Artery: Any tubular, branching vessel that carries blood from the heart throughout the body.

Arthritis: Literally means joint inflammation. It is a general term for more than 100 conditions known as rheumatic diseases. These diseases affect not only the joints but also other parts of the body, including important supporting structures such as muscles, tendons, and ligaments, as well as some internal organs. These diseases can cause pain, stiffness, and swelling in joints and may also affect other parts of the body.

Atrophy: Decrease in size or wasting away of a body part or tissue. When muscles are not used, they atrophy (get smaller and weaker).

Autoantibodies: Abnormal antibodies produced against the body's own tissues.

Autoimmune disease: A disease in which the immune system destroys or attacks a person's own tissues.

B

Benign: A mild disease or condition that is not life threatening.

Biofeedback: A technique designed to help a person gain control over involuntary (independent of the will) body functions, such as heart rate, blood pressure, or skin temperature. A way to enhance a body signal so that one is aware of something that usually occurs at a level below consciousness. An electronic device provides information about a body function (such as heart rate) so that the person using biofeedback can learn to control that function. Biofeedback can help people with arthritis learn to relax their muscles. In this case, an electronic device amplifies the sound of a muscle contracting, so the arthritis patient knows that the muscle is not relaxed

Biopsy: The removal of tissue or cells from a person to examine them for signs of disease.

Body mechanics: Correct positioning of the body for a given task, such as lifting a heavy object or typing.

C

Capillaries: Tiny blood vessels that carry blood between arterioles (the smallest arteries) and venules (the smallest veins). Capillaries form networks throughout the body's organs and tissues. They open and close in response to the organs' needs for oxygen and nutrients.

Cardiovascular: Involving the heart and the circulatory system.

Cartilage: A tough, stretchy tissue that covers the ends of bones to form a low-friction, shock-absorbing surface for joints.

Collagen: A fibrous protein that is one of the main building blocks of skin, tendon, bone, cartilage, and other connective tissues.

Connective tissue disease: A group of diseases that affect the body's connective tissues, including tissue in the joints, blood vessels, heart, skin, and other supporting structures. Some of these diseases are caused by a malfunctioning of the immune system. Connective tissue diseases are fairly common and include systemic lupus erythematosus, rheumatoid arthritis, scleroderma, polymyositis, and dermatomyositis.

Connective tissue: The supporting framework of the body and the internal organs—including bone, cartilage, and ligaments. The tissue that supports body structures and holds parts together. Some parts of the body, such as tendons and cartilage, are made up of connective tissue. Connective tissue is also the basic substance of bone and blood vessels.

Corticosteroids: Potent anti-inflammatory hormones that are made naturally in the body or synthetically (man-made) for use as drugs. They also are called glucocorticoids. The most commonly prescribed drug of this type is prednisone.

Cyanosis: Bluish, grayish, or dark purple discoloration of the skin that occurs when blood cannot circulate freely and gives up all its oxygen.

Cytokines: Chemical messengers in the body that help direct and regulate response and are involved in cell-to-cell communication.

D

Degenerative joint disease: See Osteoarthritis (OA).

Dermis: The layer of skin beneath the epidermis.

E

Emollient: A substance composed of fat or oil that soothes and softens the skin.

Endorphin: A substance produced in the brain or nervous system that stops pain naturally.

Endurance: The ability to continue a given task.

Epidermis: The outermost layer of skin.

Erythrocyte sedimentation rate (ESR): A blood test that determines how fast erythrocytes (red blood cells) settle out of unclotted blood and is used to detect inflammation in the body. Connective tissue diseases can change blood proteins, which changes how quickly red blood cells settle out of unclotted blood to the bottom of a test tube. Higher ESRs (indicating more rapid settling of red blood cells and the presence of inflammation) are found in all of the connective tissue diseases. Also referred to as the "sed rate" or ESR.

Erythrodermic psoriasis: A form of psoriasis characterized by widespread reddening and scaling of the skin often accompanied by itching or pain. Symptoms may be precipitated by severe sunburn, use of oral steroids, or a drug-related rash.

Exercise: Movement of the body designed to improve its physical condition. The goals of an arthritis exercise program are to improve physical conditioning, muscle strength, flexibility, well-being, and function.

F

Fibromyalgia: A chronic disorder characterized by widespread musculoskeletal pain, fatigue, and multiple tender points.

Fibrous capsule: A tough wrapping of tendons and ligaments that surrounds the joint.

Flare: A period of time in which disease symptoms reappear or become worse.

Flexibility: Ability to bend various joints and move freely.

G

Gangrene: A condition that occurs when tissue dies. Tissue death is usually caused by a loss of blood supply. Gangrene may affect a small area, such as a finger or toe, or a large portion of a limb.

Gene: A unit of inheritance that contains the instructions, or code, that a cell uses to make a specific product, usually a protein. Genes are made of a substance called DNA. They govern every body function and determine inherited traits passed from parent to child.

Genetics: The science of understanding how diseases, conditions, and traits are inherited.

Giant Cell Arteritis: A disease causing inflammation of the temporal arteries and other arteries in the head and neck. Inflammation causes the arteries to narrow, reducing blood flow in the affected areas. The condition may cause persistent headaches and vision loss. It is also known as cranial arteritis, temporal arteritis, or Horton's disease.

Gout: A type of arthritis caused by the reaction of the body to needle-like crystals of uric acid that accumulate in joint spaces. This reaction causes inflammation, swelling, and pain in the affected joint, most commonly the big toe.

Guttate psoriasis: A form of psoriasis characterized by drop-like lesions on the trunk, limbs, and scalp. Symptoms may be triggered by viral respiratory infections or certain bacterial (streptococcal) infections.

H

Histologic examination: The study of a tissue specimen by staining it and examining it under a microscope.

Hydrotherapy: Therapy that takes place in the water.

I

Immune response: The reactions of the immune system to foreign substances.

Immune System: A complex network of specialized cells and organs that work together to defend the body against attacks by "foreign" invaders such as bacteria and viruses. In some rheumatic conditions, it appears that the immune system does not function properly and may even work against the body.

Immune system: A complex network of specialized cells and organs that work together to defend the body against attacks by foreign substances, such as bacteria and viruses.

Incidence: The number of new cases of a particular disease that occur in a population during a defined period of time, usually one year.

Inflammation: A characteristic reaction of tissues to injury or disease. It is marked by four signs: swelling, redness, heat, and pain.

Internist: A doctor who specializes in internal medicine (not requiring surgery).

Inverse psoriasis: A form of psoriasis characterized by large, dry, smooth, vividly red plaques in the folds of skin.

Ischemic lesion: A sore or other skin abnormality caused by an insufficient supply of blood to the tissue.

Isometrics: Isometric exercises are exercises that cause a muscle to contract and do work while joints do not move, for example, pushing against a wall.

J

Joint space: The area enclosed within the fibrous capsule and synovium.

Joint: The place where two bones meet. Most joints are composed of cartilage, joint space, fibrous capsule, synovium, and ligaments.

Juvenile rheumatoid arthritis: A chronic arthritis of childhood that causes pain, stiffness, swelling, and loss of function in the joints and may also affect other parts of the body.

K

Keratolytic: A substance that promotes the softening and peeling of the epidermis.

L

Ligaments: Stretchy bands of cord-like tissue that connect bone to bone.

M

Manipulation: Trained professionals such as chiropractors or osteopaths use their hands to help restore normal movement to stiff joints.

Methotrexate: A drug often used to treat cancer that is also used in lower doses to treat some forms of arthritis.

Microwaves: Microwave therapy is a type of deep heat therapy. The electromagnetic waves pass between electrodes placed on the patient's skin. This creates heat that increases blood flow and relieves muscle and joint pain.

Mobilization therapies: A group of treatments that include traction, massage, and manipulation. When used by a trained professional, these methods can help control pain and increase joint and muscle motion.

Muscle: Tissue that can contract, producing movement or force. There are three types of muscle: striated muscle, attached to bones; smooth muscle, found in such tissues as the stomach and blood vessels; and cardiac muscle, which forms the walls of the heart. For striated muscle to function at its ideal level, the joint and surrounding structures must be in good condition.

N

Nailfold capillaroscopy: A test used to identify the primary or secondary form of Raynaud's phenomenon. The examiner places a drop of oil on the nailfold (the skin at the cuticle or base of the nail) and uses a hand-held magnifying glass or microscope to look at the capillaries in the nailfold. Certain changes in theses capillaries can be characteristic of connective tissue diseases.

Nonsteroidal anti-inflammatory drugs (NSAIDs): A group of medications, including aspirin, ibuprofen, and related drugs, used to reduce inflammation that causes joint pain, stiffness, and swelling.

NSAID: An abbreviation for nonsteroidal anti-inflammatory drug. NSAIDs do not contain corticosteroids and are used to reduce pain and inflammation. Aspirin and ibuprofen are two types of NSAIDs.

O

Occult: Disease or symptoms that are not readily detectable by physical examination or laboratory tests.

Osteoarthritis: OA (also know as degenerative joint disease) primarily affects cartilage within the joints, causing it to fray, wear, ulcerate, and in extreme cases, to wear away entirely, leaving a bone-on-bone joint. At the edges of the joint, bony spurs may form. OA can cause joint pain, loss of function, reduced joint motion, and deformity. Disability results most often from disease in the spine and in the weight-bearing joints (knees and hips).

P

Phototherapy: Use of natural or artificial light to treat a disease.

Physiatrist: A doctor who specializes in the diagnosis and management of injuries and diseases causing pain, loss of function, and disability. Treatment plans often include the use of exercise, massage, heat, electricity (TENS), relaxation techniques, splints and braces, and local injections to relieve pain.

Plaques: Patches of thickened and reddened skin that are covered by silvery scales.

Polymyalgia Rheumatica: A condition of unknown cause that affects the lining of joints, particularly in the shoulders and hips. Symptoms include pain and stiffness, typically in the neck, shoulders, and hips. It may be associated with giant cell arteritis.

Polymyositis: A rheumatic disease that causes weakness and inflammation of muscles.

Predisposition: A tendency to develop a certain disease.

Prevalence: The total number of people in a population with a certain disease at a given time.

Psoriasis vulgaris: The most common form of psoriasis, characterized by reddened lesions covered by silvery scales.

Psoriasis: A chronic (long-lasting) skin disease characterized by scaling and inflammation. Scaling occurs when cells in the outer layer of skin reproduce faster than normal and pile up on the skin's surface. Possibly a disorder of the immune system.

Psoriatic arthritis: Joint inflammation that occurs in about 5 to 10 percent of people with psoriasis (a common skin disorder).

PUVA: A treatment sometimes used for extensive or severe psoriasis that combines oral or topical administration of a medicine called psoralen with exposure to ultraviolet A (UVA) light.

R

Range of motion (ROM): The ability of a joint to go through all its normal movements. A measurement of the extent to which a joint can go through all its normal spectrum of movements. Range-of-motion exercises help increase or maintain flexibility and movement in muscles, tendons, ligaments, and joints.

Rehabilitation specialist: See physiatrist.

Relaxation therapy: People with arthritis use relaxation to release the tension in their muscles, which relieves pain.

Rheumatoid Factor: A special kind of antibody often found in people with rheumatoid arthritis.

Rheumatoid arthritis: An often chronic systemic disease that causes inflammatory changes in the synovium, or joint lining, that result in pain, stiffness, swelling, and loss of function in the joints. The disease can also affect other parts of the body.

Rheumatologist: A doctor who specializes in diagnosing and treating disorders that affect the joints, muscles, tendons, ligaments, and bones.

S

Short waves: These deliver deep heat to relieve pain. (Short waves are not used much currently because of problems in people with pacemakers.)

Smooth muscle: The muscles of the body that are not under a person's conscious control. Smooth muscle is found mainly in the internal organs, including the digestive tract, respiratory passages, urinary bladder, and walls of blood vessels.

Spasm: An involuntary, sudden muscle contraction. In Raynaud's phenomenon, involuntary contraction of the smooth muscle in the blood vessels decreases the flow of blood to the fingers or toes (which leads to color changes in the skin).

Spondyloarthropathies: A group of rheumatic diseases that affect the spine, such as Reiter's syndrome and ankylosing spondylitis.

Strengthening exercises: Exercises that build stronger muscles, for example, exercises that require movement against a force (weight lifting or isometric exercises).

Synovial fluid: Fluid released into movable joints by surrounding membranes. This fluid lubricates the joint and reduces friction.

Synovitis: Inflammation of the synovial membrane, the tissue that lines and protects the joint.

Synovium: A thin membrane that lines a joint and releases a fluid that allows the joint to move easily.

Systemic lupus erythematosus: Lupus is a type of immune system disorder known as an autoimmune disease, which causes the body to harm its own healthy cells and tissues. This leads to inflammation and damage of various body tissues. Lupus can affect many parts of the body, including the joints, skin, kidneys, heart, lungs, blood vessels, and brain.

Systemic treatment: A treatment, such as a pill, that is taken internally.

Systemic: Disease or symptoms that affect many different parts of the body.

T

T cell: A type of white blood cell that is part of the immune system and normally helps protect the body against infection and disease. In psoriasis, it also can trigger inflammation and excessive skin cell reproduction.

Temporal Arteries: Vessels located over the temples on each side of the head, that supply blood to part of the head.

Tendons: Tough, fibrous cords of tissue that connect muscle to bone.

TENS (transcutaneous electrical nerve stimulation): Passes electricity to nerve cells through electrodes placed on the patient's skin. TENS is used to relieve pain.

Topical agent: A treatment, such as a cream, salve, or ointment, that is applied to the surface of the skin.

Toxicity: The potential of a drug or treatment to cause harmful side effects.

Traction: Gentle, steady pulling along the length of body structure, for example, the spine or neck.

Transcutaneous: Through the skin.

U

Ultrasound: Sound waves that provide deep heat to relieve pain.

UVB phototherapy: An artificial light treatment used for mild psoriasis.

V

Vasodilator: An agent, usually a drug, that widens blood vessels and allows more blood to reach the tissues.

Vasospasm or Vasoconstriction: A sudden muscle contraction that narrows the blood vessels, reducing blood flow to a part of the body.

Chapter 59

Sources of Further Help and Information

ABLEDATA, A National Database of Assistive Technology Information
8455 Colesville Road,
Suite 935
Silver Spring, MD 20910-3319
(800) 227-0216

American Chronic Pain Association
P.O. Box 850
Rocklin, CA 95677
(916) 632-0922
fax (916) 632-3208
email acpa@pacbell.net

American Academy of Orthopaedic Surgeons
6300 N. River Road
Rosemont, IL 60018-4262
847/823-7186
800/346-2267
fax (847) 823-8125
World Wide Web address: http://www.aaos.org
The academy publishes several brochures on the knee, including Knee Arthroscopy and Total Knee Replacement, which doctors can obtain and give to their patients. Single copies of two other pamphlets, Arthroscopy and Total Joint Replacement, are available free to the public if a self-addressed, stamped envelope is provided.

American College of Rheumatology/Association of Rheumatology Health Professionals
60 Executive Park South, Suite 150
Atlanta, GA 30329
phone: 404/633-3777
Fax: 404/633-1870
World Wide Web address: http://www.rheumatology.org
This national professional organization can provide referrals to rheumatologists and allied health professionals, such as physical therapists. One-page fact sheets are available on various forms of arthritis. Lists of specialists by geographic area and fact sheets are also available on ACR's web site.

American Physical Therapy Association
1111 N. Fairfax Street
Alexandria, VA 22314
(703) 684-2782
800/999-APTA (2782)
World Wide Web address: http://www.apta.org
The association has published a free brochure titled "Taking Care of the Knees."

Arthritis Foundation
1330 West Peachtree Street
Atlanta, GA 30309
(800) 283-7800
(404) 872-7100
fax (404) 872-0457
or your local chapter, listed in the telephone directory
Web address: http://www.arthritis.org
The Arthritis Foundation is the major voluntary organization devoted to supporting arthritis research and providing educational and other services to individuals with arthritis. The foundation publishes a free pamphlet on rheumatoid arthritis and a magazine for members on all types of arthritis. It also provides up-to-date information on research and treatment, nutrition, alternative therapies, and self-management strategies. Chapters nationwide offer exercise programs, classes, support groups, physician referral services, and free literature. Single copies of brochures are free with a self-addresses stamped envelope.

The Foundation has several free brochures about coping with arthritis, taking nonsteroid and steroid medicines, and exercise. A free brochure on protecting your joints is titled "Using Your Joints Wisely."

Disabilities served: Arthritis, rheumatic diseases

Users served: People with arthritis and rheumatic diseases and their families, health care professionals

Description: The Arthritis Foundation is a national, voluntary health association committed to supporting research to find the cure for and prevention of arthritis and improve the quality of life for those affected by arthritis. Programs include support for scientific research, specialist training, public information and education, and help within the community for people who have rheumatic diseases. The 71 local chapters and divisions of the foundation provide basic information as well as assistance in locating treatment specialists, clinics, and other agencies to help with physical financial, and emotional problems caused by arthritis. The chapters support a variety of local services, including information and education programs, support groups, exercise classes, arthritis clinics, home care programs, and rehabilitation services.

Information services: The foundation disseminates information about arthritis care to its chapters and to professionals in the arthritis treatment field. A variety of pamphlets are available from the foundation's local chapters, including information on specific forms of arthritis, various treatments, and solutions to physical and emotional problems associated with arthritis. Some materials are available in Spanish. Chapters maintain lists of medical and community services and make referrals upon request. The foundation holds national and regional scientific meetings and continuing community education programs to advise local physicians of the latest clinical advances.

Center for Computer Assistance to the Disabled (C-CAD)
1950 Stemmons Freeway,
Suite 4041
Dallas TX 75207-3109
(214) 746-4217

Equal Employment Opportunity Commission
1801 L Street NW
Washington, D.C. 20507
(202) 663-4264

517

Fibromyalgia Alliance of America
P.O. Box 21990
Columbus, OH 43221-0990
614/457-4222
fax (614) 457-2729
Contact: Mary Anne Saathoff, R.N.

Fibromyalgia Association of Texas
Route 1, Box 106A
Edgewood, TX 75117
(903) 896-1495
Contact: Ms. Faye Wright

Fibromyalgia Association of Greater Washington (FMAGW)
13203 Valley Drive
Woodbridge, VA 22191-1531
Phone: 703/790-2324
Fax: 703/494-4103
Web: www.fmagw.org
Contact person: Tamara Liller

Fibromyalgia Network
P.O. Box 31750
Tucson, AZ 85751-1750
(520) 290-5508
800/853-2929
fax (520) 290-5550
www.fmnetnews.com
Contact: Ms. Kristin Thorson

Healthsouth Corporation
1 Healthsouth Parkway
Birmingham, AL 35243
800/768-0018
205/967-7116
205/969-4741 (fax)
www.healthsouth.com
Disabilities served: Spinal cord and head injuries, musculoskeletal trauma and orthopaedic conditions, sports and work-related injuries, stroke, arthritis, neurological and neuromuscular disabilities

Users served: Patients with the above listed disabilities, including support services for their family members

Description: HEALTHSOUTH Corporation was established in 1984 to build a national rehabilitation network of inpatient and outpatient rehabilitation facilities that are capable of providing the full spectrum of medical rehabilitation services. All HEALTHSOUTH facilities offer comprehensive medical rehabilitation services; a coordinated, interdisciplinary team approach; physician direction and supervision; top quality, highly-motivated rehabilitation professionals; state-of-the-art technology and techniques; and barrier-free physical environments.

Healthsouth operates 52 locations in 21 States, with a network of 1,400 beds and an employee base of 3,500. Since the company's founding, the comprehensive rehabilitation network has provided services to more than 100,000 patients and experienced more than a million outpatient visits.

Information services: HEALTHSOUTH publishes newsletters for medical professionals and is expanding its national, regional and local speakers' bureaus, to address medical/rehabilitation topics, current treatments, and technical innovations.

Hip Society
951 Old County Road #182
Belmont, CA 94002
(650) 596-6190
Fax: 650-508-2039
www.hipsoc.org
The Society maintains a list of physicians who are specialists in problems of the hip and provides physician referrals by geographic area.

Job Accommodation Network
P.O. Box 6080
Morgantown, WV 26506-6080
(800) 526-7234

Missouri Arthritis Rehabilitation Research and Training Center (MARRTC)
University of Missouri-Columbia
Department of Medicine, Division of Immunology and Rheumatology
MA427 Health Sciences Center
One Hospital Drive
Columbia, MO 65212
573-882-8738
fax 573-882-1380

Disabilities served: Arthritis and musculoskeletal diseases

Users served: People with arthritis, families, faculty for education of rehabilitation personnel, physicians

Description: The Missouri Arthritis Rehabilitation Research and Training Center is a project funded by the National Institute on Disability and Rehabilitation Research (NIDRR) to evaluate techniques for assessing performance; evaluate new techniques; demonstrate rehabilitation models; and provide training to professionals, persons with arthritis, and their families.

Information services: MARRTC publishes curricula and training materials, journal articles, monographs, and a newsletter.

National Arthritis and Musculoskeletal and Skin Diseases Information Clearinghouse (NAMSIC)
National Institutes of Health
1 AMS Circle
Bethesda, MD 20892-3675
Phone: 301/495-4484
TTY: 301/ 565-2966
Automated faxback system: 301/881-2731
World Wide Web address: http://www.nih.gov/niams
The Clearinghouse has additional information about some knee problems, including osteoarthritis and avascular necrosis, as well as information about total knee replacement and arthritis and exercise. Single copies of fact sheets and information packages on these topics are available free upon request.

Disabilities served: Rheumatoid arthritis, osteoarthritis, gout, systemic lupus erythematosus, scoliosis, scleroderma, sports injuries, and approximately 600 other rheumatic, musculoskeletal, and skin diseases.

Users served: Physicians, nurses, occupational and physical therapists, librarians, researchers, educators, members of the media, patients, and their families.

Description: The National Arthritis and Musculoskeletal and Skin Diseases Information Clearinghouse is a service of the National Institute of Arthritis and Musculoskeletal and Skin Diseases, a division of the National Institutes of Health.

Established in 1978, the clearinghouse is a national resource center for information about professional, patient, and public education materials; and federal programs related to rheumatic, musculoskel-etal, and skin diseases.

Information services: The clearinghouse maintains a file on the Combined Health Information Database (CHID), an online computerized database available to the public via BRS Information Technologies. Bibliographies, fact sheets, and brochures are compiled and distributed.

National Chronic Pain Outreach Association Inc.
P.O. Box 274
Millboro, VA 24460
(540) 997-5004
fax (540) 997-1305
www.chronicpain.org

National Institute of Arthritis and Musculoskeletal and Skin Diseases
Building 31, Room 4C05
Bethesda, MD 20892-2350
(301) 496-8188
fax (301) 480-6069
www.nih.gov/niams

National Institute of Neurological Disorders and Stroke
31 Center Drive
Bldg 31 Room 8A52
Bethesda, MD 20892
(302) 496-9746
fax (302) 497 0296
www.nih.gov

National Osteoporosis Foundation
Suite 500
1150 17th Street, N.W.
Washington, D.C. 20036

NIAMS Fast Facts
available 24 hours a day by fax. Using the phone on a fax machine, call NIAMS Fast Facts at (301) 881-2731. Listen to the instructions and dial; the text will print to the fax machine.

Osteoporosis and Related Bone Diseases National Resource Center
1150 17th St., N.W.,
Suite 500
Washington, D.C. 20036
(1-800) 624-BONE
TTY for hearing-impaired callers: (202) 466-4315
E-mail: orbdnrc@nof.org
World Wide Web: http://www.osteo.org

Paget Foundation for Paget's Disease of Bone and Related Disorders
120 Wall Street
Suite 1602
New York, NY
10005-4001
(1-800) 23-PAGET
E-mail: pagetfdn@aol.com
World Wide Web: http://www.paget.org

Policy Barriers that Impede Utilization of Technology to Maintain the Independence and Employment of Individuals Aging with a Disability Project (PAD)
Ethel Percy Andrus Gerontology Center
University of Southern California
Los Angeles, CA 90089-0191
213/740-6060
http://www.usc.edu/dept/gero/
Disabilities served: Rheumatoid arthritis, cerebral palsy, post-polio, stroke, and spinal cord injury.

Users served: Professionals in rehabilitation and related fields, people with disabilities, and researchers.

Description: PAD is a research project examining the responsiveness of current public policy to the dynamic needs of people "aging in" with lifelong disabilities. PAD research investigates policies affecting the availability, affordability, and accessibility of assistive technologies aimed at maintaining community-based living and the employment of middle-aged and elderly individuals with long-standing disabilities. In addition, PAD develops and critically evaluates recommendations for improving the responsiveness of current disability/aging programs.

Information services: PAD can provide general policy information to inquirers by phone or by letter. Technical publications on project research can be obtained by contacting the PAD office.

President's Committee on Employment of People with Disabilities
1331 F Street NW
Washington, D.C. 20004
(202) 376-6200

Spondylitis Association of America
14827 Ventura Boulevard
Suite 119
Sherman Oaks,
California 91403
Phone: (818) 981-1616
Toll Free: 1-800-777-8189
Fax (818) 981-9826
World Wide Web Address: http://www.spondilitis.org

Index

Index

Page numbers followed by 'n' indicate a footnote.

Page numbers in *italics* indicate a table or illustration

A

527

H

Diabetes Sourcebook, 2nd Edition

Basic Information about Insulin-Dependent Diabetes, Noninsulin-Dependent Diabetes, Gestational Diabetes, and Related Disorders, Including Diabetes Prevalence Data, Management Issues, the Role of Diet and Exercise in Controlling Diabetes, Insulin and Other Diabetes Medicines, and Complications of Diabetes Such as Eye Diseases, Digestive Disorders, Periodontal Disease, Amputation, and End-Stage Renal Disease; Along with Reports on Current Research Initiatives, a Glossary, and Resource Listings for Further Help and Information

Edited by Karen Bellenir. 800 pages. 1998. 0-7808-0224-1. $78.

Diet & Nutrition Sourcebook, 1st Edition

Basic Information about Nutrition, Including the Dietary Guidelines for Americans, the Food Guide Pyramid, and Their Applications in Daily Diet, Nutritional Advice for Specific Age Groups, Current Nutritional Issues and Controversies, the New Food Label and How to Use It to Promote Healthy Eating, and Recent Developments in Nutritional Research

Edited by Dan R. Harris. 662 pages. 1996. 0-7808-0084-2. $78.

"Useful reference as a food and nutrition sourcebook for the general consumer."
— *Booklist Health Sciences Supplement, Oct '97*

"Recommended for public libraries and medical libraries that receive general information requests on nutrition. It is readable and will appeal to those interested in learning more about healthy dietary practices."
— *Medical Reference Services Quarterly, Fall '97*

"An abundance of medical and social statistics is translated into readable information geared toward the general reader." — *Bookwatch, Mar '97*

"With dozens of questionable diet books on the market, it is so refreshing to find a reliable and factual reference book. Recommended to aspiring professionals, librarians, and others seeking and giving reliable dietary advice. An excellent compilation." — *Choice, Feb '97*

Diet & Nutrition Sourcebook, 2nd Edition

Basic Information about Nutrition, Including General Nutritional Recommendations, Recommendations for People with Specific Medical Concerns, Dieting for Weight Control, Nutritional Supplements, Food Safety Issues, the Relationship between Nutrition and Disease Development, and Other Nutritional Research Reports; Along with Statistical and Demographic Data, Lifestyle Modification Recommendations, and Sources of Additional Help and Information

Edited by Karen Bellenir. 600 pages. 1998. 0-7808-0228-4. $78.

Ear, Nose & Throat Disorders Sourcebook

Basic Information about Disorders of the Ears, Nose, Sinus Cavities, Pharynx, and Larynx, Including Ear Infections, Tinnitus, Vestibular Disorders, Allergic and Non-Allergic Rhinitis, Sore Throats, Tonsillitis, and Cancers That Affect the Ears, Nose, Sinuses, and Throat, Along with Reports on Current Research Initiatives, a Glossary of Related Medical Terms, and a Directory of Sources for Further Help and Information

Edited by Karen Bellenir and Linda M. Shin. 592 pages. 1998. 0-7808-0206-3. $78.

Endocrine & Metabolic Disorders Sourcebook

Basic Information for the Layperson about Pancreatic and Insulin-Related Disorders Such as Pancreatitis, Diabetes, and Hypoglycemia; Adrenal Gland Disorders Such as Cushing's Syndrome, Addison's Disease, and Congenital Adrenal Hyperplasia; Pituitary Gland Disorders Such as Growth Hormone Deficiency, Acromegaly, and Pituitary Tumors; Thyroid Disorders Such as Hypothyroidism, Graves' Disease, Hashimoto's Disease, and Goiter; Hyperparathyroidism; and Other Diseases and Syndromes of Hormone Imbalance or Metabolic Dysfunction, Along with Reports on Current Research Initiatives

Edited by Linda M. Shin. 632 pages. 1998. 0-7808-0207-1. $78.

Environmentally Induced Disorders Sourcebook

Basic Information about Diseases and Syndromes Linked to Exposure to Pollutants and Other Substances in Outdoor and Indoor Environments Such as Lead, Asbestos, Formaldehyde, Mercury, Emissions, Noise, and More

Edited by Allan R. Cook. 620 pages. 1997. 0-7808-0083-4. $78.

". . . a good survey of numerous environmentally induced physical disorders . . . a useful addition to anyone's library ."
— *Doody's Health Science Book Reviews, Jan '98*

". . . provide[s] introductory information from the best authorities around. Since this volume covers topics that potentially affect everyone, it will surely be one of the most frequently consulted volumes in the Health Reference Series." — *Rettig on Reference, Nov '97*

"Recommended reference source."
— *Booklist, Oct '97*

Fitness & Exercise Sourcebook

Basic Information on Fitness and Exercise, Including Fitness Activities for Specific Age Groups, Exercise for People with Specific Medical Conditions, How to Begin a Fitness Program in Running, Walking, Swimming, Cycling, and Other Athletic Activities, and Recent Research in Fitness and Exercise

Edited by Dan R. Harris. 663 pages. 1996. 0-7808-0186-5. $78.

"A good resource for general readers."
— *Choice, Nov '97*

"The perennial popularity of the topic . . . make this an appealing selection for public libraries."
— *Rettig on Reference, Jun/Jul '97*

Food & Animal Borne Diseases Sourcebook

Basic Information about Diseases That Can Be Spread to Humans through the Ingestion of Contaminated Food or Water or by Contact with Infected Animals and Insects, Such as Botulism, E. Coli, Hepatitis A, Trichinosis, Lyme Disease, and Rabies, Along with Information Regarding Prevention and Treatment Methods, and a Special Section for International Travelers Describing Diseases Such as Cholera, Malaria, Travelers' Diarrhea, and Yellow Fever, and Offering Recommendations for Avoiding Illness

Edited by Karen Bellenir and Peter D. Dresser. 535 pages. 1995. 0-7808-0033-8. $78.

"Targeting general readers and providing them with a single, comprehensive source of information on selected topics, this book continues, with the excellent caliber of its predecessors, to catalog topical information on health matters of general interest. Readable and thorough, this valuable resource is highly recommended for all libraries."
— *Academic Library Book Review, Summer '96*

"A comprehensive collection of authoritative information."
— *Emergency Medical Services, Oct '95*

Gastrointestinal Diseases & Disorders Sourcebook

Basic Information about Gastroesophageal Reflux Disease (Heartburn), Ulcers, Diverticulosis, Irritable Bowel Syndrome, Crohn's Disease, Ulcerative Colitis, Diarrhea, Constipation, Lactose Intolerance, Hemorrhoids, Hepatitis, Cirrhosis, and Other Digestive Problems, Featuring Statistics, Descriptions of Symptoms, and Current Treatment Methods of Interest for Persons Living with Upper and Lower Gastrointestinal Maladies

Edited by Linda M. Ross. 413 pages. 1996. 0-7808-0078-8. $78.

". . . very readable form. The successful editorial work that brought this material together into a useful and understandable reference makes accessible to all readers information that can help them more effectively understand and obtain help for digestive tract problems."
— *Choice, Feb '97*

Genetic Disorders Sourcebook

Basic Information about Heritable Diseases and Disorders Such as Down Syndrome, PKU, Hemophilia, Von Willebrand Disease, Gaucher Disease, Tay-Sachs Disease, and Sickle-Cell Disease, Along with Information about Genetic Screening, Gene Therapy, Home Care, and Including Source Listings for Further Help and Information on More Than 300 Disorders

Edited by Karen Bellenir. 642 pages. 1996. 0-7808-0034-6. $78.

"Provides essential medical information to both the general public and those diagnosed with a serious or fatal genetic disease or disorder." — *Choice, Jan '97*

". . . geared toward the lay public. It would be well placed in all public libraries and in those hospital and medical libraries in which access to genetic references is limited."
— *Doody's Health Sciences Book Review, Oct '96*

Head Trauma Sourcebook

Basic Information for the Layperson about Open-Head and Closed-Head Injuries, Treatment Advances, Recovery, and Rehabilitation, Along with Reports on Current Research Initiatives

Edited by Karen Bellenir. 414 pages. 1997. 0-7808-0208-X. $78.

Health Insurance Sourcebook

Basic Information about Managed Care Organizations, Traditional Fee-for-Service Insurance, Insurance Portability and Pre-Existing Conditions Clauses, Medicare, Medicaid, Social Security, and Military Health Care, Along with Information about Insurance Fraud

Edited by Wendy Wilcox. 530 pages. 1997. 0-7808-0222-5. $78.

"The layout of the book is particularly helpful as it provides easy access to reference material. A most useful addition to the vast amount of information about health insurance. The use of data from U.S. government agencies is most commendable. Useful in a library or learning center for healthcare professional students."
— *Doody's Health Sciences Book Reviews, Nov '97*

Immune System Disorders Sourcebook

Basic Information about Lupus, Multiple Sclerosis, Guillain-Barré Syndrome, Chronic Granulomatous Disease, and More, Along with Statistical and Demographic Data and Reports on Current Research Initiatives

Edited by Allan R. Cook. 608 pages. 1997. 0-7808-0209-8. $78.

Kidney & Urinary Tract Diseases & Disorders Sourcebook

Basic Information about Kidney Stones, Urinary Incontinence, Bladder Disease, End Stage Renal Disease, Dialysis, and More, Along with Statistical and Demographic Data and Reports on Current Research Initiatives

Edited by Linda M. Ross. 602 pages. 1997. 0-7808-0079-6. $78.

Learning Disabilities Sourcebook

Basic Information about Disorders Such as Dyslexia, Visual and Auditory Processing Deficits, Attention Deficit/Hyperactivity Disorder, and Autism, Along with Statistical and Demographic Data, Reports on Current Research Initiatives, an Explanation of the Assessment Process, and a Special Section for Adults with Learning Disabilities

Edited by Linda M. Shin. 579 pages. 1998. 0-7808-0210-1. $78.

Men's Health Concerns Sourcebook

Basic Information about Health Issues That Affect Men, Featuring Facts about the Top Causes of Death in Men, Including Heart Disease, Stroke, Cancers, Prostate Disorders, Chronic Obstructive Pulmonary Disease, Pneumonia and Influenza, Human Immunodeficiency Virus and Acquired Immune Deficiency Syndrome, Diabetes Mellitus, Stress, Suicide, Accidents and Homicides; and Facts about Common Concerns for Men, Including Impotence, Contraception, Circumcision, Sleep Disorders, Snoring, Hair Loss, Diet, Nutrition, Exercise, Kidney and Urological Disorders, and Backaches

Edited by Allan R. Cook. 760 pages. 1998. 0-7808-0212-8. $78.

Mental Health Disorders Sourcebook

Basic Information about Schizophrenia, Depression, Bipolar Disorder, Panic Disorder, Obsessive-Compulsive Disorder, Phobias and Other Anxiety Disorders, Paranoia and Other Personality Disorders, Eating Disorders, and Sleep Disorders, Along with Information about Treatment and Therapies

Edited by Karen Bellenir. 548 pages. 1995. 0-7808-0040-0. $78.

"This is an excellent new book . . . written in easy-to-understand language."
— *Booklist Health Science Supplement, Oct '97*

". . . useful for public and academic libraries and consumer health collections."
— *Medical Reference Services Quarterly, Spring '97*

"The great strengths of the book are its readability and its inclusion of places to find more information. Especially recommended." — *RQ, Winter '96*

". . . a good resource for a consumer health library."
— *Bulletin of the MLA, Oct '96*

"The information is data-based and couched in brief, concise language that avoids jargon. . . . a useful reference source." — *Readings, Sept '96*

"The text is well organized and adequately written for its target audience." — *Choice, Jun '96*

". . . provides information on a wide range of mental disorders, presented in nontechnical language."
— *Exceptional Child Education Resources, Spring '96*

"Recommended for public and academic libraries."
— *Reference Book Review, '96*

Ophthalmic Disorders Sourcebook

Basic Information about Glaucoma, Cataracts, Macular Degeneration, Strabismus, Refractive Disorders, and More, Along with Statistical and Demographic Data and Reports on Current Research Initiatives

Edited by Linda M. Ross. 631 pages. 1996. 0-7808-0081-8. $78.

Oral Health Sourcebook

Basic Information about Diseases and Conditions Affecting Oral Health, Including Cavities, Gum Disease, Dry Mouth, Oral Cancers, Fever Blisters, Canker Sores, Oral Thrush, Bad Breath, Temporomandibular Disorders, and other Craniofacial Syndromes, Along with Statistical Data on the Oral Health of Americans, Oral Hygiene, Emergency First Aid, Information on Treatment Procedures and Methods of Replacing Lost Teeth

Edited by Allan R. Cook. 558 pages. 1997. 0-7808-0082-6. $78.

"Recommended reference source." — *Booklist, Dec '97*

Pain Sourcebook

Basic Information about Specific Forms of Acute and Chronic Pain, Including Headaches, Back Pain, Muscular Pain, Neuralgia, Surgical Pain, and Cancer Pain, Along with Pain Relief Options Such as Analgesics, Narcotics, Nerve Blocks, Transcutaneous Nerve Stimulation, and Alternative Forms of Pain Control, Including Biofeedback, Imaging, Behavior Modification, and Relaxation Techniques

Edited by Allan R. Cook. 667 pages. 1997. 0-7808-0213-6. $78.

"The information is basic in terms of scholarship and is appropriate for general readers. Written in journalistic style ... intended for non-professionals. Quite thorough in its coverage of different pain conditions and summarizes the latest clinical information regarding pain treatment."
— *Choice, Jun '98*

"Recommended reference source."
— *Booklist, Mar '98*

Pregnancy & Birth Sourcebook

Basic Information about Planning for Pregnancy, Maternal Health, Fetal Growth and Development, Labor and Delivery, Postpartum and Perinatal Care, Pregnancy in Mothers with Special Concerns, and Disorders of Pregnancy, Including Genetic Counseling, Nutrition and Exercise, Obstetrical Tests, Pregnancy Discomfort, Multiple Births, Cesarean Sections, Medical Testing of Newborns, Breastfeeding, Gestational Diabetes, and Ectopic Pregnancy

Edited by Heather E. Aldred. 737 pages. 1997. 0-7808-0216-0. $78.

". . . for the layperson. A well-organized handbook. Recommended for college libraries ... general readers."
— *Choice, Apr '98*

"Recommended reference source."
— *Booklist, Mar '98*

"This resource is recommended for public libraries to have on hand."
— *American Reference Books Annual, '98*

Public Health Sourcebook

Basic Information about Government Health Agencies, Including National Health Statistics and Trends, Healthy People 2000 Program Goals and Objectives, the Centers for Disease Control and Prevention, the Food and Drug Administration, and the National Institutes of Health, Along with Full Contact Information for Each Agency

Edited by Wendy Wilcox. 698 pages. 1998. 0-7808-0220-9. $78.

Rehabilitation Sourcebook

Basic Information for the Layperson about Physical Medicine (Physiatry) and Rehabilitative Therapies, Including Physical, Occupational, Recreational, Speech, and Vocational Therapy; Along with Descriptions of Devices and Equipment Such as Orthotics, Gait Aids, Prostheses, and Adaptive Systems Used during Rehabilitation and for Activities of Daily Living, and Featuring a Glossary and Source Listings for Further Help and Information

Edited by Theresa K. Murray. 600 pages. 1998. 0-7808-0236-5. $78.

Respiratory Diseases & Disorders Sourcebook

Basic Information about Respiratory Diseases and Disorders, Including Asthma, Cystic Fibrosis, Pneumonia, the Common Cold, Influenza, and Others, Featuring Facts about the Respiratory System, Statistical and Demographic Data, Treatments, Self-Help Management Suggestions, and Current Research Initiatives

Edited by Allan R. Cook and Peter D. Dresser. 771 pages. 1995. 0-7808-0037-0. $78.

"Designed for the layperson and for patients and their families coping with respiratory illness. . . . an extensive array of information on diagnosis, treatment, management, and prevention of respiratory illnesses for the general reader."
— *Choice, Jun '96*

"A highly recommended text for all collections. It is a comforting reminder of the power of knowledge that good books carry between their covers."
— *Academic Library Book Review, Spring '96*

"This sourcebook offers a comprehensive collection of authoritative information presented in a nontechnical, humanitarian style for patients, families, and caregivers."
— *Association of Operating Room Nurses, Sept/Oct '95*

Sexually Transmitted Diseases Sourcebook

Basic Information about Herpes, Chlamydia, Gonorrhea, Hepatitis, Nongonoccocal Urethritis, Pelvic Inflammatory Disease, Syphilis, AIDS, and More, Along with Current Data on Treatments and Preventions

Edited by Linda M. Ross. 550 pages. 1997. 0-7808-0217-9. $78.